Stalking

Stalking

Psychiatric Perspectives
and Practical Approaches

Group for the Advancement of Psychiatry
Committee on Psychiatry and the Law

Edited by
Debra A. Pinals, MD

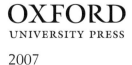

OXFORD
UNIVERSITY PRESS

2007

OXFORD
UNIVERSITY PRESS

Oxford University Press, Inc., publishes works that further
Oxford University's objective of excellence
in research, scholarship, and education.

Oxford New York

Auckland Cape Town Dar es Salaam Hong Kong Karachi
Kuala Lumpur Madrid Melbourne Mexico City Nairobi
New Delhi Shanghai Taipei Toronto

With offices in
Argentina Austria Brazil Chile Czech Republic France Greece
Guatemala Hungary Italy Japan Poland Portugal Singapore
South Korea Switzerland Thailand Turkey Ukraine Vietnam

Published by Oxford University Press, Inc.
198 Madison Avenue, New York, New York 10016

www.oup.com

Oxford is a registered trademark of Oxford University Press.

Library of Congress Cataloging-in-Publication Data
Stalking : psychiatric perspectives and practical approaches / Group for the Advancement of Psychiatry,
Committee on Psychiatry and the Law ; edited by Debra A. Pinals.
    p. ; cm.
ISBN 978-0-19-518984-1
1. Stalking—Psychological aspects. 2. Stalking. I. Pinals, Debra A. II. Group for the Advancement of
Psychiatry. Committee on Psychiatry and the Law.
[DNLM: 1. Social Behavior Disorders. 2. Crime Victims—legislation and jurisprudence. WM 600
S7825 2007]
RC553.E76S73 2007
362.2'0425—dc22   2006100850

9 8 7 6 5 4 3 2 1

Printed in the United States of America
on acid-free paper

To our families and colleagues

FOREWORD

Stalking produces social disruptions and serious psychological distress, most importantly in victims, but also in stalkers, who themselves are caught up in repetitive, and ultimately futile and self-destructive patterns of behavior (chapters 4 and 5). All too often, stalking is also a harbinger of physical and/or sexual assault (chapter 3). Stalking is now recognized as a social problem that criminal justice systems have a responsibility to control and, when possible, to prevent (chapters 6 and 7). This book represents an important milestone marking mental health professionals' acceptance of their roles in ameliorating the psychological damage in stalking victims and—equally important—in assessing and managing those who stalk (chapter 4).

Traditionally, most areas of psychiatry have focused on disorders of mental function, with behavior regarded as a mere epiphenomenon. Forensic psychiatrists have always been forced to attend to behavior, however, for it is the criminal activity of those they assess and struggle to manage that is central to forensic practice. Yet forensic mental health professionals working as clinicians and researchers have all too often succumbed to the temptation to shortcut the complex task of analyzing the social, cultural, developmental, and neurobiological contributions to crime by simply employing diagnoses that pathologize behavior.

For example, if asked why a child molester molests children, forensic clinicians often respond, "Because he has a paraphilia." If forensic clinicians are then asked how they know he has a paraphilia, they answer, "Because he keeps molesting children." This is not to say the psychological mechanisms captured in the current concepts of pedophilia do not play a role in the behavior of some child molesters. The problem is that if we simply offer a diagnostic label without engaging in a thorough analysis of the roots of the problematic behavior, we risk perpetuating half-truths and may promote faulty approaches to assessment and management.

One of the pleasures of reading this book on stalking is that it presents a model of how to approach a problem behavior. The book examines the phenomena of stalking in its many and various manifestations, then evaluates the research and theories about the nature, epidemiology, classification, and origins of stalking, and finally uses clinical experience to articulate the current evidence-based approaches to assessment and management of both stalkers and their victims. Chapters on special topics related to stalking among juveniles and cyberstalking expand on the unique contributions this book offers.

Stalking acquired its name and was swept to public prominence on a wave of fascination with those individuals who repeatedly contacted, followed, attempted to intrude upon, and occasionally attacked celebrities. Once stalking became a criminal offense, it drew the attention of law enforcement agencies, researchers, and ultimately clinicians. It then became clear that "star stalkers" represented merely the glittering tip of a previously hidden and even more sinister iceberg. Rightly, therefore, most subsequent research has focused on the stalking of ordinary people. Yet this has led to a relative neglect of celebrities and other prominent people who are at high risk of attracting unwanted attention. This book's chapter on celebrity and presidential targets is particularly welcome in redressing that imbalance in the current literature.

Stalking is a problem behavior that usually arises out of social and interpersonal conflicts. Stalking emerges most frequently in a situation in which the hopes or assumed entitlements of the stalker have been frustrated or abrogated. The deserted partner, the humiliated coworker, the dissatisfied patient, and the disappointed suitor who embark on stalking have unfulfilled expectations or grievances directed at a person who has failed to behave as they believed they had a right to expect. In my experience, stalkers talk more about rights than even UN bureaucrats or consumer advocates. This sensitivity to their own rights and prerogatives is not matched by any appreciation of the rights of those they target. Even those stalkers who recognize the illegality and destructiveness of their behavior will often justify their actions as efforts to seek justice or appropriate retribution. To be fair, these stalkers often appeal to standards that might once have received substantial support from their fellow citizens—they invoke, for example, "traditional" ideas about the sanctity and permanence of marriage, or atavistic notions about masculinity and proper female roles. This is not to suggest that stalkers are merely conservative individualists. What distinguishes them from normal citizens with old-fashioned values is that the stalkers willingly and repeatedly intrude on their targets, blind or indifferent to the fear and distress they create. Stalkers' understanding of rights is not individualistic; it is autistic. Stalking has its roots in situations of social, cultural, and interpersonal disjunction, but persistent stalkers also have specific psychological vulnerabilities or mental disorders that lead them to behave as they do (chapter 2).

The use of the term "stalking" to refer to wilful, malicious, and repeated nonconsensual contacts with and harassing of other individuals reflects both a recent social and scientific "discovery" and a growing behavioral phenomenon (chapter 1). Even if one counts only harassment that continues for months on end, a woman's lifetime risk of being stalked now approaches 10%. Stalking could, like child sexual abuse, have been a long-standing, major problem that went largely unrecognized until forced into the public's attention by advocacy groups and the media. Though this is part of the story, the phenomenon's new-found profile also reflects increasing rates of a type of behavior that has become impossible to ignore any longer. A number of social developments have contributed to the recognition and increased frequency of stalking.

The commonest form of persistent stalking is by rejected partners following the end of a relationship. Given that serial monogamy has effectively replaced one partner for life as the norm for intimate relationships in the Western world, the opportunities for asymmetrical, conflict-ridden partings have greatly increased. Similarly, the changing roles of women in the domestic and work spheres has challenged less flexible and capable men, and some have responded with various types of harassment including stalking. Systems for complaint and grievance resolution represent increasingly important methods for regulating society and guaranteeing the rights of ordinary citizens confronted with the power of government and commercial agencies. In some persons, however, failure to obtain what they regard as rightfully theirs can feed a resentment that leads to stalking.

Most of us now live in urban environments surrounded by strangers. Our culture supports notions of community in theory, but in practice, Western society all too often promotes distrust and fear of our actual neighbors. We may know little, if anything, of the man who lives next door, but we are encouraged to feel a bond with newscasters and celebrities from various media pseudocommunities. Few personal letters may arrive at our door and few visitors may enter our homes, but for some there is a world of contact with others in cyberspace and the mobile phone network. All these aspects of modernity may have their benefits, but they also carry risks—one of which is being stalked.

At one time, even scholarly books were introduced not by a preface, but by an "advertisement." In the 1827 edition of that greatest of all psychiatric texts, Robert Burton's *The Anatomy of Melancholy*, the anonymous author of the advertisement claimed the work would be "the delight of the learned, the refuge of the uninformed, and the solace of the indolent." I'm not sure about solace, but this book is certainly informative throughout. As to delight, Michele Pathé, Rosemary Purcell, and I, who work on stalking in Australia, are certainly delighted to see our American colleagues make use of our work.

Knowledge about stalking is rapidly accumulating. This is a truly first rate book that will bring both specialists and professionals with a more general interest right up to date, and leave no excuses to remain uninformed about either stalkers or their victims.

Paul Edward Mullen, MB BS, DSc., FRANZCP, FRC Psych.
Professor of Forensic Psychiatry, Monash University
Clinical Director, Victorian Institute of Forensic Mental Health

PREFACE

Stalking behavior is not a new phenomenon, but one that has increasingly received attention among mental health and legal professionals, media representatives, and the lay public. A search of the medical literature prior to 1990 for appearances of the term "stalking" yields just a handful of references, and most of these refer to the act of searching or "looking for something," as in "stalking" elusive diseases. A similar search of the literature from 1990 to the present indicates there has been an explosion in the number of publications on this topic. In addition to the attention stalking has received in scientific periodicals, several academic texts have been written on stalking and related themes. Additionally, high profile (and sometimes sensational) examples of stalkers pursuing television personalities, musicians, and movie stars are frequently cited in the popular press.

Where did all this public interest originate? The first statute addressing stalking was passed by the California legislature in 1990. Since then, each state within the United States has passed its own antistalking laws, and similar legislative responses to stalking have been seen in several other countries around the world.

Psychiatrists have for years served as treatment providers and consultants to clinical cases involving obsessional following and harassment. With the passage of antistalking laws, forensic psychiatrists and other mental health professionals now are often called upon to provide assessments related to alleged stalkers' competence to stand trial, criminal responsibility, and risk of future harm. Assessing violence risk in children and adolescents has also come under the spotlight after several high profile school shootings. In conducting such violence risk assessments, clinicians often encounter children who have obsessive interests in others, and who may engage in behavior intended to alarm or cause fear.

These forces have come into play at the same time that the field of violence risk assessment by mental health professionals has shifted in new directions, reframing prior studies looking at violence and mental illness, leaving us the hope that we might improve our capacity to assess and mitigate risk of harm to others. In an era when we are recognizing unique risks of sex offenders, fire set-ters, and perpetrators of domestic violence, we have also come to recognize that stalking can be a subtype of potentially violent behavior, and one that merits additional professional attention.

If much has already been written about stalking, what is the value of an-other volume on the subject? To answer this question, it is helpful to begin by explaining how this book has been created. The Group for the Advancement of Psychiatry (GAP) was founded in 1946 by a group of physicians specializing in psychiatry whose goals included increasing public awareness of issues related to mental health in the United States. Since its inception, GAP has had tremen-dous influence in pioneering ideas and applying psychiatric insights to many public health and interpersonal problems we face. The organization functions through individual committees of special interest, which operate as think tanks, and whose publications and other work products contribute to scientific litera-ture and mental health knowledge. The GAP Committee on Psychiatry and the Law is one of the many committees actively at work today, and one of the com-mittees responsible for publication of several influential documents in the field of forensic mental health. It is comprised of specialists in forensic psychiatry, that branch of psychiatry in which legal, risk management, and psychiatric do-mains intersect. Our committee members come from different regions in North America, and all were invited to join GAP in recognition of their individual clinical and academic accomplishments.

Several years ago, the former chair of the GAP Committee on Psychiatry and the Law, Donna M. Schwartz-Watts, MD, led our group to recognize that our collective knowledge and experience formed the basis for a valuable con-tribution to the existing literature on stalking. That knowledge and experience comes from our work with stalkers in a variety of contexts: performing evalu-ations of criminal defendants for courts and attorneys; functioning as psychi-atric administrators and as consultants to governmental agencies; assessing the potential for violence in the workplace; making risk-reduction and management recommendations to stalking victims; providing treatment to both stalkers and their victims; and acting as educators and clinical consultants when questions about violence risk have arisen. In preparing this book, our committee has spent many hours discussing and debating the nuances involved in our diverse experi-ences with stalking. Along the way several invited guests, each well-respected in the field of forensic psychiatry, has added their contributions to our discussions and ultimately, to this book.

Research on the topic of stalking is still in its early stages, and often our discussion focused on unanswered questions. Most previously published writings about stalking represent the work of clinicians and researchers who understandably are describing or commenting on their own research or distinctive theoretical outlook. One of our goals in putting forth this book was to bring together the findings and perspectives of others along with our appraisal of their work. We also wanted to produce a volume that shares with readers aspects of our discussions and reviews potential directions for future research. These aims are reflected in the unique process that we used in the development of this book. Although each chapter has listed authors, all chapters were reviewed and edited extensively by the committee as a whole, leading to the recrafting of manuscript versions that included insights from our discussions.

We have included chapters dealing with topics that have not been explored in depth in other volumes, including a chapter on forensic evaluations that examines the relationships between stalkers' mental conditions and legally relevant mental states, and a chapter on stalkers of celebrities and other high profile targets. We have also included chapters that focus on current thinking related to the epidemiology, definitions, and typological constructs of stalking, varying statutory schemes, cyberstalking, as well as risk assessment and risk management of adult and juvenile stalkers.

We hope that this book will assist mental health professionals in their work and provide important information for law enforcement, courts, attorneys, and other legal professionals, as well as members of the public who may find this work relevant to their personal situations.

ACKNOWLEDGMENTS

This book is not the sole work of the editor or the individual chapter authors. It truly represents the work of many persons, without whose efforts and ideas it would not have been conceived and realized. As noted, Donna Schwartz-Watts, MD, deserves much credit for planting the seed of the idea for the GAP Committee on Psychiatry and the Law and for nurturing it until the roots were deep enough to keep us moving forward, even after life circumstances took her in a different direction. We are grateful for her vision.

In addition to our primary authors, contributors to our discussions included Carl Malmquist, MD, Roy O'Shaughnessy, MD, Emily Keram, MD, and Victoria Harris, MD, MPH. Members of the GAP Publication Board (and especially David Adler, MD) helped shepherd the book through its layers of review, with diligence and reliability, and we are indebted for their help and thoughtful comments. Holly Andrade, MSW, was extremely helpful in reviewing our manuscript with a keen editorial eye, and her willingness to step in and make herself available as needed is very much appreciated. The administrative assistants of each contributor must be credited as well. In particular, I am indebted to Ms. Cara Sanford for her faithful assistance, patience, and organizational skills. Our editorial staff at Oxford University Press, particularly Joan Bossert, has been admirable for their professionalism, experience, and knowledge in the world of publication. And finally, we are grateful to our families and colleagues who have supported us along the way.

A NOTE ABOUT SOURCES OF CASE MATERIAL IN THIS BOOK AND CONFIDENTIALITY

In preparing this book, we have included several case vignettes to illustrate key pedagogical points about stalking. In certain instances, case examples use information available in public record documents, such as newspaper articles and court records. In other cases, vignettes are fictional portrayals. In yet others, vignettes are composites or examples of the authors' case materials with names and other personal identifiers changed to preserve individuals' anonymity.

CONTENTS

Part IV Special Issues

CONTRIBUTORS

Kenneth L. Appelbaum, MD   Professor of Clinical Psychiatry, Director, Correctional Mental Health Policy and Research, Commonwealth Medicine, University of Massachusetts Medical School, Worcester, MA

Peter Ash, MD   Associate Professor of Psychiatry, Director, Psychiatry and Law Service, Chief, Child and Adolescent Psychiatry Service, Department of Psychiatry and Behavioral Sciences, Emory University, Atlanta, GA

John R. Cooke, MD, JD   Addiction Psychiatry Fellow, University of Medicine and Dentistry and Medicine of New Jersey, Piscataway, NJ

Todd Elwyn, JD, MD   Assistant Clinical Professor, Department of Psychiatry, The University of Hawaii John A. Burns School of Medicine at Manoa, Honolulu, HI

Deborah Giorgi-Guarnieri, JD, MD   Eastern State Hospital; Director of Forensic Psychiatry Residency, Medical College of Virginia, Williamsburg, VA

Graham D. Glancy, MB, ChB, FRC Psych., FRCP (C)   Assistant Professor, Department of Psychiatry, University of Toronto; Clinical Assistant Professor, McMaster University, Toronto

David J. Kapley, JD, MD   Private Practice in Psychiatry, Child and Adolescent Psychiatry, and Forensic Psychiatry, Bowling Green, KY

James Knoll, MD	Associate Professor of Psychiatry, Director of Forensic Psychiatry, SUNY Upstate Medical University, Syracuse, NY
Douglas Mossman, MD	Professor and Director, Division of Forensic Psychiatry, Wright State University Boonshoft School of Medicine, Dayton, OH; Administrative Director, Glenn M. Weaver Institute of Law and Psychiatry, University of Cincinnati College of Law, Cincinnati, OH
Alan W. Newman, MD	Director, Residency Training Program, Medical Director, Inpatient Psychiatry, Department of Psychiatry, Georgetown University Hospital, Washington, DC
Michael A. Norko MD	Associate Professor of Psychiatry, Deputy Training Director, Forensic Psychiatry Residency, Yale University School of Medicine; Acting Director, Whiting Forensic Division of Connecticut Valley Hospital, Middletown, CT
Robert T. M. Phillips, MD, PhD, DFAPA	Adjunct Associate Professor of Psychiatry and Adjunct Professor of Law, University of Maryland Schools of Medicine and Law; Senior Consultant Psychiatrist, Protective Intelligence Division United States Secret Service, Annapolis, MD
Debra A. Pinals, MD	Associate Professor of Psychiatry, Co-Director, Law and Psychiatry Program and Director, Forensic Psychiatry Training, Department of Psychiatry, University of Massachusetts Medical School; Area Medical Director, Central Massachusetts Area, Massachusetts Department of Mental Health, Worcester, MA
Mordecai N. Potash, MD	Assistant Professor, Department of Psychiatry and Neurology, Tulane University School of Medicine, New Orleans, LA
Phillip J. Resnick, MD	Professor of Psychiatry, Case Western Reserve University; Director, Division of Forensic Psychiatry, University Hospitals of Cleveland, Cleveland, OH
Charles L. Scott, MD	Associate Clinical Professor of Psychiatry, Chief, Division of Psychiatry and the Law, Department of Psychiatry and Behavioral Sciences University of California, Davis Medical Center, Sacramento, CA

John Tennison, MD   Medical Director, Texas Psychiatry Associates, San Antonio Treatment Center and Texas Recovery and Counseling Services; Founder and Director, Texas Mental Health Institute, San Antonio, TX

PART I

Introduction

1 Stalking: Introduction, Definition, and Epidemiology

Deborah Giorgi-Guarnieri
Michael A. Norko

The 1990s witnessed the emergence of stalking as a new social construct that was recognized through the development of antistalking statutes. Simultaneously, stalking received widespread attention in the popular news media and in scholarly works by mental health professionals. Considerable variation exists among the legal, clinical, and research definitions of stalking. Large-scale epidemiological studies, conducted in Australia, Great Britain, and the United States, suggest that stalking is a relatively common behavior. Women have an 8–33% lifetime risk of being the victim of stalking, depending on the definition. For men, the lifetime risk is 2–7%. Studies on the epidemiology of stalking violence give a wide range of results: 3–46% of stalkers progress to violence. Higher rates of stalking have been reported among some populations, including college students, mental health clinicians, and celebrities. Female stalkers differ from male stalkers in their motivations and target populations. Finally, children and adolescents also exhibit stalking behaviors outside of normal developmental behaviors.

INTRODUCTION

Behavior patterns that we now call "stalking" have been described for thousands of years. Hippocrates, Galen, Plutarch, and various physicians of the Middle Ages described these behaviors (Lloyd-Goldstein, 1998). In 1837, Esquirol differentiated erotomania and nymphomania (Esquirol, 1838/1965). Both Kraepelin (1921/1976) and de Clérambault (1921) described erotomania in the 1920s. Classic literature provides several historical instances of what appears to be stalking. It has been argued that Shakespeare's last 25 sonnets reflect his obsessional attachment and spurned pursuit of the "dark lady," with evidence of obscenities, threats, paranoia, and irrationality (Skoler, 1998). Mullen, Pathé, and Purcell (2000) describe evidence of behaviors typical of stalkers in the lives and written works of Italian poets Danté Alighieri (1265–1321) and Petrarch (1304–1374), and the philosopher Søren Kierkegaard (1813–1855). Louisa May Alcott's first novel, *A Long Fatal Love Chase*, written in 1866 but discovered and published in 1993, tells the story of a young woman pursued with increasing anger, resentment, and ultimately violence by the husband she left (Mullen et al., 2000).

Two of the late twentieth century's most notorious forensic psychiatric cases arose from the mental problems and violent behavior of stalkers. The murder of Tatiana Tarasoff by Prosenjit Poddar in 1969 and the assassination attempt on President Reagan by John Hinckley in 1981 featured well-publicized examples of stalking-related behavior—the former involving two University of California students and the latter a Hollywood celebrity, Jodie Foster, and a president of the United States. Popular culture during that time provides additional examples. Several movies, such as *Play Misty for Me* (1971), *The Story of Adele H.* (1975), *Fatal Attraction* (1987), and *Enduring Love* (2004), portray stalking in a main character's pursuit of a relationship. The cartoon character Pepé Le Pew animated stalking using humorous lines such as "Eez love, my cherie" and his offer to rewrite the alphabet so "U and I are together." In 1983, Sting sang similarly disturbing lyrics in the song *Every Breath You Take*.

Despite these previous vivid events and portrayals, the current conceptualization of stalking emerged in the 1990s when a combination of news events, legal conceptualizations, and new clinical insights focused attention on behavior that we now term "stalking." The wider recognition of the phenomenon is generally attributed to the 1989 shooting death of actress Rebecca Schaeffer (a regular cast member of the television series *My Sister Sam* in the late 1980s) by an obsessed fan, Robert Bardo (Fremouw, Westrup, & Pennypacker, 1997; Saunders, 1998). The first antistalking law in the United States was thereafter enacted by the California Legislature in 1990. By 1992, 30 states had such laws, and by 1993 all the other states (with the exception of Maine, which then relied on its antiterrorism laws for such purposes) and the District of Columbia had enacted such legislation (Saunders, 1998).

Today, stalking is a crime in all state and federal jurisdictions, as well as in Canada, Australia, and Great Britain, among others (Meloy, 1999). This rapid legislative response and the significant media attention devoted to publicized events create the appearance that stalking behavior has suddenly emerged as a new phenomenon, or at least has suddenly increased in frequency. It is difficult to comment on the historical frequency of stalking behavior because there is only one study reporting empirical data on this issue (Lloyd-Goldstein, 1998). In a New York City study, court clinic referrals for stalking behaviors showed a three-fold increase between 1987 and 1993—from 0.6% of all referrals to 1.7% (Harmon, Rosner, & Owens, 1995). Of note, New York passed stalking legislation in 1992, making it unclear whether there was an actual increase in stalking behaviors or just an increase in the referral of defendants with stalking behavior to court clinics.

Mullen and colleagues (2000) argue that it has been a combination of media sensationalism of stalking and changes in the way we view human relationships in the last decade that have created the modern construct of stalking and forced its ascendancy in both science and popular culture. These authors also credit

Lowney and Best (1995) with the elucidation of the development of this social construct through three phases between 1980 and 1994. In 2001, Mullen, Pathé, and Purcell (2001) attempted an explanation of the new construct and increasing behavior. They asserted that the dramatic emergence of stalking behavior was in part due to increasing instability in relationships (for the average person) and in part due to the exposure accompanying fame (for celebrities). They emphasized that a complex society with more isolation coupled with a culture of blame guided stalking behavior. Finally, they noted celebrities struggled with the need for the public eye and the fear of their ardent fans. Mullen and colleagues (2001) marveled at how well the term "stalking" captures a variety of behaviors and social conditions.

As members of the GAP Committee on Psychiatry and the Law, we debated numerous concepts related to stalking. Although we share Mullen and colleagues' (2001) scholarly interest in stalking, we have not been as certain that the term stalking neatly packages all the obsessive attachment behaviors psychiatric clinicians observe nor are we confident that overall relationship instability contributes to stalking. Specifically, the clinical boundaries between stalking and predatory behaviors are not clear and confound the definition of stalking. (See Definition section below.) Stalking behavior also perplexes the legal system, as it is both a crime and a behavior that at times precedes more serious crimes. (See Epidemiological Studies section below and chapter 4, Risk Assessment of Stalking.) As mental health professionals, the more we learn more about stalking, the clearer it becomes that stalking behavior can lead to violence. In the view of our committee, the increase in relationship dissolution might lead to an increase in stalking. An increase in prevalence, however, is uncertain because there are no actual related data. To understand the phenomenon best, it behooves mental health practitioners, legal professionals, and those working with stalkers and their victims to have a greater understanding of the complexities of its definition.

DEFINITION

How stalking is defined often depends on whether the setting and context for examining the behavior is legal, clinical, and research oriented. Although usage of the term stalking is common, colloquial meaning can be quite different from that used among mental health and legal professionals. Meloy (1998) notes that statutory definitions of stalking generally involve the following three elements: "(1) a pattern (course of conduct) of behavioral intrusion upon another person that is unwanted; (2) an implicit or explicit threat that is evidenced in the patterns of behavioral intrusion; and (3) as a result of these behavioral intrusions, the person who is threatened experiences reasonable fear" (p. 2).

The exact legal definition varies from state to state, as does the requirement of criminal intent for prosecution. It is noteworthy that stalking behavior that is undiscovered by the victim does not constitute a basis for prosecution of stalking, though it might meet some popular or clinical and psychodynamic definitions. The crime of stalking is complicated further by the behavior of stalking. The behavior may lead to more serious crimes, such as murder and sexual assault, but the charges may not reflect the crime of stalking. (For further discussion regarding stalking laws and legal definitions of stalking, see chapter 6, Trends in Antistalking Legislation.)

From a clinical perspective, Meloy and Gothard (1995) defined stalking as "an abnormal or long-term pattern of threat or harassment directed toward a specific individual" (p. 259). Westrup and Fremouw (1998) noted the lack of a clear and consistent definition of stalking in the available literature. They proposed the following definition of stalking behavior: "one or more of a constellation of behaviors that (a) are directed repeatedly towards a specific individual (the target); (b) are experienced by the target as unwelcome and intrusive, and (c) are reported to trigger fear or concern in the target" (p. 258).

Mullen and colleagues (2000) point out that even such attempts at precise definition leave open the questions of how many intrusions are necessary to constitute stalking and what level of intrusions characterize objectionable or fear-inducing behavior. Our committee discussions have included trying to answer questions such as, at what point would persistent attempts at courtship be considered stalking behavior? Could the second phone call of an awkward or perhaps unattractive, young suitor seeking a date be considered stalking? As Mullen and colleagues (2000) say, "stalking lies in the eye of the beholder" (p. 9). In considering these dilemmas, they modify a clinical definition as "a constellation of behaviours involving repeated and persistent attempts to impose on another person unwanted communication and/or contact" (p. 7). Their further elaboration of their definition may be helpful: "Stalking is those repeated acts, experienced as unpleasantly intrusive, which create apprehension and can be understood by a reasonable fellow citizen (the ordinary man or woman) to be grounds for becoming fearful" (p. 10). Examples of stalking behaviors include phone calls, letters and cards, faxes, Internet communications, graffiti, unwanted gifts or other materials, following, approaching, maintaining surveillance, ordering goods or services for the victim, initiating legal action against the victim, spreading rumors, threats, damage to property and pets, assault, and stalking by proxy (Pathé, 2002).

In preparing this book, the GAP Committee on Psychiatry and the Law selected Mullen and colleagues' (2000) definition of stalking, except where otherwise defined by a particular law or study under discussion. We debated aspects of Mullen and colleagues' (2000) predatory stalker type. The behavior of predatory stalkers is usually unknown to the target, and thus may not have induced fear. Consequently, the behavior of the predatory stalker may not meet our definition of stalking. This issue is further discussed in chapter 2, Stalking: Classification and Typology.

Stalking is those repeated acts, experienced as unpleasantly intrusive, which create apprehension and can be understood by a reasonable fellow citizen (the ordinary man or woman) to be grounds for becoming fearful. (Mullen, Pathé, & Purcell, 2000, p. 10)

THE PSYCHODYNAMICS OF STALKING

Harold Searles (1956) authored an article titled "The Psychodynamics of Vengefulness." In it he wrote,

Vindictiveness seems to lend itself particularly well to the repression of grief and separation anxiety. It enables the person to avoid or postpone the experiencing of both of these affects, because he has not really *given up* the other person toward whom his vengefulness is directed: that is his preoccupation with vengeful fantasies about that person serves, in effect, as a way of psychologically *holding on* to him. (p. 31)

The psychodynamics of vengefulness yield some insight into one aspect of stalking in that the behavior appears often as an outgrowth of repetitive permutations of love, hate, union, and loss. Stalking activities impair the social, occupational, and psychological functions of both the stalker and the victim. Over the years, more comprehensive theories have evolved to help us further understand the psychological antecedents of stalking. Meloy (1999) and Mullen (2003) have proposed two such theories. Meloy (1999) describes a stalker's psychodynamic pattern. He highlights defense mechanisms, including projection, idealization, devaluation, projective identification, splitting, and denial. He emphasizes emotions of shame, rage, envy, and jealousy. He explains that narcissistic fantasies both fuel and excuse the stalking behavior. According to these views, a pattern of stalking begins with the narcissistic fantasy of the love object. Rejection challenges the fantasy. The stalker then defends against feelings of humiliation and shame with rage. Rage progresses to behaviors of revenge, control, and violence. These behaviors in turn restore the "narcissistic linking fantasy" (pp. 87–88).

Mullen and colleagues (2001) approach the psychodynamics of stalking by classifying stalkers according to relationship to victim, pathology, and motivation. Mullen and Pathé (1994) examine psychodynamics only in stalkers who have a delusional relationship with their victims. This group, historically known as the erotomanics, is associated with violence. They are prone to rage should the victim's rejection penetrate their psychotic defenses. The erotomanic attachment, usually romantic, can become sexualized and lead to sexual attacks on the victim.

In this section, a case example is presented that contains both the behaviors and the thought processes of a stalker. Readers here would do well to focus on the thoughts and subsequent behaviors of the stalker, which will assist in understanding other aspects of stalking described throughout the text.

CASE EXAMPLE 1.1. WALTER AND CINDY

Walter Kovacs was a 26-year-old man who pleaded guilty to aggravated murder. His crime involved the fatal shooting of Cindy Taylor, a 20-year-old college student. Mr. Kovacs first met Cindy when they were attending college classes. Cindy agreed to meet Walter at the student union building, and they eventually began to have lunch with each other on occasion. Walter enjoyed spending time with Cindy. He found her outgoing, friendly, and playful. In contrast, Walter was a loner, had few friends, and had little dating experience. Although he continued to take one or two classes per semester, he had no firm graduation plans. He lived with his parents and was unemployed.

Walter first became aware of his romantic interest in Cindy during a summer break. He began to go out of his way to spend more time with Cindy, meeting her at the library and walking her home. He chose a summer job at the student union building with Cindy so he could spend more time around her. By the end of the summer, he felt he was deeply in love with Cindy. On occasion, Cindy would hug Walter or kiss him on the cheek.

One evening, Walter spent the night at Cindy's dorm room. They engaged in some petting but neither reached a sexual climax. After they spent the night together, Cindy indicated that she felt guilty about it and was no longer interested in spending time with him. Walter was disappointed, but believed that she was "playing hard to get." When Cindy began refusing to return his calls, he began to feel hurt and angry. Walter finally confronted Cindy in person and asked her to be his girlfriend. Cindy replied that she was "sorry" but her answer was "no" and commented on their age difference. Walter had difficulty accepting Cindy's refusal and wondered whether she was playing "mind games" with him. He hoped that she would reconsider and "confess her true feelings" of love for him. When this did not happen by the end of the summer break, Walter became further saddened and distressed.

Walter began to develop the notion that Cindy had humiliated and insulted him by leading him on and "playing games" with him. Although Cindy offered her friendship to him, he rejected the offer, as he felt "used" and deceived. Back in college, Walter's grades suffered. He became depressed and eventually withdrew from college altogether. He became increasingly angry with Cindy and spent a great deal of time ruminating about how to regain his "dignity." Walter struggled with his conflicting desires to reunite with her and, conversely, to seek revenge upon her.

He began making harassing hang up phone calls to Cindy's dorm room. His behavior progressed from scratching the paint on her car to letting the air out of her tires. Later, he wrote "A Slut Lives Here" on her dorm room door with a permanent marker. When he was arrested for these acts, he openly confessed. He justified the acts as "retribution" for the "greater crime" Cindy had committed against him.

After Walter's arrest, his father persuaded him to be evaluated at a psychiatric hospital because of his anger and irritability. Walter was admitted for a 2-week stay and was diagnosed as having an adjustment disorder and a personality disorder. He was highly intelligent and skilled at downplaying any concerning symptoms, and was cautious in the information he revealed to his treatment team. However, he did agree to keep a journal of his thoughts and emotions.

Walter's journal was replete with references to Cindy and the intense feelings of jealousy, envy, and inadequacy that she evoked in him. He felt as though she was the best possible mate that he could ever attain, and her rejection made him feel hopeless. He also described fantasies of killing her. However, he was well aware that denial of any violent thoughts would result in a quicker discharge. Toward the end of his hospitalization, he told his treatment team that he was no longer having homicidal thoughts, when, in fact, he remained rather conflicted. Upon discharge, he agreed to see a therapist once to twice a week. He did not tell his outpatient therapist about his thoughts of retaliation against Cindy.

Several months after his discharge from the hospital, Walter began sending threatening and harassing e-mails to Cindy. In the e-mails, he blamed her for his arrest and subsequent hospitalization, which only served to inflame his anger. The major theme of the e-mails concerned his need to "get even" with Cindy. For example he wrote, "When I was locked up in the hospital, I learned that I have the patience necessary to store up all the hurt you gave to me and return it all to you at the proper time."

Another e-mail stated, "Why the hell shouldn't you face any consequences for your irresponsible actions? I got into tremendous amounts of trouble because of you!" Other e-mails were more directly threatening. For example, he wrote, "I have already been to your dorm and I know how easy it is to gain entrance to your room. I wonder how long it would take your dorm mates to notice you were not going to class or that your room smelled like rotting flesh." Cindy was so distressed by the threatening e-mails that she began blocking them from her e-mail server. As a result, she was not aware of the e-mails' escalating and threatening nature.

On the morning that he decided he was to kill Cindy, Walter called her several times from his cell phone. He kept his cell phone with him because he hoped that she would return his calls. He waited in an area that he knew she would pass by on her way to class. When he finally saw her on her way to class, he noticed that she was walking with a male classmate, which further enraged him.

Walter approached her from behind and shot her at close range in the back of the head with a handgun. Cindy died instantly. The campus police had been a block away and arrived at the scene within seconds. During a psychiatric evaluation after the offense, Walter said that he had been driven by a desperate sense of "love, hate, and betrayal." He said, "If she had come back to me and shown loyalty, I would have forgotten and forgiven anything."

Case Discussion

Although some of the following discussion requires speculation, the case of Walter and Cindy demonstrates some important psychodynamic aspects of stalking for the purpose of discussion, and this case will be revisited in other chapters in this book. In the beginning, Walter "loves" Cindy. Stalking often is conceptualized as pathology of love. When she refuses his calls and declines to be his girlfriend, Walter suffers from anxiety and narcissistic injury. The separation anxiety progresses to depression and functional school failure upon his return to college. Instead of grieving his loss, Walter becomes increasingly angry. His vengeful fantasies and actions escalate as Cindy continues to ignore and reject him. Her death represents the ultimate separation or reunion.

Reflecting on the words of Harold Searles, it seems Walter and Cindy would have suffered less if he had worked through the separation anxiety and grieved the loss at the time of the break-up and his return to college. According to Meloy's (1999) dynamic theories related to stalking, the narcissistic fantasy that joins Walter to Cindy is broken with the rejection, and the feelings of shame and humiliation turn into rage. The energy of these emotions becomes the driving force that leads to Walter's eventual deadly actions, and he becomes eternally linked to Cindy. One could argue that a point of intervention and prevention could well have been at the time he entered mental health treatment. Had he been more forthcoming, and had his risk management involved a more aggressive specific approach for stalking behaviors, the mental health professionals may have been more successful in interpreting his dysfunctional defenses and guiding him toward a healthier expression of his grief and separation anxiety. Yet, Walter's choice to stalk and eventually kill Cindy represents a prominent mode of vengefulness.

EPIDEMIOLOGICAL STUDIES

Our knowledge of the prevalence of stalking in the community is based on the few epidemiological studies done to date. This information is summarized in Table 1.1. The first study (Australian Bureau of Statistics, 1996) involved

Table 1.1. Overview of Findings From Epidemiological Studies of Stalking Victims

Study/Year	Sample/ Method	Frequency of Stalking	Stalker	Duration of Stalking
Australian Bureau of Statistics (ABS), 1996	6,300 women in Australia by survey	Women: 15% over lifetime	Most strangers to victim	30% > 1 month 25% = 6 months to 2 years 15% > 2 years
National Institute of Justice (NIJ) and the Centers for Disease Control and Prevention (CDC), 1998	8,000 adult men and 8,000 women in the United States by telephone interview	Women: 8% over lifetime Men: 2% over lifetime	59% former intimate	50% < 1 year 25% = 2–5 years 10% > 5 years
British Crime Survey (BCS), 1998	10,000 men and women by face-to-face interviews	Women: 16% over lifetime Men: 7% over lifetime; 3% both men and women in prior year	29% former intimates 33% unknown to victim	26% 1–3 months 19% > 1 year
Louisiana, 1998	1,171 females by telephone interview	Women: 15% over lifetime; 2% in current year	51% ex-intimates 33% acquaintances 13% strangers	15% lifetime 2% current
Purcell, 1999	3,700 adults by survey	Men and women: 33% over lifetime; 2.9% in prior year	57% known to victim	10% > 1 year
Germany, 2005	1,000 men and 1,000 women; 400 women and 200 men by mail response	Men and women: 11.6% Women over lifetime: 17% Men over lifetime: 4%	76% known to the victim	17% = 1 month 24% > 1 year

a random and representative sample of 6,300 adult women, who were asked whether a man had ever stalked them. Stalking was defined as follows: being followed or watched; having a man loiter outside the home, workplace, or places of leisure; being phoned or sent mail; receiving offensive material; or experiencing property interference or damage. In the survey, 15% of women reported being stalked at some time in their lives. Most women reported being stalked by a stranger. In 30% of subjects the stalking lasted less than 1 month, in approximately 25% of cases the stalking lasted 6 months to 2 years, and in 15% the stalking lasted longer than 2 years.

In the United States, the National Institute of Justice (NIJ) and the Centers for Disease Control and Prevention (CDC) commissioned a study to examine domestic violence against women (Tjaden & Thoennes, 1998). Although the data were collected not solely for the purpose of further understanding stalking, the authors reported findings that looked at the prevalence of stalking. Data were collected by telephone interviews conducted with 8,000 adult women and 8,000 adult men, asking subjects specific behavioral questions. The questions included whether anyone had ever followed or spied on them, sent unsolicited mail or correspondence, made unsolicited phone calls, stood outside their home, school, or workplace, showed up at the same places even though they had no business being there, left them unwanted items, tried to communicate with them against their will, vandalized their property, or destroyed something they loved. These behaviors were considered stalking according to this study if they occurred on two or more occasions and if they caused the victim significant fear or fear of bodily harm.

The findings of NIJ/CDC study revealed that 8% of women and 2% of men experienced the study's definition of stalking at some time in their lives. The 12-month prevalence of stalking was 1% for women and 0.4% for men. When respondents who reported being only "somewhat frightened" were added to the sample, the lifetime risks were 12% for women and 4% for men, and the 12-month prevalence were 6% for women and 1.5% for men. There were no differences in stalking victimization between white and minority groups, although among minority groups, women from Native American Indian and Alaskan backgrounds were at higher risk than women from other minority groups.

Among female victims of stalking, the stalker was male in 94% of the cases, and a current or former intimate in 59% of the cases. Among women stalked by an intimate, 80% reported being assaulted by the stalker. Among male victims, the gender of stalkers was evenly split, with an even three-way split of stalkers being current or former intimates, strangers, or acquaintances.

In terms of duration, 50% of victims were stalked for less than 1 year, 25% for 2 to 5 years, and 10% for more than 5 years.

One half of the victims reported the stalking to the police. The police prosecuted less than 20% of the reported cases, and one-half of the prosecuted cases resulted in conviction.

In another significant epidemiological study related to stalking, the British Crime Survey (BCS) of 1998 enrolled about 10,000 persons in England and Whales (Budd & Mattinson, 2000). According to the findings, 3% reported being stalked in the prior year, whereas 16% of women and 7% of men were subjected to persistent and unwanted attention sometime in their life. Using the respondents as a representative sample, the BCS estimated that 2.9% of adults (aged 16 to 59), or 880,000 victims, experienced stalking in the previous year.

Purcell, Pathé, and Mullen (2002) conducted a random community survey in Melbourne, Australia, in 1999. The subject sample was 3,700 adults registered to vote, 74% of whom responded. One in four respondents reported being a victim of repeated behaviors that met the legal definition of stalking. One in 10 reported victimization lasting greater than 1 month. Those who reported victimization in the previous year constituted 2.9%. A third of those ages 18–35 had been subjected to stalking behaviors in their lifetime.

In this study, more victims (75%) were female than male. Most of the victims were in a relationship and employed. Fifty-seven percent knew their stalker, and 24% of the victims had same-sex perpetrators.

Purcell and colleagues (2002) also showed that explicit threats (including physical, reputation, or child harm) accompanied 29% of stalking behaviors. Third-party threats (family members, friends, and current partners) totaled 16%. Eighteen percent of victims gave an account of assaults; 23%, property damage; 2%, sexual assaults; 10% third party; and on three occasions, the family pet was killed. Half of the threats progressed to assaults. Sixty-three percent of victims changed their lifestyle to increase security.

From July 1, 1998, to June 30, 1999, the Louisiana Office of Public Health (Centers for Disease Control and Prevention, 2000) collected telephone data concerning stalking incidence and prevalence from 1,808 Louisiana residents. The study findings included only women respondents (1,171, or 65%). The findings showed that 15% of women had been stalked sometime in their life and 2% were being stalked currently. Seventy-five percent of the victims believed they were in danger at the time they were stalked, and 67% reported the stalking behavior to the police. Seventy percent of the victims changed their behavior, 51% of the stalkers were ex-intimates, 33% were acquaintances, and 13% were strangers. Thirty-two percent reported physical injuries, and 55% reported stress in connection with the stalking.

In a more recent study out of Germany, a randomly selected group of people from Mannheim, Germany (a mid-sized city) were sent via mail a stalking questionnaire and a scale of well being (Dressing, Kuehner, & Gass, 2005). In this study, the authors chose to define stalking as consisting of multiple episodes of harassing behaviors that had to be present for at least 2 weeks, involving more than one form of intrusive behavior, and having provoked fear. Of the 679 respondents, 11.6% reported having been stalked at some point in their life. Women were stalked more frequently than men were (17% vs. 4%). Most victims (87%) were women, and most (86%) stalkers were men. In about three-quarters of the cases (76%), the victim knew the stalker.

The above named studies report widely disparate values for the prevalence of stalking. Although definitions of stalking and methods of data collection make comparisons difficult, trends in the literature have emerged indicating that stalking is an important problem in our society and one worthy of further research attention. For women, the studies report an 8–33% lifetime risk of being the victim of stalking; for men, the reported lifetime risk is 2–7%. In a review article, Dressing, Kuehner, and Gass (2006) find similar lifetime prevalence rates of 12–16% among women and 4–7% among men. In our discussions among members of the GAP Committee on Psychiatry and the Law, we interpreted the disparities as reflecting differences in definitions of stalking used in each study, differences in survey questions and methods, and (possibly) increased public recognition of and attention to stalking. Dressing, Kuehner, and Gass (2006) reach a similar summation: "Increased social and political awareness and expanded research funding are prerequisites to realize sound and well-designed studies" (p. 395). Increased public recognition of and attention to stalking may mean that stalking cases are increasingly being recognized, or it may mean that the increased attention to this phenomenon has led to a rise in its prevalence. Although the latter is theoretically of interest, there are no current definitive data to verify this.

EPIDEMIOLOGY OF STALKING VIOLENCE

The epidemiology of stalking violence has been studied even less than the epidemiology of stalking. Reported rates of stalking leading to violence (broadly defined) vary from 3% to 47% (see Table 1.2; Mullen & Pathé, 2002). Zona, Sharma, and Lane (1993) reviewed 74 cases from the Threat Management Unit

Table 1.2. Reported Rates of Violence Against Victim by Stalker

Study	Violence Against Victim Reported (%)	Source of Data
Zona, Sharma, and Lane (1993)	3	Stalker
Harmon, Rosner, and Owens (1995)	21	Stalker
Harmon, Rosner, and Owens (1998)	46	Stalker
Hall (1998)	25–35	Victim
Mullen, Pathé, Purcell, and Stuart (1999)	36	Stalker
Brewster (2000)	46	Victim
Mohandie, Meloy, McGowan, and Williams (2006)	46	Prosecutorial agency, entertainment security department, and police agency, authors' files

(TMU), the majority of which were referred from the entertainment industry. They reported that 2 of their 74 stalkers had assaulted their victim. Harmon and colleagues (Harmon, Rosner, & Owens, 1995) studied the Forensic Psychiatry Clinic evaluations. They reported that 21% (of 48 stalkers) had committed assault. In 1998, Harmon Rosner, and Owens reviewed 10 years of clinic evaluations. They reported that 47% (of 81 stalkers) had committed assaults. Hall (1998) surveyed victims, who are considered a more reliable source. Of the 145 victims, 38% were hit or beaten and 22% were subjected to sexual assaults. Two subjects were victimized with arson attacks.

In the 1998 *Third Annual Report to Congress Under the Violence Against Women Act*, stalking was defined as "harassing or threatening behavior that an individual engages in repeatedly," and stalkers were noted to be violent toward their victims in 25–35% of the cases (from Merschman, 2000). Mullen, Pathé, Purcell, and Stuart (1999) studied the rate of violence in 145 stalkers referred to a psychiatric clinic with special interest in stalking. In this study, over one-third of victims were assaulted and 6% of stalkers attacked a third party. In all of these studies, the data focused on a select group of stalkers or victims.

In 2000, Brewster (2000) assessed the relationship of verbal threats to physical violence in ex-intimate stalkers. The National Crime Victimization Survey (NCVS) conducted by the Department of Justice in 1995 provided the data. The NCVS uses household survey instruments, including its Basic Screen Questionnaire, Crime Incident Report, and Police Public Contact Survey. The sample consisted of 187 victims of ex-intimate stalkers. Brewster found that 46% reported physical violence. Of the victims of physical violence, 52.9% were directly threatened, 19.8% received implied threats, and 27.3% were not threatened physically prior to the physical violence.

Mechanic, Weaver, and Resick (2000) studied the relationship of stalking behavior and ex-intimate violence in battered women. The sample consisted of 114 battered women, 94% of whom reported that they were threatened with harm. In the same sample, 89% experienced physical harm; 88%, attempts to harm; and 61%, stolen mail. Half of the women reported that the ex-intimate had violated a restraining order in the previous 6 months. The results supported the high rate of stalking violence and harassment among battered women. Emotional and psychological abuse predicted stalking behaviors during and after the relationship, with higher frequencies occurring with longer time from the end of the relationship.

In a study of risk factors for femicide in abusive relationships, stalking was among the characteristics of intimate partner violence associated with intimate partner femicide (Campbell et al., 2003). Intimate partners perpetrated high rates of assault in connection with stalking of female victims in this study.

In a related article, Rosenfeld (2003) focused on recidivism. The New York City Forensic Psychiatry Clinic of Bellevue Hospital provided the data, including forensic clinic evaluations, court documents, criminal complaint forms, and records from the Department of Probation. Reoffenders included clients who renewed harassment or were arrested a second time. The recidivism rate was about 50%. The combination of personality disorder and a history of substance abuse raised the risk of reoffending. These results overlap the findings in studies of violent stalkers.

Rosenfeld (2004) summarized risk factors in stalking violence. Noting that fear of violence is common among victims, he reviewed the existing literature on stalking violence. He found several risk factors, but no definitive numbers. Several complications to epidemiological conclusions included data samples that over- or underidentified the offenders, the definition of violence used in the studies, and failure to separate minor and serious violence. Yet, Rosenfeld still found risk factors corresponding to stalking violence. The risk factors were threats, mental disorders, past violence, and victim-offender relationship. Interestingly, the mental disorders with the greatest association to violence included substance abuse and antisocial or paranoid personality disorders. Finally, Rosenfeld notes the paucity of comparable data and the need for continued research on stalking violence. (For a detailed discussion of violence among stalkers and risk assessment, see chapter 4, Risk Management of Stalking.)

In January 2006, Mohandie, Meloy, McGowan, and Williams published the RECON typology of stalking. The study included 1,005 stalking cases. The files came from the authors' files, prosecutors' offices, a police department, and an entertainment corporation security department. Stalking was defined as "two or more unwanted contacts by a subject toward a target that created a reasonable fear in that target" (p. 148). Violence included "acts of intentional physical aggression toward a person or object" (p. 149). Both threats and violence were investigated. Threats, most often made to the target (94%), occurred in 60% of cases. In comparison, the stalkers acted violently in 46% of the cases. Violence was directed toward the victim in 30%, toward a third party in 7%, and toward an animal in 2%. Assault occurred more often than other violent acts. Homicide or mass murder happened at a rate of 0.50%. Mohandie and colleagues also noted that weapons were used for threats or violence in 20% of cases.

Testing the reliability of research on stalking violence is the next step. The potential for a stalker to become violent comprises the essence of law enforcement and the victim's fears. These studies vastly differ in data, definitions, and focus. Victim reports are considered more accurate than stalker reports because of stalker incentives to underreport violence. Reviewing forensic clinic evaluations or court cases may underestimate stalking behavior as a precursor to violence. The definitions of stalking and violence differ among the studies. The classification of stalkers and/or the occurrence of a threat prior to violence were important foci of some, but not all, studies. The variation in data collection, definitions used, and study focus made direct comparisons of results difficult. Reliable research would certainly allow for more accurate definitions in laws and counseling for victims.

SPECIAL POPULATIONS

Some epidemiological studies have focused on special populations, such as college students, therapists, celebrities, and victims of women stalkers (see Table 1.3). Celebrity and special target stalking is dealt with in chapter 10 in this book. Further information on childhood and adolescent stalking can be found in chapter 8.

College Students

Two studies account for much of our knowledge about the prevalence of stalking among college students. Fremouw and colleagues (1997) surveyed 600 college students recruited from a psychology class in West Virginia. Study I contained a 29-behavior questionnaire, and Study II contained a revised 22-item questionnaire. They found that 30% of female students and 17% of male students reported being stalked, when stalking was defined as "having someone knowingly and repeatedly following, harassing, or threatening you" (p. 667). This definition was used because it corresponded to the legal definition in the jurisdiction of the university. In one part of the study, a group of respondents were asked whether they had ever stalked someone else. No female students responded affirmatively, but 3 of 129 male students (2.3%) did so.

Bjerregaard (2000) examined stalking and its victims in the college population. Noting previous rates of 4–40% victimization (Spitzberg, Nicastro, & Cousins, 1998), she surveyed 788 undergraduate students at UNC–Charlotte. Twenty-five percent of females and 11% of males reported having been stalked.

Table 1.3. Stalking Prevalence Reported by College Students

Study	Source of Data	Stalking Victimization (%)	Types of Stalking
Fremouw and colleagues, 1997	College students (Victim report)	Women: 30 Men: 17	Following, harassing, threatening
Bjerregaard, 2000	College students (Victim report)	Women: 25 Men: 11	Calling, harassing, threatening

Females reported being stalked for an average of 83 days and males for 99 days. Most offenders were the opposite sex. The most common stalker was unmarried, white, a student, and an acquaintance. Most victims were contacted by letter, phone, or in person; 2.5% of female victims reported a death threat or threat to their family through the mail. By phone, 24% of females and 14% of males were threatened with physical violence. Over half of the females, compared to 21% of the males, expressed victim fear.

Mental Health Professionals

Four studies have examined rates of stalking mental health care professionals (see Table 1.4). Taken together, the data suggest that health-care professionals report having been stalked at rates higher than the general population. In a study of 178 counseling center staff members, Romans, Hays, and White (1996) reported that 5.6% of the staff said a current or former client had stalked them. Stalking was defined as "willfully, maliciously, and repeatedly following or harassing another person and making a credible threat" (p. 595). The study also assessed harassing behavior, defined as a "willful course of conduct directed at a specific person which seriously alarms or annoys the person, and which serves no legitimate purpose" (p. 595). A much higher percentage (64%) of staff responded affirmatively to that inquiry. In response to other questions, approximately 8% of staff members reported that a family member or other close person had been

Table 1.4. Stalking Prevalence Among Studies of Mental Health Professionals

Population	Studies	Rates of Reported Stalking or Harassment (%)	Types of Stalking
Mental health professionals (Staff report)	Romans and colleagues (1996)	5.6 (staff)	Willfully, maliciously, repeatedly followed
		64 (staff)	Conduct that seriously alarmed
Forensic psychiatrists (Victim report)	Miller (1985)	42 (doctors) 3 (doctors)	Harassed Physically assaulted
Psychologists (Victim report)	Gentile, Asamen, Harmell, and Weathers (2002)	10 (psychologists) 0	Not defined Physically harmed
Clinicians in Italy (Victim report)	Galezzi, Elkins, and Curci (2005)	11 (mental health professionals)	Unwanted contacts

stalked or harassed by a client, and 9.6% reported that they supervised another person who had been stalked by a client.

Pathé, Mullen, and Purcell (2002) described patients who stalk their doctors. The authors define stalking as harassing behaviors extending beyond 2 weeks. They reported a survey of 850 forensic psychiatrists as subjects with 480 respondents (Miller, 1985). Overall, 42% of respondents reported having been harassed. Three percent had been physically assaulted. Threats of physical harm occurred in 17%, and threats such as a lawsuit occurred in 13%. Pathé and colleagues (2002) reviewed two other studies: one conducted at the Oregon Psychiatric Society (Lion & Herschler, 1998) and the other a self-referred victim survey including health-care professionals (Pathé & Mullen, 1997). Pathé and colleagues (2002) also noted that the two major motivations for stalking were resentment and romantic/childlike attachments. They concluded that better psychiatric education about stalking could improve treatment and reduce the occurrence.

Gentile, Asamen, Harmell, and Weathers (2002) also studied stalking of mental health professionals, focusing on psychologists. Two hundred and ninety-four psychologists returned the survey. Roughly 10% reported being stalked. Clients stalked more male than female psychologists. Male and female clients stalked female psychologists almost equally. Primarily female clients stalked male psychologists.

Galeazzi, Elkins, and Curci (2005) looked at stalking of clinicians in Italy, where the media has not focused much attention on stalking. They surveyed 475 mental health professionals. Stalking was defined as 10 or more unwanted contacts occurring for 4 or more weeks. Eleven percent met the criteria for stalking. Male professionals were more likely to be stalked. The professionals most likely to be stalked were psychologists and psychiatrists. Although the rate of stalking was less than in the previous studies, stalking of mental health professionals occurred even in a country where stalking has not dominated the media.

Conclusions Related to Stalking Epidemiology Among Special Victim Populations

These studies suggest that among the general population, individuals at greater risk of being stalked include college students, mental health professionals, and women. (As noted above, this assessment does not include celebrities and/or child and adolescent stalking.) The committee questions whether the college student data are comparable to the other special population data. The college-age population may be more aware of stalking than the average adult. This age group may also be more likely to report stalking. Finally, the college studies use slightly different definitions. The rates of stalking in all three populations range from 5%

to 62%, as compared to a range of 2–33% in the general population. Specific research could help these populations treat and manage stalking.

MALE AND FEMALE STALKERS

Two articles focus on how female stalkers differ from male stalkers. (Data obtained from these articles appears in Table 1.5.) Purcell, Pathé, and Mullen (2001) studied the question of whether female stalkers differ from male stalkers. The sample consisted of 40 female and 150 male stalkers referred to a forensic mental health clinic. The study results demonstrated similar demographics except that male stalkers had more criminal offenses and higher rates of substance abuse. The duration and frequency of stalking was similar for males and females, as was the intrusiveness and potential for danger. Most female stalkers were motivated to attain intimacy with the victim. Male stalkers had a broader range of motivations. Females were less likely to stalk strangers and more likely to stalk same-sex victims. The target profile of female stalkers was someone previously known and cast in the role of professional helper.

Meloy and Boyd (2003) reviewed demographic, clinical, and forensic characteristics of female stalkers. The database consisted of 82 cases of female stalkers from the United States, Australia, and Canada. The demographics of female stalkers were similar to male stalkers except that one-third of female stalkers were raising children. Violence toward the victim occurred in 55% of relationships with prior intimacy. In the remaining sample, violence occurred at a rate of 15%. Most female stalkers had Axis I and Axis II diagnoses. Female stalkers were less likely to follow and more likely to intrude, vandalize, use surveillance, and steal from the victim. They threatened their victims at the same rate as male stalkers. The frequency of violence with prior intimates was 55%, with an overall assault rate of 22.5% for all female stalkers. Two of the female stalkers in this study killed their victims. The victims were mostly males and the stalking behaviors persisted for 1 to 5 years.

Table 1.5. Stalking Rates of Male and Female Stalkers

Population	Studies	Numbers of Stalkers	Demographics
Male and female stalkers (Stalker report)	Purcell, Pathé, and Mullen (2001)	40 female 150 male	Similar demographics among male and female stalkers
Female stalkers (Stalker report)	Meloy and Boyd (2003)	82 females	Similar demographics when compared to studies of male stalkers

CONCLUSION

A review of the epidemiology literature clearly indicates that stalking is not a rare phenomenon and may be on the rise. Studies have lacked consistency in methods and populations, making comparisons of results difficult. Results available show only a range. Existing literature suggests that women have an 8–33% lifetime risk of being the victim of stalking, depending on the definition of stalking used to gather the results. For men, the lifetime risk is 2–7%. Studies on the epidemiology of stalking violence also yield a wide range of results: 3–46% of stalkers progress to violence. Special populations at greater risk of being stalked include college students, mental health professionals, and women. Continued research is necessary to thoroughly understand stalking and its victims. We believe that greater education and training about stalking can address and decrease this phenomenon and related mortality and morbidity in today's society.

REFERENCES

Australian Bureau of Statistics. (1996). *Woman's safety Australia* (Cat. No. 4128.0). Canberra: Australian Bureau of Statistics.

Bjerregaard, B. (2000). An empirical study of stalking victimization. *Violence and Victims, 15*(4), 389–406.

Brewster, M. P. (2000). Stalking by former intimates: Verbal threats and other predictors of physical violence. *Violence and Victims, 15*(1), 41–53.

Budd, T., & Mattinson, J. (2000). *The extent and nature of stalking: Findings from the 1998 British Crime Survey.* London: Home Office Research, Development and Statistics Directorate.

Campbell, J. C., Webster, D., Koziol-McLane, J, Block, C., Campbell, D., Curry, M. A., et al. (2003). Risk factors for femicide in abusive relationships: Results from a multisite case control study. *American Journal of Public Health, 93*(7), 1089–1097.

Centers for Disease Control and Prevention. (2000). Prevalence and health consequences of stalking—Louisiana. *JAMA, 284*(20), 2588–2589.

de Clérambault, G. G. (1921). Les délires passionnels: Erotomanie, jalousie. *Société Clinique de Médicine Mentales, 1–2*, 62–71.

Dressing, H., Kuehner, C., & Gass, P. (2005). Lifetime prevalence and impact of stalking in a European population. *British Journal of Psychiatry, 187*, 168–172.

Dressing, H., Kuehner, C., & Gass, P. (2006). The epidemiology and characteristics of stalking. *Current Opinion in Psychiatry, 19*(4), 395–399.

Esquirol, J. E. D. (1965). *Mental maladies: A treatise on insanity* (R. de Saussure, Trans.). New York: Hafner Press. (Original work published 1838)

Fremouw, W. J., Westrup, D., & Pennypacker, J. (1997). Stalking on campus: The prevalence and strategies for coping with stalking. *Journal of Forensic Science, 42*(4), 666–669.

Galeazzi, G. M., Elkins, B. A., & Curci, P. (2005). The stalking of mental health professionals by patients. *Emergency Psychiatry, 56*(2), 137–138.

Gentile, S. R., Asamen J. K., Harmell, P. H., & Weathers, R. (2002). The stalking of psychologists by their clients. *Professional Psychology: Research and Practice 33*(5), 490–494.

Hall, D. M. (1998). The victims of stalking. In J. R. Meloy (Ed.), *The psychology of stalking: Clinical and forensic perspectives* (pp. 113–137). San Diego: Academic Press.

Harmon, R., Rosner, R., & Owens, H. (1995). Obsessional harassment and erotomania in a criminal court population. *Journal of Forensic Sciences, 40*(2), 188–196.

Harmon, R., Rosner, R., & Owens, H. (1998). Sex and violence in a forensic population of obsessional harassers. *Psychology, Public Policy, and Law, 4*(1/2), 236–245.

Kraepelin, E. (1976). *Manic-depressive insanity and paranoia* (R. M. Barclay, Trans.; G. M. Robertson, E. Edinburgh, and S. Livingstone, Eds.). New York: Arno Press. (Original work published 1921)

Lion, J. R., & Herschler, J. A. (1998). The stalking of clinicians by their patients. In J. R. Meloy (Ed.), *The psychology of stalking: Clinical and forensic perspectives* (pp. 163–173). San Diego: Academic Press.

Lloyd-Goldstein, R. (1998). De Clérembault on-line: A survey of eratomania and stalking from the old world to the World Wide Web. In J. R. Meloy (Ed.), *The psychology of stalking: Clinical and forensic perspectives.* San Diego: Academic Press.

Lowney, K. S., & Best, J. (1995). Stalking strangers and lovers: Changing media typifications of a new crime problem. In J. Best (Ed.), *Images of issues: Typifying contemporary social problems* (pp. 33–57). New York: Aldine DeGruyter.

Mechanic, M., Weaver, T., & Resick, P. (2000). Intimate partner violence and stalking behavior. *Violence and Victims, 15*(1), 55–72.

Meloy, J. R. (Ed.). (1998). *The psychology of stalking: Clinical and forensic perspectives.* San Diego: Academic Press.

Meloy, J. R. (1999). Stalking: An old behavior, a new crime. *The Psychiatric Clinics of North America, 22*(1), 85–99.

Meloy, J. R., & Boyd, C. (2003). Female stalkers and their victims. *Journal of the American Academy of Psychiatry and Law, 31,* 211–219.

Meloy, J. R., & Gothard, S. (1995). Demographics and clinical comparison of obsessional followers and offenders with mental disorders. *American Journal of Psychiatry, 152*(2), 258–263.

Merschman, J. C. (2000). The dark side of the web: Cyberstalking and the need for contemporary legislation. *Harvard Women's Law Journal, 24,* 255–292.

Miller, R. D. (1985). The harassment of forensic psychiatrists outside of court. *Bulletin of American Academy of Psychiatry and Law, 13,* 337–343.

Mohandie, K., Meloy, J. R., McGowan, M. G., & Williams, J. (2006). The RECON typology of stalking: Reliability and validity based upon a large sample of North American stalkers. *Journal of Forensic Science, 51*(1), 147–155.

Mullen, P. E. (2003). Multiple classifications of stalkers and stalking behavior available to clinicians. *Psychiatric Annals, 33*(10), 651–656.

Mullen, P. E., & Pathé, M. (1994). Stalking and the pathologies of love. *Australian and New Zealand Journal of Psychiatry, 28*(3), 469–477.

Mullen, P. E., & Pathé, M. (2002). Stalking. *The University of Chicago Crime and Justice,* 273–315.

Mullen, P. E., Pathé, M., & Purcell, R. (2000). *Stalkers and their victims* (pp. 6–15). Cambridge, UK: Cambridge University Press.

Mullen, P. E., Pathé, M., & Purcell, R. (2001). Stalking: New constructs of human behavior. *Australian and New Zealand of Psychiatry, 35*(1), 9–16.

Mullen, P. E., Pathé, M., Purcell, R., & Stuart, G. (1999). Study of stalkers. *The American Journal of Psychiatry, 156,* 1244–1249.

Pathé, M. (2002). *Surviving stalking* (pp. 9–13). Cambridge, UK: Cambridge University Press.

Pathé, M., & Mullen, P. E. (1997). The impact of stalkers on their victims. *British Journal of Psychiatry, 170,* 12–17.

Pathé, M. T., Mullen, P. E., & Purcell, R. (2002). Patients who stalk their doctors: Their motives and management. *Medical Journal of Australia, 176,* 335–338.

Purcell, R., Pathé, M., & Mullen, P. E. (2001). A study if women who stalk. *American Journal of Psychiatry, 158,* 2056–2060.

Purcell, R., Pathé, M., & Mullen, P. E. (2002). The prevalence and nature of stalking in the Australian community. *Australian and New England Journal of Psychiatry 2002, 36,* 114–120.

Romans, J. S. C., Hays, J. R., & White, T. K. (1996). Stalking and related behaviors experienced by counseling center staff members from current or former clients. *Professional Psychology: Research and Practice, 27,* 595–599.

Rosenfeld, B. (2003). Recidivism in stalking and obsessional harassment. *Law and Human Behavior, 27*(3), 251–265.

Rosenfeld, B. (2004). Violence risk factors in stalking and obsessional harassment: A review and preliminary meta-analysis. *Criminal Justice and Behavior, 31*(1), 9–36.

Saunders, R. (1998). The legal perspective on stalking. In J. R. Meloy (Ed.), *The psychology of stalking: Clinical and forensic perspectives* (pp. 28–51). San Diego: Academic Press.

Searles, H. F. (1956): The psychodynamics of vengefulness. *Psychiatry* 19, 31–39.

Skoler, G. (1998). The archetypes and psychodynamics of stalking. In J. R. Meloy (Ed.), *The psychology of stalking: Clinical and forensic perspectives* (pp. 85–112). San Diego: Academic Press.

Spitzberg, B. H., Nicastro, A. M., & Cousins, A. V. (1998). Exploring the interactional phenomenon of stalking and obsessive relational intrusion. *Communication Reports, 11,* 33–47.

Tjaden, P., & Thoennes, N. (1998). *Stalking in America: Findings from the National Violence Against Women Survey* (Research in Brief Series, Publication

NCJ 169592). Washington, DC: National Institute of Justice and Centers for Disease Control and Prevention.

Westrup, D., & Fremouw, W. J. (1998). Stalking behavior: A literature review and suggested functional analytic assessment technology. *Aggression and Violent Behavior, 3*(3), 255–274.

Zona, M. A., Sharma, K. K., & Lane, J. (1993). A comparative study of erotomanic and obsessional subjects in a forensic sample. *Journal of Forensic Science, 38*(4), 894–903.

PART II

Clinical Aspects of Stalking

2   Stalking: Classification and Typology

Debra A. Pinals

Stalking, as currently conceptualized, is a complex phenomenon, and individual stalking cases can be quite distinct. Several authors have proposed classification schemes in an effort to discern and understand common themes among cases of stalking. These stalking "typologies" reflect both theoretical considerations and empirical examinations of persons whose behaviors have shaped the definition of stalking. Typologies have been constructed from clinical and law enforcement perspectives. Classification schemes to date have been broadly based on factors such as the motivation of the stalker, psychiatric symptoms among stalkers, the nature of the relationship between the pursuer and the victim, victim characteristics, and harm to the victim. These classifications have been conceptualized to assist with risk assessment, risk management, and treatment considerations in stalking cases. This chapter describes some historical underpinnings of classification categories, compares existing typologies of stalkers, and explicates the typological scheme adopted throughout this book.

INTRODUCTION

Over the last 15 years, stalking has become increasingly recognized as a distinctive form of potentially criminal behavior that may come to the attention of mental health professionals. At the same time that the criminal justice system has grappled with defining stalking for legal purposes, clinicians who encounter stalking behavior have attempted to create useful classifications of stalking behaviors. Attempts have also been made to develop taxonomies of stalking types that might guide law enforcement professionals. Taxonomic classifications are common in science and, when they are successful, they help us organize and identify unique aspects of information and refine our understanding of the given phenomenon under study.

Setting up a system of classification of stalking, a behavior that is difficult to define and codify, has several advantages. Once established, a useful taxonomy of stalkers could improve communication among professionals and could help them better appreciate aspects of stalking, including the natural course of the behavior and prognosis of particular stalkers. In addition, taxonomic categorization can facilitate case comparisons and improve clinicians' abilities to assess risks, manage risks, and provide treatment. Stalking typologies may also enlighten decisions about social policy and legal regulation related to the phenomenon.

Although the science of classifying stalking is still relatively young, a growing number of publications have begun to tease out types and nuances of stalking behavior. As a result, clinicians can now choose from an array of typological schemes that can be useful for general clinical practice and case management. Yet the typological schemes that have been described vary markedly. This chapter reviews theoretical foundations for understanding stalking behavior in a categorical framework and describes several of the classification models proposed to date.

After reviewing the existing classification models, our GAP Psychiatry and the Law Committee decided to use the system developed by Mullen and colleagues (Mullen, Pathé, & Purcell, 2000; Mullen, Pathé, Purcell, & Stuart, 1999) in this book. A separate section in this chapter is devoted to an examination of Mullen and colleagues' classification system, to which we will refer throughout much of this volume. Therefore, readers may wish to focus on the section of this chapter (see pp. 45–51) that reviews Mullen and colleagues' typology. The number and variety of proposed classification schemes can be confusing. To help readers digest the existing published works in this area, this chapter concludes with a discussion of several systems' advantages, disadvantages, and limitations.

HISTORICAL BACKGROUND TO STALKING CLASSIFICATION

Before stalking gained its social and legal contemporary definitions, depictions of stalking in popular media often portrayed the behavior as stemming from obsessive pathological love linked to psychological problems and emotional instability. In a sense, this represented an informal way of classifying or categorizing stalking behavior as a manifestation of psychopathology. The concept of erotomania has emerged from cases of preoccupying love and false beliefs of being loved that have been described for centuries. Often, people think that those engaged in stalking behavior must have a type of "erotomanic" delusion, and early research positing typologies of stalking attempted to explore this issue (Harmon, Rosner, & Owens, 1995; Zona, Sharma, & Lane, 1993). Although studies over the last 15 years have shown that only a minority of stalking behaviors are driven by such delusional states, the development of stalking classifications began with attempts to examine forms of erotomania. A review of the historical clinical conceptualizations of erotomania is therefore a good place to begin our discussion of the evolution of stalking taxonomies.

Erotomania: Origins and Evolving Conceptualizations

The term erotomania has several connotations. It has, at times, been confused with nymphomania, which describes the person who repeatedly engages and seeks amorous encounters, generally driven by lust (Enoch & Ball, 2001). The writer most frequently credited with a detailed description erotomania is the French psychiatrist Gaëtan Gatian de Clérambault, although Segal (1989) suggests that Emil Kraepelin was the first to systematically describe erotomania in the clinical literature.

In the early 1920s, de Clérambault described a syndrome called "psychose passionelle" (de Clérambault, 1942) which became known as de Clérambault's syndrome (Leong, 1994; Enoch & Ball, 2001; Lerner, Kapstan, & Witztum, 2001). De Clérambault's description included a pure form of erotomania, sometimes referred to as "primary erotomania," and a more general, or "secondary," form (de Clérambault, 1942; Lloyd-Goldstein, 1998). More recent clinical definitions of the term erotomania overlap with de Clérambault's syndrome in certain respects, though not completely.

The revised third edition of the American Psychiatric Association's *Diagnostic and Statistical Manual* (*DSM-III-R*; American Psychiatric Association [APA], 1987) was the first of the DSMs to include erotomania, which marked a major step in incorporating the concept into modern nosological terms. In the *DSM-III-R*, a person who had erotomanic delusions without other marked symptoms of mental disorders was regarded as having a type of a delusional disorder. A person experiencing a delusional disorder of the erotomanic type (see Table 2.1) would be experiencing a condition close to de Clérambault's primary erotomania, whereas a person whose erotomanic delusion was only one feature of a larger symptom complex (such as part of mania or schizophrenia) would have what de Clérambault described as secondary erotomania (de Clérambault, 1942; Lloyd-Goldstein, 1998).

Table 2.1. General Features of Delusional Disorder, Erotomanic Type (*DSM IV-TR*; APA, 2000)

1. Nonbizzare delusions lasting at least one month.
2. Delusion(s) involves the belief that "another person, usually of higher status, is in love with the individual."
3. Functioning may not appear impaired, apart from functioning revolving around the delusion.
4. Any mood episodes are brief in relation to the time period in which the individual has experienced delusional beliefs.
5. The individual would not meet the criteria for schizophrenia and symptoms would not be caused by substance use or a medical condition.
6. Hallucinations (tactile and olfactory), if they are present, must be related to the delusion belief.

In the *DSM-III-R*, an erotomanic delusion was one in which "the predominant theme . . . is that a person, usually of higher status, is in love with the subject" (APA, 1987, p. 202), similar in part to what de Clérambault specified. Although Segal (1989) argued that the syndrome described by de Clérambault was essentially no different from the conditions that Kraepelin and the *DSM-III-R* described, others (Leong, 1994; Lloyd-Goldstein, 1998) point out nuanced differences. For example, the 1987 *DSM* description of an erotomanic delusional disorder did not adopt de Clérambault's propositions that the patient would believe that the object of their preoccupation was the first to fall in love, that there would typically be an explosive onset of symptoms, or that other symptoms (including hallucinations) would be totally absent.

The definition of an erotomanic delusion has remained essentially the same in later revisions of the diagnostic manual, including the most recent edition, *DSM-IV-TR* (American Psychiatric Association, 2000; see also *DSM-IV,* 1994), and this definition remains the one most generally accepted by American mental health professionals.

For our purposes, we should note that language in *DSM-III-R* provided an important link between stalking and erotomania several years before anti-stalking laws came into existence in the United States. For example, *DSM III-R* stated that a person with an erotomanic delusional disorder might make numerous efforts to contact the object of the delusion through "telephone calls, letters, gifts, visits, and even surveillance and stalking . . . though occasionally the person keeps the delusion a secret" (APA, 1987, p. 199). *DSM-III-R* also commented that persons with the disorder (especially men) might come afoul of the law because of their efforts to pursue their victim or to save the victim from some falsely anticipated harm.

Two years after the publication of *DSM III-R*, Meloy (1989) described a nondelusional type of erotomania, which he labeled "borderline erotomania." In this form of pathological attachment, the pursuer develops an obsessional, perceived link to the pursued, but the pursuer holds no unrealistic beliefs about being loved in return. The borderline erotomanic stalker may have feelings for the victim that vacillate between love and hate. The capacity for healthy attachment is significantly disrupted, which contributes to the stalking-type behaviors and the potential for the feelings to change to hostility and aggression. Persons displaying what Mullen and Pathé (1994) later called "morbid infatuation" exhibit qualities similar to persons whom Meloy characterizes as having borderline erotomania.

DEVELOPMENT OF STALKING TYPOLOGIES

In general, recent stalking classification schemes have been developed using both empirical and theoretical approaches. As Boon and Sheridan (2001) note, stalking typologies have also been developed with different goals. For example, some typologies have been set forth to generally guide assessment and management of stalkers, whereas others have been described as being specifically aimed to assist law enforcement (see, e.g., Boon & Sheridan, 2001, and Sheridan & Boon, 2002). Some typologies are based on retrospective examinations of a cohort of persons who have engaged in behaviors with an obsessional focus on particular victims (often including threats or harassment), or examinations of victim reports. In these approaches, typologies are generally posited at the outset, and empirically gathered descriptive data is organized around the stalker types. Other authors (e.g., De Becker, 1997; McAnaney, Curliss, & Abeyta-Price, 1993) have approached the problem of classifying stalkers from more theoretical or impressionistic perspectives, without an empirical examination of their typological construct. Table 2.2 describes some of the rationales for stalking classifications, prototypical methods used for categorical divisions, and typical aspects of stalkers examined. Models utilizing the above approaches have derived from clinical observations, from work with law enforcement officials or from security-type case consultations.

Stalker typologies generally include a variety of factors, including the motivation of the stalker, the nature of the relationship of the stalker and the victim, victim characteristics, the psychiatric diagnosis of the stalker, and the harm done to the victim. Studies utilizing typologies based on these factors sometimes compare each type across other variables, such as stalker age, gender, age, race, level of education, marital status, criminal history, and duration and modalities of obsessional, threatening, and assaultive behaviors (see, for example, Harmon et al., 1995; Mullen et al., 1999; Zona et al., 1993).

Table 2.2. Development of Stalking Typologies

---

1. Typical Rationale for Various Stalking Classifications
   a. Clinical management
   b. Law enforcement
   c. Legal considerations

2. Prototypes of Methodologies Used for Stalking Typologies
   a. Theoretical categories derived from existing publications and experience
   b. Stalking file case review based on proposed typological schema
   c. Review of victim reports and categorization of proposed typologies

3. Typical Aspects of Stalker Subtypes
   a. Motivation of the stalker
   b. Nature of the relationship of the stalker and the victim
   c. Victim characteristics
   d. Psychiatric diagnosis of the stalker
   e. Risk of harm to the victim

The reliability and validity of existing classification schemes is limited by the methodology employed to date, which is discussed in greater detail below. A small number of studies have purported to utilize more empirical approaches categorizing stalking behaviors (Coleman, 1997; Del Ben & Fremouw, 2002; Mohandie, Meloy, McGowan, & Williams, 2006), but these have not clearly been replicated across samples. As Westrup (1998) notes, existing descriptive typologies will be able to answer only limited questions, and new avenues of research, such as an exploration of functional analyses of the antecedents and consequences of stalking behavior, may provide a direction that offers additional practical utility.

CLASSIFICATION SCHEMES

Data Derived From Evaluations of Stalkers

The empirical studies that have been conducted to develop stalking typologies have used a variety of subject populations and numbers of subjects examined. These studies have provided building blocks for other more theoretical classifications of stalkers. Dietz and colleagues (Dietz, Matthews, Martell, et al., 1991; Dietz, Matthews, Van Duyne, et al., 1991), for example, attempted to gain a greater understanding of those individuals who targeted celebrities and members of the United States Congress. Their work represents an early effort to examine individuals based on who they pursued. Almost a decade later, Meloy (2001) similarly focused on whether the target was a private or public figure.

Around the time that antistalking statutes began to be passed, Zona and colleagues (1993) developed one of the first and most influential classifications of stalking. Their model uses data gathered from examining case files of the Los Angeles Police Department Threat Management Unit, which had been created to focus exclusively on persons who had "an obsessional, or abnormal long-term pattern of threat or harassment directed toward a specific individual" (Zona et al., 1993, p. 896). Zona and colleagues described this obsessional pattern as ego-syntonic, as opposed to the ego-dystonic obsessional thinking found in some anxiety disorders. Because the Los Angeles area has a high concentration of celebrities, many of the case files of Zona et al. involved stalking of high-visibility individuals. Thus, their study findings would not be representative of all stalkers or stalkers in other regions.

Regardless of its limitations, the study remains widely cited, and represented a first major step at classification of stalkers. In an attempt to examine what proportion of stalkers had erotomania, their group compared stalking behaviors by persons with and without erotomania, as the term was defined in *DSM-III-R* (Zona, Palarea, & Lane, 1998; Zona et al., 1993). They also examined stalking behaviors by evaluating the dyadic relationship between the stalker and victim. In their 1993 report, Zona and colleagues ultimately classified their cohort of 74 cases into three types of stalkers, whom they labeled as *erotomanic*, *love obsessional*, and *simple obsessional*. (See Table 2.3.) Subsequent data analysis looking at additional cases revealed a fourth group of stalkers, whom Zona and colleagues regarded as manifesting a *false victimization syndrome* (Zona et al., 1998, p. 79; further discussion of false victimization can be found in chapter 5 of this volume).

Zona and colleagues' (1993, 1998) erotomanic stalkers typically did not know their victims (as in the case of celebrity victims) or did not know them well, but were distinguished from the other types of stalkers by their erotomanic beliefs that their victims were in love with them. The love obsessional stalkers had many features in common with the erotomanic stalkers. They most frequently included persons who did not personally know their victims, although they may have had knowledge of the victims through the media or because of the victims' political positions. Many of the love obsessional stalkers had erotomanic delusions. However, the stalkers were designated as love obsessional rather than erotomanic type when their erotomanic delusions were just a part of their symptom picture, such as seen in those individuals who had multiple types of delusions simultaneously, those that had other psychiatric symptoms, and those whose delusions involved the idea that the victim might love them if they made their presence known.

Other persons classified as love obsessional stalkers were obsessed with love for their victims but did not have erotomanic delusions that their victims loved them. Zona et al. (1993) noted that these individuals had been referred to as those with borderline erotomania, which connoted significant personality disorganization that led to the preoccupying love for the victim. However, they specifically avoided the term borderline in an effort to decrease confusion. Simple obsessional stalkers were persons who had preexisting relationships with their victims. Generally, the stalking behavior in this subgroup followed a disruption of the relational bond, for example, after a break-up in a romantic relationship or the stalker's perception of being treated poorly. The victims

Table 2.3. Zona and Colleagues' (1993) Typology

Typology	Focus of Typology	Empirical Case Review	Comments
1. Erotomanic 2. Love obsessional 3. Simple obsessional	Psychiatric diagnosis	Yes	1. Study sample included high numbers of celebrities 2. Subsequent publication (Zona, et al., 1998) yielded a fourth group, labeled "false victimization" syndrome

of simple obsessional stalkers included acquaintances, neighbors, professional contacts, and former intimate partners.

The decision to include any manner of acquaintance into one category has been criticized (Westrup, 1998). After gathering additional data, Zona and colleagues (1998) commented that they found it useful to divide the simple obsessional group into stalkers who had and had not been intimate with their victims.

Of the 74 subject cases reviewed in Zona and colleagues' (1993) report, 7 (9.5%) involved stalkers with erotomania and 32 (43.2%) cases were classified as love obsessional. Simple obsessionals, especially those with a prior intimate relationship with their victim, comprised almost half of the cases Zona and colleagues (1993) encountered in this analysis (35 out of 74, or 47.3%).

As more cases were reviewed (Zona et al., 1998), the group of simple obsessionals appeared with an even higher frequency, a result that appears consistent with findings from epidemiologically based studies (see chapter 1). Percentages of subtypes seen in their 1998 data analysis looking at 341 cases are presented in Figure 2.1. The erotomanic perpetrators were more frequently women, whereas in the other subtypes, most perpetrators were men. In the erotomanic cases, most of the victims were men, whereas most victims of the other two subgroups of stalkers were women. Of the 52 out of 74 subjects whose case files had data sufficient to support or refute a psychiatric disorder, almost two-thirds of subjects carried a mental illness diagnosis. Although Zona and colleagues made no distinction between personality disorders and other mental illnesses in their original study, in their 1998 analysis they noted that the majority of stalkers had Cluster B personality diagnoses (antisocial, borderline, histrionic, and narcissistic).

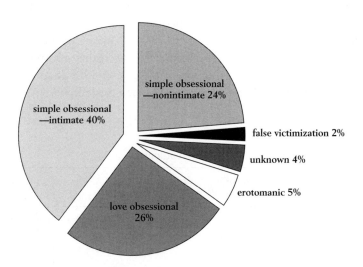

Figure 2.1. Frequency of Subtypes in Zona and Colleagues' (1998) Classification System

By definition, 100% of the erotomanic type subjects had a diagnosable mental illness. Many of the love obsessionals carried diagnoses of schizophrenia or bipolar disorder. The simple obsessional type of stalkers had the highest rates of substance abuse and personality disorders.

Meloy and Gothard (1995) validated and extended the findings of Zona et al. (1993) by looking at psychiatric diagnoses among 20 individuals in custody whom they termed "obsessional followers." They defined these subjects as those who had engaged in more than one overt act of unwanted pursuit that was felt by the target to be harassing. Comparing these subjects to 30 other offenders with mental disorders in custody, they found that obsessional followers were "older, smarter, and better educated," and more likely to have erotomanic delusional disorder and personality disorders other than antisocial personality disorder. However, the range of Axis I psychiatric conditions between the two groups did not differ significantly (Meloy & Gothard, 1995, p. 261). This suggests that psychiatric diagnosis alone may be an inadequate factor for categorizing persons who engage in stalking-like behavior.

Beyond making diagnostic and demographic comparisons, Zona and colleagues (1993) used their stalking typology to explore whether patterns would emerge in their subjects' behaviors. The erotomanic subjects seemed to maintain contact for twice as long as the love obsessional group and more than three times as long as the simple obsessionals. Interestingly, the duration of the obsession, regardless of the duration of contact, was longer than 10 years for both the erotomanic and love obsessional groups. The two subjects who caused bodily harm to their victims belonged to the simple obsessional group. In the later data analysis (Zona et al., 1998), the simple obsessionals continued to show the shortest duration of stalking and the highest rates of harm to property and to victims.

Utilizing a different data set, Harmon, Rosner, and Owens (1995) characterized stalking behavior along two axes, which represented a novel approach to stalking classifications (see Table 2.4). This effort stretched the ideas raised

Table 2.4. Harmon and Colleagues' (1995) Typology

Typology				
Affective Spectrum	Nature of Relationship	Focus of Typology	Empirical Case Review	Comments
1. Affectionate/ amorous 2. Persecutory/ angry	1. Personal 2. Professional 3. Employment 4. Media 5. Acquaintance 6. None 7. Unknown	Type of prior relationship and emotional valence of stalker	Yes	Early example of using more than one axis for classification

by Zona et al. (1993) to capture factors outside of diagnosis and included an examination of the relationship between the stalker and the victim. The first axis of the Harmon et al. (1995) classification describes the attachment between stalker and victim as either *affectionate/amorous* or *persecutory/angry*. The second axis refers to the *nature of any previous relationship between victim and perpetrator* (i.e., personal, professional, employment, media, acquaintance, none, unknown). The authors used this conceptualization to review 48 cases of persons referred to the Forensic Psychiatry Clinic of the Criminal and Supreme Courts of New York who had engaged in harassing or menacing behavior.

According to Harmon et al. (1995), the affectionate/amorous type describes persons who initially pursue another individual for amorous reasons. The feelings may change to hostility or aggression if there is a perceived rejection, leading to a modification of the rationale for pursuing the victim. Persecutory/angry attachment occurs when a person is pursued after the perpetrator senses a real or imagined injury related to a business or professional relationships. Stalkers in this group may pursue multiple individuals associated with the obsession. Similar to findings of prior research, a small proportion of those engaged in obsessional harassment had erotomania, but a variety of other psychiatric diagnoses were found. The authors concluded that behavioral patterns appeared to be more important than psychiatric diagnoses in understanding obsessional harassing.

A subsequent analysis of a larger data set ($N = 175$) revealed a similar pattern of a broad range of psychiatric diagnoses among the subjects of stalkers and obsessional harassers (Harmon, Rosner, & Owens, 1998), including about one third (32%) who were found to have a personality disorder, whereas about 20–25% of the sample carried diagnoses of schizophrenia, alcohol and substance use disorders, and/or mood and adjustment disorders (Harmon et al., 1998). Delusional disorder was seen in only 15% of the sample, although in the previous examination of their smaller sample size (Harmon et al., 1995) it had been more prevalent with 14 (29%) of the sample diagnosed with delusional disorder (6 of whom had the erotomanic type, 3 had the persecutory type, and 5 displayed an unspecified type).

Using a dichotomous classification system, Kienlen, Birmingham, Solberg, O'Regan, and Meloy (1997) divided stalking into *psychotic* and *nonpsychotic* behavior (see Table 2.5). Interestingly, a law enforcement typology proposed by Geberth (1992) had previously divided stalkers into similar categories, which utilized nonclinical labels of the psychopathic personality stalker and the psychotic personality stalker. The study by Kienlen and colleagues (1997) used archival data from the forensic examinations of 25 persons who met Missouri statutory criteria for stalking. Of the 23 individuals for whom diagnostic information was reported, 78% had an Axis I diagnosis, yet only 8 (32%) of the total sample were psychotic. Of the psychotic stalkers, only one was diagnosed with delusional disorder with erotomanic features, replicating the relatively low

Table 2.5. Select Additional Typologies Based on Reviews of Stalker Case Files

Authors	Typology	Empirical Case Review	Comments
Kienlen et al. (1997)	1. Psychotic 2. Nonpsychotic	Yes	1. Dichotomous classifications are straightforward but may be oversimplified. 2. Unclear whether psychosis alone accounts for the variance in outcomes.
Schwartz-Watts & Morgan (1998)	1. Violent 2. Nonviolent	Yes	1. Dichotomous classifications are straightforward but may be oversimplified. 2. Distinction between violent and nonviolent in this classification was based on local statutes.

incidence of erotomanic delusions found in other studies (Harmon et al., 1995; Meloy & Gothard, 1995; Zona et al., 1993). Of the stalkers with nonpsychotic disorders, the majority (67%) did have Axis I diagnoses, which included major depression, adjustment disorders, and substance use disorders. The psychotic stalkers were not diagnosed with personality disorders, whereas the majority of the nonpsychotic stalkers were diagnosed with an Axis II personality disorder, especially from Cluster B. Individuals in both the psychotic and nonpsychotic groups often had histories of substance abuse or dependence, but this was more common in the nonpsychotic group.

Placing all stalkers with psychotic disorders into one group was a novel design, especially given the findings described above that individual psychiatric diagnoses could not adequately capture patterns in stalking behavior. However, as Westrup (1998) noted, the study has limitations, including its small sample size and design as an archival study without a comparison group. Furthermore, no data suggest that the presence or absence of psychosis itself accounts for the most variance within stalking behavior, and thus it may not be the most productive way of classifying individuals who engage in stalking.

Schwartz-Watts and Morgan (1998) used a different dichotomous classification scheme to categorize the behavior of 42 pretrial detainees charged with stalking in South Carolina. (See Table 2.5.) Stalkers in this study were divided into defendants charged with violent acts (if they had charges related to bodily harm to victims or if they met criteria for a South Carolina charge of aggravated stalking [$n = 20$]), and those who were not accused of violent acts ($n = 22$).

Victims who were previously involved with the stalker were more likely to be assaulted than those who were only casually acquainted with the stalker. Notably, for both groups, ex-wives and former girlfriends were particularly at risk for being stalked, although former girlfriends comprised the larger groups of victims for the nonviolent group. In this study, violence was defined by specific criteria, related to criminal charges based on the South Carolina stalking statute. Given the disparate nature of stalking statutes, this study's findings, although offering an important advance in our conceptualization of stalkers and their risk of violence, would be difficult to apply across jurisdictions.

Building on existing work coming primarily out of the psychiatric literature, Mullen et al. (1999) proposed a classification scheme based on one of the larger databases of stalking cases. This classification scheme has gained widespread attention, and because we believe it remains a key typology, it will be discussed in greater detail below.

Finally, the most recent rigorously prepared classification of stalkers comes from an examination of a 1,005-member sample of North American stalking cases, derived from a collection of sources, including an entertainment company security department, files from the authors, and files from a police department and prosecutorial agencies (Mohandie et al., 2006). (See Table 2.6.) Known as the RECON (*R*elationship and *Con*text-based) Typology of Stalking, the authors examined relationships between the stalker and the victim and the context within which the stalking took place. The authors sought to develop a simple typological scheme that would be stable over time despite evolving motives of a stalker; they also wanted their classification system to reflect behavioral phenomena and to avoid limitations of prior typological schemes. For example, the authors commented that using mental health labels as typological categories (as Zona and colleagues, 1993, had used) could present difficulties, such as making labeling more complicated and confounding aspects of research due to some redundancy in categories (for example, they noted that erotomania became a type of stalking but is also a diagnosis). In developing their typology,

Table 2.6. RECON Typology of Stalking (Mohandie et al., 2006)

Typology	Focus of Typology	Empirical Case Review	Comments
Type I: Prior relationship a. Intimate b. Acquaintance *Type II: No prior relationship or limited contact* a. Public figure b. Private stranger	Focus is on the relationship between stalker and victim and the context (public or private)	Yes	Large sample size (*N* = 1,005) Data included multiple sources in North America

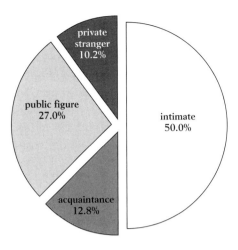

Figure 2.2. Frequency of Subtypes in the RECON Classification System (*N* = 1,005; Mohandie et al., 2006)

they sought to posit a scheme that would have utility across disciplines (rather than focused on mental health or law enforcement goals separately, for example) and that could be used for research purposes.

Four groups are included in the RECON typology (Mohandie et al., 2006; see Figure 2.2). *Intimate* and *acquaintance* groups make up Type I, which includes those stalkers who had a prior relationship with the victim, but the victim is a private figure. Type II stalkers are those who have had no prior relationship or only limited contact with the object of their pursuit. The group is divided into two subtypes, *public figure* and *private stranger*, depending on whether the stalking target was a public or private figure.

When Mohandie and colleagues (2006) classified their data set using Zona and colleagues' (1993) typology, 62% fell into the simple obsessional group, 35% in the love obsessional group, and 3% in the erotomanic group. These proportions, which differ somewhat from those seen in Zona et al.'s (1993, 1998) data, reflect Mohandie et al.'s more heterogeneous sample and probably are more representative of the proportions that most clinicians and law enforcement professionals would encounter outside the setting and context in which Zona and colleagues obtained their cases. As was the case in earlier studies, Mohandie and colleagues (2006) found that stalkers in the intimate group showed the greatest risk for threats and violence. The lowest risk of threats and violence was seen in the public figure stalkers.

The authors identify several advantages of their typology: it is clear, it does not require assumptions related to mental disorders, it avoids redundancy of categories, and it is not affected as the dynamics of the stalking situation change. In this way, it may hold much promise. More time will be needed to see how it stands up to practical application across users, but it will be important to see whether and how future studies using and provide validation for this typology.

Empirical Data Examining Victim Perspectives

Another approach to stalking classification relies in large measure upon examining the perspective of stalking victims (Sheridan & Boon, 2002; Wright et al., 1996). Looking at stalking from the target's vantage point may allow researchers to examine a broader array of stalking behaviors than is available from stalkers' self-reports of their behavior, stalkers' diagnosis, or whether their behavior had led to a referral for forensic evaluation. A recent interesting study in this regard came from Sheridan and Boon (2002), which examined data from 124 British stalking victims (see Table 2.7). The authors hoped their findings would prove especially useful for law enforcement purposes.

In developing their typology, Sheridan and Boon (2002; see also Boon & Sheridan, 2001) gathered victim reports through questionnaires that asked about basic demographics, details of the history of the stalking situation, and details regarding what helped, what made matters worse, and the victims' emotions across time. Descriptions of each stalker type include typical stalker characteristics, case management implications, and a case example. The authors use mental health terms in their descriptions of various stalker types, though from a clinical standpoint, the terms are not always utilized with clear or precise clinical meaning. Nevertheless, Sheridan and Boon (2002) have approached their classification in a way that appears relatively easy to understand for the non–mental health professionals for whom the classification is geared.

Sheridan and Boon (2002) identified four stalker typology categories, two of which were divided into subtypes (see Figure 2.3 and Table 2.7). The first type, *ex-partner harassment/stalking*, comprised 50% of the cases and was associated with a high risk of violence. The second type, *infatuation harassment* made up 18.5% of the sample. This group of subjects focuses on their victims with

Table 2.7. Sheridan and Boon's (2002; Boon & Sheridan, 2001) Typology of Stalking

Typology	Focus of Typology	Empirical Case Review	Comments
1. Ex-partner harassment/stalking 2. Infatuation harassment 　a. Young love 　b. Midlife love 3. Delusional fixation stalking 　a. Dangerous 　b. Less dangerous 4. Sadistic stalking	Focus is primarily on the motives of the stalkers.	Yes	Data derived in large measure from victim perspectives.

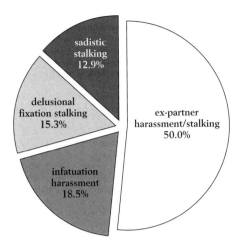

Figure 2.3. Frequency of Subtypes in Sheridan and Boon's (2002) Classification System

positive sentiments and yearning. To further assist with management of this group, the authors divided it into *young love* and *midlife love* subtypes.

Sheridan and Boon (2002) labeled their third stalker category *delusional fixation stalking*, and 15.3% of the stalkers in their study met the characteristics of this group overall. The first subtype within this group was identified as *dangerous*, because these stalkers—who often had presentations of borderline personality disorder or "episodic schizophrenia" (Sheridan & Boon, 2002)—usually had already come to the attention of police and mental health providers. These individuals held a firm belief that a relationship existed between themselves and the object. As occurs in erotomania, the object was generally from a higher status, such as a treatment provider, a professor, or a celebrity. Sheridan and Boon (2002) believed that the stalkers in this group were at high risk to become physically violent and sexually assaultive toward the objects of their attention because these stalkers typically had a history of sexual problems and other criminal offenses, and some had prior stalking convictions. With regard to implications for case management, Boon and Sheridan (2001) believed that this type would not be responsive to reason or rejection and should be referred to a forensic psychiatrist.

Within the *delusional fixation stalking* type, Sheridan and Boon (2002; Boon & Sheridan, 2001) posited a second subtype, which they labeled *less dangerous*. These stalkers had fixed, false beliefs that there was an idealized relationship between them and their objects of their attention, though these stalkers may hardly know the stalked individuals or may not know them at all. This type of stalker does not engage in threats, but believes the victim wants to be with him or her. Although deemed less dangerous, someone who attempts to stop the relationship, especially if believed by the stalker to be a potential risk to his or her idealized object, may become a target of violent behavior.

Finally, the fourth type of stalking in the Sheridan and Boon (2002) taxonomy, *sadistic stalking,* comprised 12.9% of their sample. This construct looked at the victim in particular, identifying the victim as someone worthy of "spoiling" (Sheridan & Boon, 2002), and as someone who would not understand why they were targeted. The target and stalker begin as low-level acquaintances, but eventually the stalker's motive is to frighten or demoralize the victim. For example, the stalker might reorder or remove private papers, or leave notes inside the victim's car, leaving the victim with some evidence that the stalker has had contact with their personal property. As the behavior progresses, these stalkers attempt to take full control of their victims' lives. Their behavior may include implied threats (e.g., pictures of tombstones) and sexual communications that intimidate or humiliate but would avoid directly pointing to the perpetrator. There may be reprieves from the behavior, which may later resume after a hiatus. These types of stalkers may work hard to defy police.

Typologies Based on Theoretical Considerations

Several stalking typologies are based on theory and impressions (see Table 2.8). These impressionistic classification schemes are derived out of existing scientific publications related to stalking and/or direct experience with a population of stalkers, and they are not based on a systematic study of a particular group of stalkers.

In 1993, McAnaney, Curliss, and Abeyta-Price offered a theoretical stalking typology based on their review of the then-available writings. Stalkers were divided into persons who fit *erotomanic delusional* descriptors, persons with *borderline erotomania,* persons whose behavior involved *former intimates,* and *stalkers with sociopathic traits.* The borderline erotomanic group reflected Meloy's (1989) description. The category of former intimate stalkers refers to findings from the FBI's 1990 Supplemental Homicide Report, which noted that 30% of female homicide victims were killed by intimate partners (such as husbands or boyfriends). McAnaney and colleagues (1993) also note that many victims of domestic violence were stalked by their significant other before a murder took place. These authors point out similarities between their "former intimate" category and the Los Angeles Police Department "simple obsessionals" and "casual acquaintance stalkers." They describe perpetrators of this type as unwilling to be rejected. These stalkers are described as jealous, controlling, and emotionally dependent but ambivalent about their dependence. Finally, their sociopathic stalker type includes those individuals who were not attempting to engage in an ongoing relationship with the victim, but who had other motives, such as serial murder and serial rape. These stalkers seemed to be searching for people who fulfilled some preconceived criteria for what they desired in their victims.

Based on his years of security consulting experience, De Becker (1997) divided stalkers into two broad categories—*unwanted pursuit by strangers* and *unwanted pursuit when the stalker is known by the victim.* De Becker (1997)

Table 2.8. Select Stalking Typologies Posited Based on Nonempirical Observations

Author	Typology
McAnaney et al. (1993)	1. Erotomanic delusional 2. Borderline erotomanic 3. Behavior involving "former intimate(s)" 4. Stalkers with sociopathic traits
De Becker (1997)	*Relationship Between Stalker and Victim* 1. Pursuit by stranger 2. Pursuit when stalker is known by the victim *Stalker Motivation* 1. Attachment seeking 2. Identity seeking 3. Rejection based 4. Delusion based

Sapp (1996) as cited in
    Davis & Chipman (1997, 2001)
	Stalker Target
	    I. Random
	    II. Celebrity
	    III. Single issue/ Single agenda
	    IV. Casual acquaintance
	    V. Coworker
	    VI. Intimate partner
	    VII. Domestic violence

articulated four motivations for stalking: attachment seeking, identity seeking, rejection based, and delusion based, which were further described in a book by psychiatrist Doreen Orion (1997), herself a victim of stalking. Attachment seekers pursue an attachment even when there may be no real basis for a relationship. A stalker in this category may act as a "naïve pursuer," that is, a person "who simply does not realize the inappropriateness of his behavior" (De Becker, 1997, p. 205). Unlike the rejection-based stalker, who may have a higher degree of narcissistic investment that generates anger at the thought of rejection, the naïve pursuer will not generally be enraged by rejection and thus may respond to clear limits that his pursuit is not acceptable.

According to De Becker (1997), an identity-seeking stalker may try to control the other person so that he can maintain his identity as part of the desired dyad. Whereas attachment seekers may respond to clear limits, identity seekers and rejection-based stalkers may be more likely to respond violently to rejection. De Becker's (1997) delusion-based stalkers are individuals who act and react based on false beliefs that can be attributed to their mental illnesses. Consistent with what is seen among persons with general delusional psychiatric symptoms, these persons tend to retain their beliefs despite others' attempts to dispel them (Orion, 1997, pp. 216–217).

Although other developers of typologies generally do not comment on whether an individual can move between subtypes, Orion (1997), in describing

De Becker's work, suggests that attempts at stopping stalkers might lead to changes in motives, and therefore, a change in classification. She noted, for example, that "care must be taken not to move [the delusion-based stalkers] into the rejection-based group" (p. 217). This suggested fluidity highlights the complexity of these relationships, but presents obstacles to studying an individual typology. This issue is discussed further below.

Another classification scheme was presented by Sapp in 1996, as reported by Davis and Chipman (1997, 2001). This scheme was developed from a criminal justice perspective, with an aim to help law enforcement assess the credibility of threats, and thus may not be as readily applied in clinical settings. It is premised on the idea that one can look at stalkers along two axes on a continuum that inversely determine the risk of violence in a stalking context. In this model, they posited that the closer the relationship to the victim, the greater the chance of violence. On the second axis, increasingly "problematic" mental dysfunctions (e.g., more acute delusional disorders) correspond to less risk of violence (Davis & Chipman, 2001).

Davis and Chipman (1997) detailed seven categories, based on the continuum described by Sapp (1996, as cited in Davis & Chipman, 2001), which relate to the Zona and colleagues (1993) typology. Moving from no relationship to the victim to having an extended or intimate relationship with the victim, the seven categories include *random-targeting talkers, celebrity-targeting stalkers,* and *single issue–targeting stalkers* (i.e., stalkers whose victims are involved with specific political, economic, or social issues). These three types fall under the erotomania-type stalker described by Zona et al.'s (1993) group. Davis and Chipman (1997) equate the next two categories, *casual acquaintance stalkers* and *co-worker-targeting stalkers,* with love obsessional-type stalkers. Their final two types, *intimate partner–targeting stalkers* and *domestic violence–targeting stalkers,* are identified with the simple obsessional stalker in Zona and colleagues' categorization. The domestic violence–targeting stalker differs from the intimate partner–targeting stalker only in that in the former there had already been prior violence in the context of the relationship. These categorizations are aimed at assisting with threat management (Davis & Chipman, 1997, 2001). Others typologies designed from a criminal justice perspective include one by Holmes (1993, 2001), who proposed categories of *celebrity stalkers, lust stalkers, hit stalkers, love scorned stalkers, domestic stalkers,* and *political stalkers.*

Although the categories described by Davis and Chipman (1997, 2001) appear relatively easy to distinguish, they do not specifically address motivation or behavior (other than the domestic violence-targeting stalker). Furthermore, the notion of placing mental disorders along a continuum of seriousness may seem questionable to mental health professionals, who understand subtleties of and variety within disorders, and who therefore might have a hard time agreeing upon a ranking of "seriousness." Similarly, the construct proposed by Holmes (1993, 2001) may have less utility in clinical settings.

Typological Constructs Specific to Domestic Violence

As noted in chapter 1 and elsewhere in this book, repeated harassment by a formerly intimate partner accounts for a significant proportion of stalking. Typological constructs of stalking typically include a recognition of this phenomenon. Although a detailed discussion of domestic violence lies beyond the scope of this chapter, it is worth mentioning that some studies of male batterers have also involved attempts to develop typological schemata. Notable in this regard are Holtzworth-Munroe's efforts, which have been reviewed in several studies (Hamberger, Lohr, Bonge, & Tolin, 1996; Holtzworth-Munroe & Stuart, 1994; Holtzworth-Munroe, Meehan, Herron, Rehman, & Stuart, 2000; Waltz, Babcock, Jacobson, & Gottman, 2000).

For example, the typological schema described by Holtzwort-Munroe and Stuart (1994) identified three subtypes of batterers: those who battered within family only, those who fell within a dysphoric/borderline spectrum, and those who were more generally violent/antisocial. Within ex-intimate partner stalking, these further classifications may be useful in assessing risk, generalizability of violence, and the prognosis in a given situation. For example, once a stalker is identified as falling within the context of a former intimate relationship wherein the stalker has a history of battering, variables related to batterer subtype may inform risk assessments and treatment. Specific knowledge related to battering and domestic violence is useful to understand stalking within these contexts.

The Stalking Typology of Mullen and Colleagues

Taken together, the typological models of stalking thus far described help shape our understanding of stalking motivation and the relationship between stalkers and their victims. Based upon their clinical experience, Mullen and colleagues (1999, 2000) provide a classification of stalkers that represents a major contribution to existing works related to stalking classification. They posit a unique typology incorporating three axes, with the first being primary. These axes are (1) the stalker's predominant motivation and the developmental context for the commencement of the stalking behavior, (2) the nature of the stalker's original relationship with the victim, and (3) the psychiatric diagnosis (Mullen et al., 2000). This classification scheme builds upon prior typologies, and according to Mullen et al. (1999), overlaps with those of Zona et al. (1993), Harmon et al. (1995), and that described by Orion (1997).

Case records of 145 stalkers formed the basis for Mullen and colleagues' original review (1999). In this study, 30% of the stalkers had previously been partnered with their victims, whereas 23% had had what was referred to as a professional relationship with the object of their pursuit. Of note, most often the professional relationship involved someone in the medical profession. In 11%

of the cases, the stalker and victim knew each other through work interactions (such as with coworkers or as customers). Stalkers had no prior contact with the victims in 14% of the cases, and victims were only casual acquaintances in 19% of the total sample. The subjects had been referred to a forensic psychiatry clinic known to have an interest in stalkers and their victims. Mullen's group utilized a specifically focused definition of stalkers as persons who engaged in "repeated (at least 10 times) and persistent (lasting for at least 4 weeks) unwelcome attempts to approach or communicate with the victim" (Mullen et al., 1999, p. 1245). Case reviews led these investigators to discern five types of stalkers: *rejected, intimacy seeking, incompetent, resentful,* and *predatory* (see Table 2.9 and Figure 2.4). In a later publication, the subject group included 168 stalkers (Mullen et al., 2000).

In our view, the typologies developed by Mullen and colleagues (1999) represent the most useful, comprehensive scheme available to clinicians for classifying stalking behavior. Because this classification will be referred to throughout this book, we next provide readers with detailed descriptions and a case example of each type. Each case example pieces together facts that reflect both fiction and various aspects of actual cases.

CASE EXAMPLE 2.1: THE REJECTED STALKER

A 42-year-old man has been romantically involved with a woman for 2 months. Although he senses that she feels very positively toward him, she stops returning his phone calls, seemingly out of the blue. He begins to telephone her with increased frequency in the hope that she will return his calls. After several weeks of daily phone calls, he drives to her place of work with a gift in hand for her. She tells him she is no longer interested in a relationship with him. He walks away but continues to call her several times a day. Eventually he begins to call her at work as well as at home, and also begins to write her numerous letters. He follows her home from work on occasion and surveys her apartment. His messages become increasingly threatening to her.

Table 2.9. Mullen and Colleagues' (1999, 2000) Typology

Typology					
Primary Axis: Motivation and Context	Additional Axis	Additional Axis	Focus of Typology	Empirical Case Review	Comments
1. Rejected	Stalker-victim relationship	Psychiatric diagnosis	Multiaxial	Yes	Rigorous classifica-
2. Intimacy seeking					tion, very
3. Incompetent					useful
4. Resentful					clinically
5. Predatory					

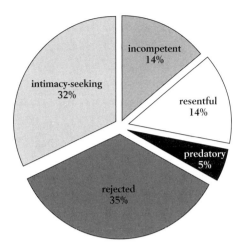

Figure 2.4. Frequency of Subtypes in Mullen and Colleagues' (2000) Classification System (N = 168)

Those stalkers who fall into Mullen and colleagues' (1999) *rejected* group are described in many of the victim-based publications as being quite prevalent. In Mullen and colleagues' (2000) series, rejected stalkers accounted for 58 (35%) of the 168 subjects. They engaged in stalking behavior following rejection by an ex-partner or a disruption in another relationship, which included relationships with parents, friends, and work associates. Jealousy and possessiveness were prominent feelings that fueled the actions of rejected stalkers, whose stalking behavior was motivated by desires to achieve reunion or to exact revenge. Not surprisingly, the motives often shifted between the two extremes. The stalking behavior allowed the stalker to maintain some relationship with the victim regardless of where the perpetrator was on the emotional spectrum.

Rejected stalkers in many ways are similar to the simple obsessional type in the Zona et al. (1993) typology, though Mullen et al. (1999) felt that some of the simple obsessional stalkers were better categorized as resentful types (see below). Personality disorders or traits (primarily with narcissistic or dependent features) were seen in most rejected stalkers, although in the 1999 study, 9 of 52 subjects had delusional disorders, 5 of which involved what Mullen and colleagues termed morbid jealousy or infatuation, that is, a "morbid exaggeration of love in all its aspects" (Mullen et al., 1999, p. 1245; see also Mullen & Pathé, 1994). This term was used because these individuals would not have been classified as having delusional disorders of the erotomanic type according to DSM diagnostic criteria, which as reviewed above, require the belief of being loved by another. In most cases, the rejected stalkers could recognize, when sufficient sanctions were in place, the losses they themselves would face if their behavior persisted.

CASE EXAMPLE 2.2: THE INTIMACY SEEKER

A man who frequented a local bar began to believe that he and a female bartender had a romantic relationship. When the woman gave him a drink without his asking, the man took this to mean that she was trying to tell him that she loved him. He suspected that this gesture was her way of communicating with him because she was too afraid to actually say anything to him. He became convinced that she was romantically interested in him and that they were "soul mates" with the same ideologies. He began to write her love letters. Although the bartender told the man she was not interested, the man was sure that she was. He interpreted many of her seemingly irrelevant actions as having significance to their relationship. The woman quit working at the bar after the man's letters began to be delivered daily. The man, having learned her phone number, began to call her at home. When she did not respond to him, he viewed her failure to respond as being more proof that she was in love with him. When she brought forward charges of stalking, he saw this as her attempt to secretly get to see him in court, so that they could be in the same place together.

In Mullen et al.'s (2000) series, 54 (32%) of the 168 subjects were classified as intimacy seeking. This group was typified by the desire to have intimacy with a particular object of love. Erotomanic delusions were seen in 27 (60%) of the 49 intimacy-seeking stalkers seen in Mullen et al.'s 1999 study, 20 of whom had delusional disorder of the erotomanic type, 5 had schizophrenia, and 2 had manic symptoms. Twenty-two subjects in the intimacy-seeking group had "morbid infatuations" or personality disorders. The intimacy-seeking stalkers seemed to be among the most persistent and harassed their victim for longer periods than all other types except the rejected stalkers. The intimacy seekers' motivations for stalking were their genuine desire to achieve relationships with their victims, whom they often perceived as already being in love with them, or who was someone with whom the intimacy seekers were in love. Negative responses, including legal sanctions, at times only fueled the belief that their relationship was meant to be. However, given the intensity of the intimacy seekers' desires for amorous relationships, jealousy, and anger due to their would-be partners' lack of reciprocation were noted in several cases. In reality, the perpetrators were often socially isolated and sometimes spent much of their time thinking about their desired relationship. Mullen et al. (2000) noted that the desired relationship was not necessarily one of sexual intimacy, and that close friendship, parental, or filial relationships could also be the goal of this type of stalker.

CASE EXAMPLE 2.3: THE INCOMPETENT STALKER

A man with mild mental retardation who lived in an institutional setting became romantically interested in a young female staff member. He wrote her several letters stating that he was in love with her. She told him that she was not interested in him romantically and that such a relationship would not be appropriate because she was a staff member at the facility. The man, who truly felt that this woman was someone special, did not heed her limit setting and continued to write her letters. He eventually learned her license plate number and put notes on her car. He followed her out to the parking lot on several occasions.

Out of the sample of 168 stalkers examined by Mullen et al. (2000), 24 (14%) fell into the incompetent group. The incompetent stalkers hoped to achieve intimacy and were aware that the person in whom they were interested might not have similar sentiments toward them. However, they had lacked the capacity to initiate appropriate social contact and had poor knowledge of usual courting behaviors. Most of the subjects had cognitive limitations and/or deficits in social functioning. In addition, some men in this group acted out of a sense of entitlement to the victim and had little willingness to start a relationship through smaller steps. This group of incompetent stalkers demonstrated a more "cavalier indifference" as an "assertive, overbearing, insensitive egoist who cannot conceive that every [woman or man] is not simply waiting to fall into their arms" (Mullen et al., 2000, p. 123).

Mullen et al. (1999) comment that although the incompetent stalkers had attributes that make them similar to intimacy seekers, incompetent stalkers constitute a distinct category because of the "differences in the imagined relationship to the victim, the pattern of stalking, and the response to treatment" (p. 1248). Specifically, the authors point out that intimacy seekers identified the object of their attention as their true love and sometimes felt the love was reciprocated, whereas the incompetent stalkers hoped to achieve an eventual intimate relationship as a result of their behaviors. The pattern of stalking was typically longer for intimacy seekers compared to incompetent stalkers, who seemed to harass for the shortest periods of time; incompetent stalkers generally more easily abandon their pursuit, but more frequently move on to other victims. As such, previous stalking behavior was noted more often in the incompetent stalkers. The psychiatric diagnoses of incompetent stalkers also differed from the diagnoses of intimacy seekers, in that the former were more likely to have cognitive deficits or certain personality disorders as opposed to psychotic disorders.

CASE EXAMPLE 2.4: THE RESENTFUL STALKER

A woman interviewed for a job as a sales clerk and thought she did well. When she learned that she did not get the job, however, she wrote to the head of the department asking why she was not hired. The department head responded kindly but stated the job had been offered to someone else. The woman continued to write letters, then began calling the department head. Eventually, she called and wrote repeatedly, making increasingly threatening remarks to the department head.

Mullen and colleagues (2000) found that 24 (14%) of their 168 subjects fell into the category of resentful stalkers. The resentful stalkers pursued targets with the purpose of frightening and distressing them, acting out of a sense of having been harmed. Some stalkers chose victims who were previously unknown to them but who represented persons or organizations that, the stalkers believed, had humiliated, embarrassed, or mistreated them. Sometimes the stalker experienced a sense of resentment toward a particular institution or company and the person who became the victim somehow symbolized the entire entity. On the other hand, the resentful stalker sometimes pursued random victims out of a general sense of grievance or paranoia. The motivation was generally considered to be one of anger or a desire for vindication. Often the resentful stalkers acted as a means of experiencing control or power over in a context in which they perceived that they had been victimized. Because they felt they had been wronged, the resentful stalkers almost always expressed a sense of justification in their actions. Mullen et al. (2000) found that paranoid personalities and even paranoid delusions occurred frequently in their group of resentful stalkers.

CASE EXAMPLE 2.5: THE PREDATORY STALKER

A man had an interest in having sexual relations with short-haired girls who appear to be in their early adolescent years. He went to a field at a nearby high school, stood where he could not be observed, and selected a girl whom he decided to rape. He waited until school was dismissed and followed her bus home to learn where she lived. Over the next weeks, he surreptitiously followed her to learn her routines, intending eventually to find or create an opportunity to sexually assault her. He noticed that she was alone for a half hour each day when she walked her dog after school. He picked a particular day, and when she was walking her dog, he forced her into his car and raped her.

The predatory stalkers, who constituted 8 (5%) of the 168 stalkers (Mullen et al., 2000), were so classified because they had been preparing for some type of attack, characterized as predominantly sexual in nature. They were motivated by a desire for sexual gratification and control through their stalking and found gratification and a sense of power in watching, practicing, and gaining familiarity with their victim's routines. Mullen et al.'s (1999) study found this group to have a high frequency of paraphilias and they often had previous arrests or convictions for sexual offenses. Their victims may be totally unaware that they are being followed and without fear, although in some cases they may suspect that they are being followed. However, one could assume that if the victim were made aware of the preparations for a sexual assault on them, they would reasonably experience fear. Mullen et al. (1999) found that all members of this stalker group were male and half had assaulted their victim. Most were not in a relationship, and data from the 1999 and 2000 studies showed that 40 to 50% were unemployed.

Comparison of Stalkers in the Mullen et al. Typology

Mullen et al. (1999, 2000) examined whether typology and/or diagnosis of the stalker would be associated with particular patterns. Interestingly, rejected and resentful stalkers seemed to employ multiple (approximately five) means of making contact with their victim, whereas stalkers of other typologies used fewer types of approaches. There was also an association between the numbers of methods of establishing contact and harassing victims and diagnosis, with persons with personality disorders utilizing the greatest number of stalking methods. Specific stalker type correlated with length of stalking behavior, but psychiatric diagnosis did not. Stalking duration was the longest among those in the rejected and intimacy-seeking groups. Mullen and colleagues (2000, 2006) also examined the stalking categories in depth in an attempt to understand the risk of harm to victims and how to manage stalkers. Further information related to risk assessment and risk management as they relate to various types of stalking appears in chapters 3 and 4.

Comparing Classifications Schemes

CASE EXAMPLE 2.6: THE DISHEVELED MAN
A disheveled man approached a young woman he had not seen before outside her place of employment and made sexual remarks to her. Although she ignored him, he stood outside her workplace each day thereafter, asking her to engage in sexual relations with him. He ultimately began following her home and would behave bizarrely outside her home (for example, by making strange noises). The man later told clinicians that he believed that the world was about to end and that "his only hope of salvation was to be with [the woman] when Armageddon came." When, on one occasion, she tried to reason with him and asked him to leave, he did not listen and instead attempted to sexually assault her. Police were called to intervene and ultimately the man was admitted to a psychiatric hospital, where he was diagnosed with schizophrenia. (Adapted from Sheridan & Boon, 2002, pp. 74–75.)

As an exercise, it is useful to apply various typologies to a case example. The vignette above is described by Sheridan and Boon (2002) as a delusional fixation stalker, dangerous type. In the Zona et al. (1993) classification scheme, this man might be construed as a love obsessional. He does not meet criteria for an erotomanic delusional disorder, as he does not believe the young woman is in love with him. He does, however, have delusions related to sexual desires, and he did not previously have a relationship with the woman. He thus would not likely qualify as a simple obsessional. He certainly would qualify as a psychotic type stalker according to Kienlen et al. (1997). In the RECON typology (Mohandie et al., 2006), because the relationship was based on limited or incidental contact (i.e., he had never worked with the woman or even been a customer of hers) and because the victim was a private figure, the stalker would be categorized as a private stranger stalker.

If one were to look at this case from the perspective of the Mullen et al. (1999) typology, one would start by considering the motivation that instigated the behavior. It appears that the stalker is seeking sexual intimacy with the woman and believes he needs this union to avoid harm. He is not angry with her, nor did he sense her rejection before his stalking behavior. He is not secretly lying in wait in order to attack her sexually, as he spends numerous evenings howling and engaging in other disorganized behavior, of which she is aware, before moving toward an assault. It seems that in his mind, had she willingly accepted his awkward attempts to unite with her, the assault would have been avoided, making him not qualify as the predatory type. Although he shows clear clumsiness around how to achieve his goal, and thus has aspects of an incompetent stalker, his behavior is not just a manifestation of a clumsy courting technique, and his motivation goes beyond a simple hope for union. His primary motivation is to establish intimacy with the woman. Thus, he best is described as an intimacy seeking stalker. Though he does not have an erotomanic delusion, he is psychotic. He might benefit from hospitalization and psychotropic medicine to treat the disorder that includes delusional beliefs about the woman and about the impending end of the world.

Viewed from the standpoint of the Sheridan and Boon (2002) typology, the case presents a high risk of assault. According to Mullen and colleagues (2000), however, the intimacy seekers as a group generally present a lower risk of assault, although the authors note that some intimacy seekers will become assaultive and engage in extreme violence. Further, Mullen et al. (1999, 2000) also maintain that membership in a specific stalking category does not solely predict a particular level of violence risk, as prior criminal convictions and substance use were also important in this regard (a topic covered in more detail in chapter 3). Regarding frequency of contact, Mohandie and colleagues (2006) note that private stranger stalkers engaged in contact much more frequently than public figure stalkers, although they were less likely to be hospitalized and more likely to be charged criminally compared with public figure stalking types. Violence in the private stranger group occurred with less frequency than was the case with intimate and acquaintance stalkers, but more frequently than with public figure stalkers.

The authors of the various proposed typologies do not share the same perspectives or goals; for example, Mullen and colleagues are clinicians, and Sheridan and Boon (2002) have aimed their work at assisting law enforcement. Nevertheless, an appreciation of the various typologies can be useful in understanding how they may be applied to individual cases. The stalker in this case winds up in psychiatric care, and a clinician caring for him would benefit from a comprehensive understanding of his presentation to best approach his treatment. From the clinical perspective that Mullen and colleagues share with the psychiatrists who make up our committee, an understanding of stalkers' motivations, their relationship to their victims, and their psychiatric diagnoses helps to inform us about their clinical management.

ANALYSIS OF CURRENT CLASSIFICATION APPROACHES

There are now multiple extant descriptions of stalking classifications in the literature. Although the preceding review is not exhaustive, it should serve to provide the reader with some sense of the wide variety of and aims behind recently published typologies of stalking. Existing classification schemes have both helped shape our understanding of stalking behavior and have allowed some common themes to emerge.

First, not all stalkers are the same, and their psychiatric diagnosis is just one aspect of how they may differ. Some stalkers have erotomanic delusions, but most do not. Second, whether the stalker and victim had a prior intimate relationship is often an important factor in distinguishing different types of stalkers, and the existence of a prior intimate relationship portend a higher likelihood of violence. Third, motivation for stalking behavior is another factor that can help distinguish stalkers. Finally, currently available classification schemes reflect descriptive efforts to categorize a group of complex and diverse behaviors. Because these typologies emerge from and reflect various interests, largely of criminal justice and mental health professionals, their usefulness in various situations differs. Though some features of these typologies overlap with each other, the diversity of the numerous proposed classifications has left the scientific and practical waters a bit muddied.

Research efforts to construct stalking typologies also suffer from several methodological limitations. Existing typologies have not used similar definitions of stalking, if they provide definitions at all. Prospective, comparison studies examining the relationship between typologies and outcomes are lacking. Unique populations, such as adolescent stalkers, cyberstalkers, and celebrity and special target stalkers (discussed later in this volume in chapters 8, 9, and 10) may have characteristics that differ from other populations of stalkers, making it difficult to apply some of the current typological schemes to their behaviors.

Several authors (Sheridan, Blaauw, & Davies, 2003; Sheridan & Boon, 2002; Mohandie et al., 2006) have noted these and other problems with many of the current classification schemes:

- Inability of some current typologies to adequately capture the heterogeneity of stalkers
- Use of ambiguous categorizations

- Questionable reliability of the classifications, especially those based on theory
- Actual samples and reported numbers often represent small data sets
- Classification terms are hard to interpret, so that often a stalker may seem to fit into more than one category
- Wide range in the number of stalker categories (from two to more than seven within the various classifications)
- Nonrandom or atypical study populations (e.g., celebrity stalkers, victims seen in individual clinics or arrested via particular statutes)
- Stalkers' motivations may change over time, lessening the reliability of typologies based on motivation (Mohandie et al., 2006).

Even with the best scientific approaches, it is difficult to capture the breadth of those who engage in stalking behaviors. Moreover, only a portion of stalkers—typically, those who somehow attract attention and are detected—come to the attention of and have their stalking behaviors identified by researchers, law enforcement officials, or mental health professionals. An unknown fraction of individuals are convicted of rape or murder without their stalking behavior becoming known, in some cases because their victims are not available to describe the progression of prearrest stalking. Some stalking victims may be reluctant to refer perpetrators to authorities or simply may not interpret persistent contacts and following as stalking. Although some stalkers may experience distress about their preoccupations, they rarely would voluntarily enter treatment because of their stalking or report their own stalking behavior to treaters unless it is court mandated. Treatment providers may be overly trusting that some romantic relationships described by patients are genuine and be unaware that their patients are actually stalking individuals who do not reciprocate their patients' feelings. In all these situations, stalkers and their behavior may go unrecognized.

Limitations of research aside, classifying an individual within a specific typological framework is not always straightforward. Mullen and colleagues (1999) note that their classifications are not mutually exclusive groups, such that determining the appropriate classification of a stalker would be a matter of judgment. Existing writings on stalking classifications usually are not clear about whether individuals move between stalker types, although Mohandie et al. (2006) seek to avoid this conundrum in their classification scheme by creating categories that are based on relationships and contexts rather than motivation.

As an illustration of the classification challenges with other typologies, consider a stalker who begins as someone searching for intimacy, only to be rejected. This individual may cross boundaries and change his primary motivation from love seeking to revenge seeking, and might thus seem to move among classification types. The typology proposed by Harmon et al. (1995) specifically requires an examination of the initial feelings of a stalker, though the authors recognize that a stalker may later develop different feelings at some point. Mullen and colleagues (1999) point out that most intimacy seekers are delusional and most will not become violent. Yet they recognize that a small percentage of intimacy seekers shift their major emotion from love to anger if they feel rejected, at which point their risk of violence increases.

In our committee's view, however, it would not make sense to change the stalker's classification type because the purpose of the original classification (to understand stalkers within a context of existing data for a particular type, to be able to understand the natural course of the stalking phenomenon, etc.) construct would then be lost. Instead, we believe that the stalker's initial motive should determine his classification, regardless of the evolution of the relationship. This fixed-category approach, based on the initial relationship and motivation of the stalker is principally relevant in employing any classification scheme in which there may be an evolution in the emotions and motives of the stalker (e.g., Harmon et al. 1995, 1998; Mullen et al., 1999). Utilizing a classification based on the original motivation for stalking allows a fixed reference point and a comparison to existing data that can be used to help understand a stalker's risk, likely behavior, and response to interventions. Further, use of a fixed classification approach does not preclude those working with stalkers to learn information about the stalker's feeling states and motivations as they emerge, which may further assist with management.

As we prepared this volume, our committee felt that choosing and applying one scheme for classifying stalkers would best allow readers to understand the broad range of assessment issues, treatment interventions, victim management strategies, and legal considerations associated with stalking. After examining the available candidates, we selected the classification scheme developed by Mullen and colleagues (1999, 2000) because we felt it offers several advantages:

- It is the most clinically useful classification scheme. Although Mullen and colleagues (1999, 2000) use a stalker's motivation as the primary factor in categorization, their system also considers psychiatric diagnosis and the relationship between stalker and victim. To clinicians, diagnoses and relationships are features that make a typology useful when one is assessing prognosis and in following up efforts at intervention.
- Attachment-based classifications, exemplified by Meloy (1989), are very helpful in linking stalking to psychodynamic constructs and unconscious motivations but are difficult to apply objectively through operational criteria.
- The scheme developed by Zona and colleagues (1993) came from a study population that contained an unusually large number of celebrity stalkers. By contrast, Mullen and colleagues' (1999, 2000) typology derives from a broad-based Australian sample and thus may be better representative of the population of stalkers that most clinicians and legal systems will encounter.

- Mullen and colleagues' (1999, 2000) descriptions of stalking and stalking categories reflect their understanding of the interweaving of interpersonal and intrapersonal dynamics, as well as psychiatric diagnosis. As later chapters in this book will show, these descriptions can help practitioners assess risk and apply management strategies that incorporate a psychiatric understanding of the stalker.
- We believe that the deliberate decision to not include motivation makes Mohandie and colleagues' (2006) RECON typology straightforward and is likely to allow greater interrater reliability. Yet, despite the difficulties in making bright-line judgments about motivation in some cases and the potential for changing motivations over time, we think that for clinicians, the motivation and rationale for a person's stalking represents a critical element in understanding the behavior and approaching its management.
- Several other stalking classifications use dichotomous variables to create categories of stalkers, but we can think of no a priori reason why a stalking typology should be created this way. Mullen and colleagues' (1999, 2000) classification implicitly recognizes that stalkers' behavior may fall into several meaningful categories, just as do many other human behaviors—a feature that is advantageous for clinicians whose work requires a nuanced appreciation of multiple aspects of stalking and the complexity of human behavior and relationships.

Our adoption of Mullen and colleagues' (1999, 2000) typology is not without some reservations, however. In particular, we are concerned about some fundamental differences between the motives and behavior of the "predatory" stalkers and the stalkers who fall into Mullen and colleagues' (1999, 2000) other four categories. Indeed, anticipating this weakness, Mullen and colleagues (1999) commented on the appropriateness of including predatory individuals among stalkers. They noted that many sex offenders engage in some stalking behaviors, and they acknowledged the need for more data to assess whether their predatory subtype was a reliable and useful classification for predicting behavior (especially future violence).

An additional problem with the predatory category is that it emphasizes persons whose motive involves desire for power and control culminating largely in sexual attack, thereby seemingly excluding persons who furtively stalk their human prey for nonsexual reasons, such as those with an intent to kill. In any of these scenarios, the victim, if aware of being followed for the purpose of some harm, might well become as frightened, as would a victim of Mullen and colleagues' (1999, 2000) predatory-but-sexually-motivated stalker. Although such behavior could be conceptualized as nonsexual predatory stalking, doing so might cast too wide a net as to what constitutes stalking. Also, the preoccupied, obsessional component of most other stalkers' thinking and behavior is usually lacking in the predatory group of stalkers, who are simply following a future victim to carry out an antisocial act.

Despite these concerns, we must acknowledge the usefulness of including predatory stalking in a classification system. Although it is distinct from the other types, predatory stalking has several elements in common with more general stalking, such as the existence of a fixation on a particular person, repetitive behaviors intended related to the object of pursuit, and the notion that the behavior would cause fear in the victim if the victim were aware of it. Moreover, predatory perpetrators might well be identified as stalkers when they come to the attention of mental health professionals (as Mullen and colleagues, 1999, 2000, found) or law enforcement officials. To that end, we suggest that if some predatory behaviors continue to be classified as a type of stalking, it might be more useful to categorize the phenomenon as "stalking in preparation for a crime," with sexual and nonsexual subtypes.

CONCLUSION

Numerous stalking classification schemes have appeared in publications geared toward mental health and law enforcement professionals. Individuals who work with stalkers would do well to have an understanding of the various typologies, how they were developed, and their advantages and limitations. In reviewing studies looking at cohorts of stalkers, one begins to appreciate the complexity of stalking as a phenomenon related to the preoccupying, pathological attachments seen among a wide spectrum of perpetrators. Existing typological frameworks have improved our ability to approach stalkers by increasing our awareness of who engages in stalking behavior, what degree of risk they may present to their targets, and how specific types of stalkers might best be managed. Although stalking will likely continue as a burgeoning area of research interest, the application of the currently available typologies can have practical value in clinical and criminal justice settings. Future research will undoubtedly capitalize on existing typologies and will help further improve our understanding of stalking over time.

REFERENCES

American Psychiatric Association. (1987). *Diagnostic and statistical manual of mental disorders* (3rd ed., revised). Washington, DC: Author.

American Psychiatric Association. (1994). *Diagnostic and statistical manual of mental disorders* (4th ed.). Washington, DC: Author.

American Psychiatric Association. (2000). *Diagnostic and statistical manual of mental disorders* (4th ed., Text Rev.). Washington, DC: Author.

Boon, J. C., & Sheridan, L. (2001). Stalker typologies: A law enforcement perspective. *Journal of Threat Assessment, 1,* 75–97.

Coleman, F. (1997). Stalking behavior and the cycle of domestic violence. *Journal of Interpersonal Violence, 12,* 420–432.

Davis, J. A., & Chipman, M. A. (1997). A forensic psychological typology of stalkers and other obsessional types. *Journal of Clinical Forensic Medicine* (U.K.), *4,* 166–172.

Davis, J. A., & Chipman, M. A. (2001). Stalkers and other obsessional types: A review and forensic psychological typology of those who stalk. In J. A. Davis (Ed.), *Stalking crimes and victim protection: Prevention, intervention, threat assessment and case management* (pp. 3–18). Boca Raton, FL: CRC Press.

De Becker, G. (1997). *The gift of fear: Survival signals that protect us from violence.* Boston: Little, Brown.

de Clérambault, G. G. (1942). Les psychoses passionelles. *Oeuvres psychiatriques.* Paris: Presses Universitaires de France.

Deitz, P. E., Matthews, D. B., Martell, D. A., Stewart, T. M., Hrouda, D. R., & Warren, J. (1991). Threatening and otherwise inappropriate letters to members of the United States Congress. *Journal of Forensic Sciences, 36,* 1445–1468.

Deitz, P. E., Matthews, D. B., Van Duyne, C., Martell, D. A., Parry, C. D. H., Stewart, T., Warren, J., & Crowder, J. D. (1991). Threatening and otherwise inappropriate letters to Hollywood celebrities. *Journal of Forensic Sciences, 36,* 185–209.

Del Ben, K., & Fremouw, W. (2002). Stalking: Developing an empirical typology to classify stalkers. *Journal of Forensic Sciences, 47,* 152–158.

Enoch, M. D., & Ball, H. N. (2001). *Uncommon psychiatric syndromes* (4th ed.). London: Arnold Press.

Geberth, V. (1992). Stalkers. *Law and Order, 40,* 138–143.

Hamberger, L. K., Lohr, J. M., Bonge, D., & Tolin, D. F. (1996). A large sample empirical typology of male spouse abusers and its relationship to dimensions of abuse. *Violence and Victims, 11,* 277–292.

Harmon, R. B., Rosner, R., & Owens, H. (1995). Obsessional harassment and erotomania in a criminal court population. *Journal of Forensic Sciences, 40,* 188–196.

Harmon, R. B., Rosner, R., & Owens, H. (1998). Sex and violence in a forensic population of obsessional harassers. *Psychology, Public Policy, and Law, 4,* 236–249.

Holmes, R. M. (1993). Stalking in America: Types and methods of criminal stalkers. *Journal of Contemporary Criminal Justice, 9,* 317–327.

Holmes, R. M. (2001). Criminal stalking: An analysis of the various typologies of stalking. In J. A. Davis (Ed.), *Stalking crimes and victim protection: Prevention, intervention, threat assessment and case management* (pp. 19–29). Boca Raton, FL: CRC Press.

Holtzworth-Munroe, A., Meehan, J. C., Herron, K., Rehman, U., & Stuart, G. L. (2000). Testing the Holtzworth-Munroe and Stuart (1994) batterer typology. *Journal of Consulting and Clinical Psychology, 68,* 1000–1019.

Holtzworth-Munroe, A., & Stuart, G. L. (1994). Typologies if male batterers: Three subtypes and the differences among them. *Psychological Bulletin, 116,* 476–497.

Kienlen, K. K., Birmingham, D. L., Solberg, K. B., O'Regan, J. T., & Meloy, J. R. (1997). A comparative study of psychotic and nonpsychotic stalking. *Journal of the American Academy of Psychiatry and Law, 25,* 317–334.

Leong, G. B. (1994). De Clérambault syndrome (erotomania) in the criminal justice system: Another look at this recurring problem. *Journal of Forensic Sciences, 39,* 378–385.

Lerner, V., Kapstan, A., & Witztum, E. (2001). The misidentification of Clerambault's and Kandinsky-Clerambault's syndromes. *Canadian Journal of Psychiatry, 46,* 441–443.

Lloyd-Goldstein, R. (1998). De Clérambault on-line: A survey of erotomania and stalking from the old world to the World Wide Web. In J. R. Meloy (Ed.), *The psychology of stalking* (pp. 193–212). San Diego: Academic Press.

McAnaney, K., Curliss, L., & Abeyta-Price, C. (1993). From imprudence to crime: Anti-stalking laws. *Notre Dame Law Review, 68,* 819–909.

Meloy, J. R. (1989). Unrequited love and the wish to kill: Diagnosis and treatment of borderline erotomania. *Bulletin of the Menninger Clinic, 53,* 477–492.

Meloy, J. R. (2001). Communicated threats and violence toward public and private targets: Discerning differences among those who stalk and attack. *Journal of Forensic Sciences, 46,* 1211–1213.

Meloy, J. R., & Gothard, S. (1995). Demographic and clinical comparison of obsessional followers and offenders with mental disorders. *American Journal of Psychiatry, 152,* 258–263.

Mohandie, K., Meloy, J. R., McGowan, M. G., & Williams, J. (2006). The RECON typology of stalking: Reliability and validity based upon a large sample of North American stalkers. *Journal of Forensic Sciences, 51,* 147–155.

Mullen, P. E., Mackenzie, R., Ogloff, J. R. P., Pathé, M., McEwan, T., & Purcell, R. (2006). Assessing and managing the risks in the stalking situation. *Journal of the American Academy of Psychiatry and Law, 34,* 439–450.

Mullen, P. E., & Pathé, M. (1994). The pathological extensions of love. *British Journal of Psychiatry, 165,* 614–623.

Mullen, P. E., Pathé, M., & Purcell, R. (2000). *Stalkers and their victims.* Cambridge, UK: Cambridge University Press.

Mullen, P. E., Pathé, M., Purcell, R., & Stuart, G. W. (1999). Study of stalkers. *American Journal of Psychiatry, 156,* 1244–1249.

Orion, D. (1997). *I know you really love me.* New York: Macmillan.

Sapp, A. (March, 1996). *Stalking typologies.* Conference presentation at the Academy of Criminal Justice Sciences, Las Vegas, NV. Cited in Davis & Chipman (2001).

Schwartz-Watts, D., & Morgan, D. W. (1998) Violent versus nonviolent stalkers. *Journal of the American Academy of Psychiatry and Law, 26,* 241–245.

Segal, J. H. (1989). Erotomania revisited: From Kraepelin to *DSM-III-R. American Journal of Psychiatry, 146,* 1261–1266.

Sheridan, L. P., Blaauw, E., & Davies, G. M. (2003). Stalking: Knowns and unknowns. *Trauma, Violence, and Abuse, 4*, 148–162.

Sheridan, L., & Boon, J. (2002) Stalker typologies: Implications for law enforcement. In J. Boon & L. Sheridan (Eds.), *Stalking and psychosexual obsession: Psychological perspectives for prevention, policing and treatment* (pp. 63–82). West Sussex, UK: Wiley.

Waltz, J., Babcock, J. C., Jacobson, N. S., & Gottman, J. M. (2000). *Journal of Consulting and Clinical Psychology, 68*, 658–669.

Westrup, D. (1998) Applying functional analysis to stalking behavior. In J. R. Meloy (Ed.), *The psychology of stalking: Clinical and forensic perspectives* (pp. 275–294). San Diego: Academic Press.

Wright, J. A., Burgess, A. G., Burgess, A. W., Laszlo, A. T., McCrary, G. O., & Douglas, J. E. (1996). A typology of interpersonal stalking. *Journal of Interpersonal Violence, 11*, 487–502.

Zona, M. A., Palarea, R. E., & Lane, J. C. (1998). Psychiatric diagnosis and the offender-victim typology of stalking. In J. R. Meloy (Ed.), *The psychology of stalking: Clinical and forensic perspectives* (pp. 69–84). San Diego: Academic Press.

Zona, M. A., Sharma, K. K., & Lane, J. C. (1993). A comparative study of erotomanic and obsessional subjects in a forensic sample. *Journal of Forensic Sciences, 38*, 894–903.

3   Stalking Risk Assessment

Phillip J. Resnick

This chapter examines the frequency of recidivism, threats, and violence in male and female stalkers. The risk factors associated with ordinary violence are distinguished from the risk factors for severe violence and homicide in stalkers. Common risk factors for ordinary violence among stalkers include substance abuse, prior criminal offenses, making threats, suicidality, and a prior intimate relationship to the stalking victim. Risk factors for stalkers committing severe violence or homicide include appearing at the victim's home, prior violence, major depression, threats to harm the victim's children, and placing threatening messages on the victim's car. Celebrity stalkers have a different set of risk factors for violence. Distinctions are made between those stalkers who make threats and those who pose threats, and between affective and predatory violence by stalkers. The overlap between domestic violence and stalking is explained. An approach to evaluating stalking situations for dangerousness is offered. Increased vigilance is necessary when events humiliate or anger the stalker. Finally, the chapter discusses how to assess threats by stalkers and when to consider seeking restraining orders.

INTRODUCTION

Stalking and violence are two separate phenomena, but they often occur together. Because stalking is defined as a pattern of harassment that induces fear of harm in the victim, it is not surprising that some stalking victims are indeed violently assaulted by their stalkers (Meloy, 2002).

The science of assessing stalkers for violence risk is still in its infancy. Because stalking has been defined as a crime for only the last approximately 15 years, a limited number of research studies regarding stalking and violence have been completed. The majority of early studies were based on referrals to court psychiatric clinics. These studies had an overrepresentation of subjects with mental illness and were more often serious cases than random stalking in the community.

Of the adult participants in the National Violence Against Women Survey (NVAWS) whose experiences fulfilled their criteria of stalking, only 55% of women and 48% of men reported their experiences to the police (Tjaden & Thoennes, 1998, 2000a). Reasons for not reporting stalking behaviors to law enforcement included fear of reprisal from the stalker and beliefs that stalking was not a police matter and that the police could not do anything to stop the behavior (National Institute of Justice, 1998). Later research studies have explored stalking in the community, stalking of college students, the relationship between stalking and domestic violence, and stalking associated with murder and attempted murder.

Little research has been done on the frequency of stalking recidivism in persons arrested for stalking. Rosenfeld (2003) found that about half the stalkers reoffended during a several-year follow-up; 80% of those who did reoffend did so during the first year. The strongest predictors of stalking recidivism were the presence of a personality disorder (in particular, antisocial, borderline, or narcissistic personality disorders) and a combination of both a personality disorder and a history of substance abuse. Stalkers with a prior intimate relationship with the victim were also at significantly greater risk of resuming their stalking behavior. Stalkers with a delusional attachment to a stranger were found to have a lower rate of reoffending. One explanation for this surprising finding is that psychotic stalkers may have been more likely to receive aggressive psychiatric treatment.

Currently, there are no actuarial instruments that have been validated to assess the risk of violence in stalkers. Rosenfeld and Lewis (2005) applied a regression tree approach to risk assessment for violence in stalkers. They identified subgroups of stalkers with differing probabilities of violence. They used models with 5, 9, and 13 variables. The regression tree models compared favorably with traditional logistic regression. The model using only 5 variables (age under 30; education less than high school; threatened victim; prior intimate relationship; revenge motivation) had the advantage of being usable without the availability of a clinical examination of the stalker (Rosenfeld & Lewis, 2005). The authors advised not applying this actuarial model if a thorough clinical evaluation was available because important individualized risk and protective factors could not be considered. This study is an important first step in ultimately developing a reliable and valid assessment tool for violence in stalkers. Valid instruments will require a long period of time to develop, and they will need to be tailored to the various subtypes of stalkers (Kropp, Hart, & Lyon, 2002). However, clinicians who evaluate stalkers may currently assess their violence risk by "structured professional judgment" (Kropp et al., 2002), a method of decision making that employs guidelines based on empirical knowledge and professional practice (Borum, 1996).

In approaching an evaluation of a stalker's risk of harm, the examiner must first separate the risk of continued stalking from the risk that the stalker will commit a violent act. Sometimes an effort to discourage continued stalking may increase the risk that the stalker will become violent. This phenomenon is called the intervention dilemma (see chapter 4 for details). The GAP Committee on Psychiatry and the Law will give special emphasis in this chapter to the rejected type of stalker because they are at highest risk for serious assaults and homicide. Details regarding stalker typologies are described in chapter 2.

FREQUENCY OF THREATS AND VIOLENCE IN STALKING

Studies of stalking report that threats of violence occur in 17–74% of cases, and that 34–55% of the stalkers were physically violent to their victims (Hall, 1998; Meloy, 1996; Mullen, Pathé, Purcell, & Stuart, 1999; Tjaden & Thoennes, 1998, 2000a). Meloy (1996, 1999) reached several conclusions about the relationship between threats and assaults in stalkers. Approximately one-half of all stalkers threaten their victim. The incidence usually exceeds 50% among stalkers with a prior intimate relationship with the victim (Meloy, 2002).

One-half (Mullen et al., 1999) to three-fourths (Meloy, 1999) of stalkers who made threats were not subsequently violent toward a person or property. In approximately 15% of cases, however, male and female stalkers were violent without prior threats (Meloy & Boyd, 2003).

Violence occurred in approximately a third of cases, yet infrequently resulted in serious physical injury (Meloy, 1999). Weapons were generally used by stalkers to intimidate and control, rather than physically injure their victims. Violence was usually limited to a physical assault and battery without a weapon, the victim being grabbed, punched, struck, or fondled by the stalker. Not surprisingly, victims of the violence were the object of stalking pursuit approximately 80% of the time. Violence toward third parties occurred in fewer than 20% of stalking cases. When it occurs, it is usually directed at individuals perceived to be impeding access to the stalking victim (Meloy, 1999).

Property violence in stalking cases occurred at about half the rate of personal violence toward the victim (Meloy, 1999). Objects damaged were usually owned by the victim (e.g., the victim's automobile) or symbolically represent the victim (e.g., the victim's clothing or personal photographs). Mullen et al. (1999) found the automobile of the victim the most common object of property damage.

Mullen and his colleagues (1999) studied 145 court referred stalkers in Australia. They found that 64% of all the stalkers made threats. Table 3.1 reports the frequency of threats and violence by category of stalker as described by Mullen and colleagues.

In the Mullen et al. (1999) study, the rejected and predatory stalkers were most likely to commit assaults, but the resentful and rejected stalkers were most likely to damage property and make threats. Resentful stalkers made threats and were prone to damage the victim's property, but less often proceeded to overt assaults. In predatory stalkers, there is a troubling lack of warning of the danger because they are the least intrusive stalkers.

Table 3.1. Frequency of Threats and Assaults by Category of Stalker

Category	Threats (%)	Assaults (%)
Rejected	71	54
Intimacy seeker	50	23
Incompetent	32	27
Resentful	87	25
Predator	33	50

Source: Mullen et al., 1999.

Most of Meloy's data and the Mullen et al. (1999) study were based on forensic cohorts, that is, stalkers referred for evaluation after they had come to the attention of law enforcement officials. The rates of threats and assaults among forensically referred stalkers may be much higher than rates of such behavior in stalkers in the general population (Bjerregaard, 2000; Logan, Leukefeld, & Walker, 2000). For example, Langhinrichsen-Rohling, Palarea, Cohen, and Rohling (2000) studied college students who had a breakup of an intimate relationship. Although 99% of the students reported that they had experienced at least one episode of unwanted pursuit behavior, only 12% of the women reported that an ex-partner had threatened them.

Because about 80% of stalking is done by men, most studies have focused on male stalkers. Meloy and Boyd (2003), however, studied 82 female stalkers. The targets of these stalkers were mostly men. Sixty-five percent of the female stalkers threatened their victims. Twenty-five percent of the female stalkers were physically violent toward the victims. The injury to the victim usually did not require medical care, but there were three homicides among this nonrandom cohort of 82 female stalkers.

Meloy and Boyd (2003) also found that the presence of a threat was positively and significantly related to subsequent acts of violence by female stalkers toward the victim. Initiating contact with the female stalker by the victim increased subsequent pursuit but not violence in 68% of the cases. As in male stalkers, prior sexual intimacy markedly increased the likelihood of physical assault.

In 2002, Meloy reported that even when a woman is a victim of domestic violence stalking, her risk of being killed by her intimate partner is, at most, 1 in 400. This risk may appear low, but when compared to the annual U.S. homicide base rate of 7/100,000, it implies a 36-fold increase in the likelihood of being killed (McFarlane, Campbell, & Watson, 2002). Mullen, Pathé, and Purcell (2000) point out that homicide rates in stalking cannot conceivably approach such rates because they would be daily occurrences given the prevalence estimates of stalking in the community.

Putting the data together, it is evident that threats of violence are common in stalking and are clearly associated with violence. However, violence can also occur in the absence of threats. Careful assessment analyzing risk factors in each

Table 3.2. Risk Factors for Violence

Substance abuse
History of crimes
Threats
Suicidality
Ex-intimate of victim
Personality disorder
Erotomanic delusions
Social isolation
Escalation of behavior

individual case is therefore necessary. Risk factors for violence by stalkers are listed in Table 3.2, and are discussed in the following sections.

RISK FACTORS FOR VIOLENCE BY STALKERS

Substance Abuse

Substance abuse increases the probability of assaultive behavior by persons with mental disorders (Eronen, Hakola, & Tiihonen, 1996; Soyka, 2000; Steadmanet al., 1998; Wallace et al., 1998). This association has also been reported in multiple studies of stalking (Brewster, 2000; Harmon, Rosner, & Owens, 1998; Logan et al., 2000; Mullen et al., 1999). Substance abuse increases the risk of violence among stalkers because it can impair impulse control, lead to paranoid thoughts, and heighten emotionality, all of which may lead to aggressive behavior (Zona, Palarea, & Lane, 1998). Those stalkers who are abusing alcohol and/or drugs are more likely to threaten, damage property, and attack their victims (Mullen et al., 2000; Rosenfeld, 2004).

History of Criminal Offenses

In offender populations, the nature and extent of prior convictions is one of the most robust predictors of future recidivism (Reiss & Roth, 1993). Studies of stalkers have revealed a similar association between a history of criminal convictions and subsequent assault (Kienlen, Birmingham, Solberg, O'Regan, & Meloy, 1997; Menzies, Fedoroff, Green, & Isaacson, 1995; Mullen et al., 1999; Sandberg, McNiel, & Binder, 1998). Violent or sexual offending in the past carries the highest risk, but any significant past criminal history increases the probability of assault in a stalking situation (Mullen et al., 2000; Rosenfeld, 2004). However, when assessing the risk of serious violence, different risk factors are more relevant (see below).

Making Threats

As outlined above, most stalkers who assault give warnings of their intentions by making threats (Harmon et al., 1998; Meloy, 1999; Mullen et al., 1999; Pathé & Mullen, 1997). Several authors have found that threats are predictive of violence in intimate relationships (Brewster, 2000; Meloy & Boyd, 2003; Meloy, Davis, & Lovette, 2001; Meloy et al., 2000; Palarea, Zona, Lane, & Langhinrichsen-Rohling, 1999; Sheridan & Davies, 2001). Negative affect (perceived anger/hatred toward the victim) based on threats and verbal abuse was correlated with the likelihood of violent behavior in one study (Morrison, 2001). A significant proportion of stalkers who promise to injure the victim keep their promises. Although Meloy (1996) found that 75% of stalkers who made threats did not carry out violent acts, threats in the stalking context should always be taken seriously and should be regarded as commitments to act (Mullen et al, 2000).

Suicidality

Suicidality of the stalker is a risk factor for attackers and near lethal approachers who have stalked public figures (Mullen et al., 2000). It is also a risk factor in domestic violence situations because of its association with incidents in which the batterer kills himself and his partner in response to her attempt to leave the relationship (Walker & Meloy, 1998). A suicidal stalker intent on killing his ex-girlfriend or ex-wife is extremely dangerous because he has no fear of the consequences for himself.

Stalking by an Ex-Intimate

Though news media tend to sensationalize high-profile cases of stalking due to erotomania by strangers, the majority of women's stalking incidents are perpetrated by previous romantic partners (Tjaden & Thoennes, 1998, 2000a). Rejected stalkers are often filled with a combination of self righteousness and overwhelming entitlement. Both states of mind are conducive to violent behavior (Mullen et al., 2000). Violence may also reduce feelings of shame or humiliation in the rejected stalker.

   In the survey by Tjaden and Thoennes (1998, 2000a), 81% of the women who were stalked by a former partner were also physically assaulted by that partner. Tjaden and Thoennes also reported that 59% of the women were stalked by an intimate partner and 30% of the male victims were stalked by an intimate partner. Husbands or cohabiting partners who stalked their partners were four times more likely than husbands or cohabiting partners in the general population to have physically assaulted their partners.

Men are much more likely than women to see stalking as a way of continuing to control and intimidate an ex-partner. This may reflect some vestiges of patriarchal ideology in which men feel more entitled to control a woman who was once "theirs" (Davis & Frieze, 2000). Women stalkers seem more intent on forming an attachment to assuage feelings of loneliness, dependency, depression, and anger, rather than to restore a narcissistically idealized relationship, a dynamic that often characterizes male stalkers (Meloy & Boyd, 2003). Furthermore, rejected stalkers may be unaware of the negative effects of their pursuit behaviors on their victims (Langhinrichsen-Rohling et al., 2000). Such men may be surprised when charges are filed.

Research studies almost unanimously indicate that targets being stalked by an ex-intimate are at a higher risk of being attacked than are targets pursued by acquaintances or strangers (Brewster, 2000; Douglas & Dutton, 2001; Farnham, James, & Cantrell, 2000; Harmon et al., 1998; James & Farnham, 2003; Kienlen et al., 1997; Mullen et al., 1999; Palarea et al., 1999; Rosenfeld, 2004; Rosenfeld & Harmon, 2002; Schwartz-Watts & Morgan, 1998; Zona, Sharma, & Lane, 1993). Ex-wives are at higher risk for violence by stalkers than ex-girlfriends. This can be explained by greater distress in the stalkers due to the threatened loss of a longer, more intense relationship.

Psychological abuse during the relationship was the strongest predictor of subsequent stalking of a serious and potentially dangerous sort (Davis, Ace, & Andra, 1999; Logan et al., 2000; Mechanic, Weaver, & Resick, 2000). Coleman (1997) found that in undergraduate college women who had broken up with a former male partner, those men who had been physically abusive during the relationship were most likely to pursue their former female partners in a harassing or violent manner after the relationships ended.

Sheridan and Davies (2001) compared the frequency of violent acts perpetrated by (1) ex-intimate stalkers, (2) acquaintance stalkers, and (3) stranger stalkers in a sample of British self-defined stalking victims. Ex-intimate stalkers were the most aggressive of the three groups. Ex-partners were also the most likely to threaten and assault third parties as well as their principal stalking target.

Palarea et al. (1999) found that stalkers with a prior intimate relationship were more likely to threaten their stalking victims and property, to commit violence against persons and property, and to "make good" on threats through some form of violent behavior. Finally, in a study of persons charged with stalking and related offenses in San Diego, prior sexual intimacy with the victim resulted in an 11-fold increase in the likelihood of violence (Meloy et al., 2001).

In examining rejected stalkers, violence predictors from the domestic violence literature are helpful. Kropp, Hart, and Lyon (2002) note the following:

These (predictors) include past evidence of physical or sexual assault in relationships, past violence in the context of sexual jealousy, past use of weapons or credible threats of death, past violations of no contact orders, recent escalation in the severity or frequency of violence, extreme minimalization or denial of violence history, and attitudes that support or condone the use of violence in relationships. (p. 610; see also Campbell, 1995; Dutton & Kropp, 2000; Kropp, Hart, Webster, & Eaves, 1999)

In summary, the evidence for a high probability of violence by stalkers of former intimates is consistent and unequivocal: the longer and more intense the prior relationship, the greater the risk of violence.

Personality Disorder

A number of studies indicate that those stalkers with psychosis are less likely to become assaultive than nonpsychotic stalkers with personality disorders (Harmon et al., 1998; Kienlen et al., 1997; Mullen et al., 1999, 2000; Rosenfeld, 2004; Rosenfeld & Harmon, 2002). Stalkers who are strangers and overtly mentally ill produce the most fear in victims. However, consistent with that described above, Farnham et al. (2000) found that the greatest danger of serious violence from stalkers in the United Kingdom was not from strangers or from people with psychotic illness, but from nonpsychotic ex-partners.

Narcissistic, paranoid, and borderline traits are common in the personalities of stalkers (Meloy, 2002). Harmon et al. (1998) found that the stalkers most likely to act aggressively were those diagnosed with both a personality disorder and substance abuse.

Erotomanic Delusions

As described in chapter 2, stalkers with erotomania have a delusional belief that the stalking victim loves them. The targets of persons with erotomanic interests usually are persons of higher social status. Erotomanic stalkers are largely impervious to judicial sanctions and often regard court appearances and imprisonment as the "price of true love." Though the overall risks are low, erotomanics can occasionally be responsible for extreme violence (Mullen et al., 1999).

Menzies et al. (1995) defined dangerous behavior in persons with erotomania as threats or violence. He was able to accurately predict dangerous behavior in 88% of cases by the presence of two variables: (1) multiple concurrent objects of pursuit; and (2) unrelated serious antisocial behavior, usually including a history of violent convictions. This study has significant limitations because it includes threats as dangerous behavior and it tested an excess of predictor variables given the small sample size (Meloy, 2002).

Stalkers who delusionally believe a relationship already exists with the target may become jealous over what, from their peculiar perspective, is seen as infidelity (Mullen et al., 2000). Morbid jealousy has a dangerous reputation because of the frequency with which it is associated with violence directed against the partner believed to be unfaithful (Mowat, 1966; Mullen & Maack, 1985; Shepherd, 1961; Silva, Ferrari, Leong, & Penny, 1998; White & Mullen, 1989). Any person, including a mentally ill stalker, will behave in accord with how he perceives reality. It does not matter whether the motives are unrealistic or self destructive (Fein & Vossekuil, 1998). Thus, concern about future assault is realistic in stalkers with a paranoid illness if their preoccupations are centered on the infidelity of their ex-partners or the infidelity of their supposed lovers (Mullen et al., 2000).

Being Socially Isolated

Socially isolated stalkers are at greater risk of using violence. Risk of assault may be reduced by being certain that the stalker is connected to a social support system (Mullen et al., 2000), which may include mental health agencies, social service agencies, religious organizations, family, and friends. Being unemployed increased the risk of assault in one cohort (Mullen et al., 2000), but this was not true of stalkers who committed very serious assaults (James & Farnham, 2003).

Escalation of Stalking Behavior

Undergraduate female psychology students who reported significantly more verbal and physical abuse during their relationships were more likely to be stalked by their former partners after the relationships ended. The pursuit may become progressively more violent when these efforts are not successful in reunifying the relationship (Coleman, 1997). Burgesset al. (1997) studied batterers who stalked and found an escalation in the types of behaviors by stalkers as the stalking progressed. They suggest that the escalation "from clandestine (e.g., anonymous hang up phone calls) to open behavior (e.g., breaking into the victim's residence) . . . may be predictive of lethal actions" (p. 402).

RISK FACTORS FOR SEVERE VIOLENCE IN STALKING

Most earlier studies of violence in stalking have focused on all types of violence. James and Farnham (2003) did an important study to ascertain whether the risk factors associated with serious violence in stalking are the same as those associated with general violence in stalking. They examined records of 85 stalkers referred to a forensic psychiatric service in England and compared those who had committed serious violence (homicide and serious assaults) with those who had not.

About one-third of the stalking cases fulfilled the criteria for serious violence, including 7 cases of homicide, 5 of attempted murder, 7 of grievous bodily harm, and 8 of assault resulting in actual bodily harm. Thirty-five percent used weapons in the incident that brought them to the attention of the police. Verbal or written threats were made to the victim in 71% of all the cases of serious violence (James & Farnham, 2003).

Using Mullen and colleagues' (1999) classification scheme, James and Farnham (2003) found that 45% of their subjects were intimacy seekers, 35% were rejected, 18% were resentful, and 2.5% were in the incompetent category. As in other studies, rejected stalkers were most likely to engage in serious violence. The most significant indicator of major violence was a previous sexual relationship between the victim and the stalker.

James and Farnham (2003) also found that indicators of serious violence differed from indicators of general violence. Previously appearing at the victim's home during the period of stalking increased the odds of serious violence by a factor of 52. Among stalkers in general, posing a threat (e.g., visiting the victim's home) was a more important predictor of violence than making a threat by oral or written means (see Fein & Vossekuil, 1999). Serious violence was associated with previous violence against people or property during the stalking period. The presence of major depression in stalkers was also associated with serious violence (James & Farnham, 2003). Table 3.3 lists risk factors found to be associated with severe violence or homicide.

Whereas a history of previous convictions and unemployment are significantly associated with general violence in stalking, they were not associated with serious violence in this study (James & Farnham, 2003). No association was found between serious violence and substance abuse, previous convictions for violence against a person, or the presence of a personality disorder. Schwartz-Watts and Rowell (2003) point out that the James and Farnham (2003) study does not contradict research findings regarding general violence in stalkers, but instead reveals very specific risk factors in a small but important cohort.

The James and Farnham (2003) research suggests that serious assaults by stalkers appear likely to be singular catastrophic events, involving those with no history of convictions or of violence predating the stalking. These stalkers are outwardly socially integrated in areas such as employment. This contrasts with

Table 3.3. Risk Factors for Severe Violence or Homicide

Appearing at the victim's home
Previous violence
Major depression
Threats to harm children
Threatening messages on car

Source: James & Farnham, 2003; McFarlane et al., 2002.

the perpetrators of less serious assaults, for whom violence is more likely to be their habitual style of social interaction. Furthermore, because the duration of stalking was significantly shorter in cases of serious violence, early intervention may be of particular importance in prevention. This type of violence may be very difficult to predict because it is often due to overwhelming rage or rejection in people with no previous indicators of violence.

In a 10-city national study of risk factors for femicide (killing of women) by men in violent intimate relationships, McFarlane et al. (2002) examined intimate partner stalking and threatening behaviors that occurred within 12 months prior to a major assault or attempted or completed femicide. McFarlane and colleagues (2002) compared victims of femicide or attempted femicide to a control group of women reporting physical abuse by intimate partners within the last year but with no attempt on their life.

The McFarlane et al. study (2002) found that 68% of attempted/actual femicide victims and 51% of abused controls experienced stalking within 12 months of the attempted/actual murder or most severe abuse incident. The most frequent types of stalking were following or spying, unwanted phone calls, and surveillance by the perpetrator from a car. Stalking was significantly associated with assault.

Women who reported that the perpetrator followed or spied on them were more than twice as likely to become victims of attempted or completed femicide. If threatening messages were left on their car, the risk was increased fourfold over the control group of abused women. Finally, women were nine times more likely to be victims of attempted/actual femicide if the perpetrator made threats to harm their children (McFarlane et al., 2002).

Dietz (1994) reported that the following features were associated with stalkers who are likely to kill celebrity and stranger targets: (1) the stalkers have a mental disorder; (2) they believe themselves to be unique; they have an exaggerated sense of self importance or (especially) a destiny; (3) they identify with other stalkers and cut out newspaper articles about stalkers; (4) they keep a diary or record of their stalking; (5) they research their target victims; (6) they may show up uninvited at the homes or businesses of their victims; (7) they switch targets often (which makes it is useful to find out why they stopped following previous victims); (8) they may purchase a weapon for the specific occasion of an assassination. See chapter 10 for more information on celebrity stalking.

CASE EXAMPLE 3.1: EXAMPLE OF A RISK ASSESSMENT

In chapter 1, pages 8–10, we gave a detailed case example of stalking followed by homicide of the stalking victim. Here, we will illustrate some of the risk factors for violence by discussing this example. Rereading the chapter 1 case example will be helpful in understanding this analysis.

Walter Kovacs was a 26-year-old man when he was rejected by 18-year-old Cindy Taylor. He thus falls into the category of a "rejected" stalker, which creates the highest risk of violence among Mullen's five categories. As is common in rejected stalkers, Walter was seeking both reconciliation and revenge during his stalking. Although Walter shared quite limited intimacy with Cindy, he fell deeply in love with her. When he was rejected, he felt used and deceived by her. His perception that she betrayed him fueled his anger.

Walter did not have the risk factors for violence of (1) being a substance abuser or (2) prior criminal conduct except in relation to his stalking and property destruction of the stalking victim. However, he was so upset by Cindy's rejection that he felt the only way he could regain his "dignity" was either to win her back or to kill her.

Walter had the risk factor of escalation in his stalking behavior. He began with hang-up calls and went on to damaging Cindy's property and making threats toward her. He felt justified in his vandalism of her car because of his belief that Cindy had committed a "greater crime" in her unfair rejection of him.

Walter made explicit threats by e-mail to kill Cindy. Cindy was so upset by these e-mails that she stopped opening them after a while. Walter engaged in specific preparation for the homicide by attempting to purchase a handgun. When this came to the attention of his family, his father responded by having him admitted for psychiatric care. His fantasies of homicidal revenge were shared early in his hospitalization. They were then falsely disavowed when Walter realized that he would not obtain his freedom if he continued to admit such violent thoughts. He consistently falsely denied his homicidal thoughts to his outpatient therapist. However, Walter regularly recorded his sadistic fantasies of revenge toward Cindy on his computer. Had his hard drive been searched, his persistent thoughts of killing her would have been discovered.

The fact that Walter appeared at Cindy's dormitory prior to killing her is consistent with the research that identifies such conduct as a risk factor for severe violence and homicide by stalkers. Although Walter was not frankly suicidal at the time he killed Cindy, he was indifferent to the consequences for himself because of his feelings of hopelessness. He did not believe that he could ever be happy without Cindy. Walter was at greater risk for violence by having a personality disorder rather than a psychotic disorder. He had dated no one beside the victim and was socially isolated. He became so preoccupied with the stalking victim that he dropped out of college. As an unemployed stalker he was at greater risk of violence than stalkers who hold a job.

After Walter was arrested and placed on probation for stalking, he was among the 50% of stalkers who persist in their stalking behavior. In Walter's case, his upset about being arrested and forced into a psychiatric hospital increased his rage at Cindy. He blamed her for the trouble that he had brought upon himself by his stalking behavior. Although he was mandated to have outpatient mental health care, the fact that he did not report his violent fantasies precluded his therapist from helping him with his continued preoccupation with Cindy. Finally, on the day of the homicide, he became further inflamed by seeing Cindy walking with another man.

DOMESTIC VIOLENCE AND STALKING

Mechanic et al. (2000) studied a sample of acutely battered women to assess the interrelationship of emotional abuse, physical violence, and stalking in battered women. Stalking can be seen as representing a severe form of psychological abuse. One theme in emotional abuse is consistent reference to coercive and controlling tactics that instill fear, as well as surveillance behaviors that monitor a partner's freedom of movement. Emotional and psychological abuse are strong predictors of stalking (Mechanic et al., 2000).

Battering, stalking, and some aspects of emotional abuse appear to be motivated by attempts to control and intimidate the victim, and these behaviors may increase in severity in the context of perceived threats to the integrity of the relationship. Mechanic and colleagues (2000) found that stalking was more closely linked with psychological abuse than it was with physical violence in their sample of acutely battered women. Most (94%) of the battered women in this study reported being threatened by their partners. The experiences of stalking and emotional abuse create a climate of fear that remained with battered women even after they separated from their abusive partners. Physical violence served to legitimize their fears that stalking behavior might escalate into serious, life-threatening violence.

Stalking in a domestic context can be viewed as a continuation of intimate violence toward a partner after the relationship ends (Logan et al., 2000). Tjaden and Thoennes (1998, 2000a) found that 21% of women stalked by husbands or cohabiting partners reported that stalking occurred before the relationship ended, and 36% reported that the stalking occurred both before and after the relationship ended. Tjaden and Thoennes (1998, 2000a) also found that ex-husbands who stalked their partners were significantly more likely than ex-husbands who did not stalk to have engaged in emotionally abusive (e.g., shouting or swearing) and controlling (e.g., limiting contact with others, jealousy, possessiveness, and denying access to family income) behavior.

A study of FBI homicide data found that of 16,552 murders of intimate partners and spouses committed by men, the most common precipitant for the murder was the woman's leaving an abusive relationship (Kellerman & Mercy, 1992). A woman who leaves an abusive spouse is at great risk of getting unwanted attention and harassment from the estranged partner as he tries to win her back (Edelson, Eiskovits, Guttman, & Sela-Amit, 1991). The attention, such as stalking, may become progressively more violent when his efforts are not successful. When the man realizes that his partner intends to abandon him, he is more likely to resort to more extreme acts of violence, including murder (Adams, 1990; Pagelow, 1992). Bachman and Saltzman (1995) found that women separated from their husbands were 3 times more likely to be victimized by spouses than divorced women, and were 25 times more likely to be victimized by spouses than married women.

Tjaden and Thoennes (2000b) studied 1,285 domestic violence crime reports from the Colorado Springs Police Department in 1998. In one out of six cases, either the victim or the police officer mentioned that the suspect had stalked the victim or had engaged in stalking-like behaviors. However, only one case resulted in the police officer formally charging the suspect with stalking. The variable that was most often associated with stalking allegations was whether the victim and suspect were former, rather than current, intimate partners.

EVALUATION OF STALKERS FOR RISK OF VIOLENCE

Mental health professionals may perform a stalking evaluation as a court-ordered assessment, as a request from a victim, or in other forensic contexts. One approach to risk assessment recommended by the GAP Committee on Psychiatry and the Law is to develop a multidisciplinary team. A stalking assessment team might include the victim, a mental health professional, a local police officer, a local prosecutor, and sometimes, a private security guard or investigator (Meloy, 1996).

Ideally, the risk assessment should not be done by the treater of either the stalking victim or the stalker because of the potential for countertransferencial bias. This is also discussed in chapter 5. Periodic violence risk assessments should be done of the stalker in chronic cases because of the ebb and flow of dynamic risk factors (Meloy, 1999).

When approached by a stalking victim for advice regarding the risk of being harmed, the clinician's first step should be to assess the evidence of stalking to rule out the possibility of false victimization syndrome. A false allegation of stalking may be due to error, a delusional misperception, or malice (see chapter 5 for additional details). For example, a female law student approached the author for advice about a "stalker" that she believed was sending repeated veiled messages and pornographic material to her through her computer. She had had a male friend assist her in setting up her new computer. She was convinced that he was now sending harassing material to her. After I examined the computer and found no evidence other than pop-up ads for sexual material, I obtained the victim's permission to speak with the alleged stalker. He explained his puzzlement about the allegations against him. The "victim" was referred for psychiatric treatment for paranoia. Although she remained doubtful that she was mentally ill, she did note an end to the "stalking" messages after she began taking antipsychotic medication.

In evaluating what to do about a stalking case from the vantage point of the victim, careful thought should be given before acting. On occasion, not intervening at all is the best way to avoid a violent outcome (De Becker, 1997). In considering steps to bring a stalker into contact with the criminal justice system, the clinician should try to anticipate whether such actions would cause the stalker to escalate his conduct or to retreat from it (White & Caywood, 1998). For example, if a stalker is put under surveillance, it creates the risk that discovery of the surveillance by the stalker will cause him to commit a violent act sooner than he otherwise would have.

Increased vigilance is necessary when events humiliate or anger the stalker. Such events include the initial rejection, contact by a third party warning the stalker to stop the behavior, receipt of a restraining order, and court appearances (Meloy, 1999). For further information about risk management strategies, see chapter 4.

In cases in which a clinician will personally evaluate a stalker, it usually is best for the clinician to try to gather preliminary information about the stalker's background before conducting the interview. Police records, mental health records, medical records, and employment files of the stalker are often quite useful. The stalker's writings and computer hard drive may be studied if they are available. The clinician may also consider interviewing victims, relatives, friends, employers, and neighbors. The clinician should also give consideration to whether to involve family members of mentally ill stalkers. For example, if a psychotic stalker lives with his parents, family contact could be quite helpful.

Psychiatric interviews give stalkers the opportunity to tell their stories, to be heard, and to reassess whether their behavior should continue (Fein & Vossekuil, 1998). The initial interview allows the stalker both to express resentment and to provide an account of events (Mullen et al., 2000). Often such accounts are characterized by self justification and minimizing of their harassing behaviors. The examiner should make a detailed inquiry into the context from which the stalking arose and the factors that tend to sustain the behavior (Mullen et al., 2000). A good nonjudgmental question is, "What drove you to these actions?"

The evaluator should pay attention in the interview to whether the nature of violence associated with stalking is affective or predatory. Affective violence is preceded by autonomic arousal, accompanied by anger or fear, unplanned, and reactive (Meloy, 2002). Predatory violence is unemotional, planned, purposeful, and carried out in the absence of any imminent threat. Violence by stalkers of public figures is likely to be predatory, whereas most violence by stalkers toward former intimate partners is affective. Most (90%) stalkers of public figures do not communicate a threat before an intended violent act because doing so would decrease their probability of success. On the other hand, stalkers of prior sexual intimates are more likely to threaten and to engage in affective violence which is usually unplanned, highly emotional, and impulsive (Meloy, 2002).

The clinician should obtain a full account of a stalker's objectives (Mullen et al., 2000). How much time is occupied by the stalking behaviors? How long is spent thinking about the target? How long does the stalker think he can continue to pay the price of this behavior in terms of time, money, and emotional turmoil?

The evaluator should explore all the prior relationships of the stalker. It is important to examine physical and psychological abuse in prior relationships to determine whether stalking is an extension of intimate violence (Logan et al., 2000). Information about prior stalking history, including telephone harassment, should be obtained. Data should also be gathered about menacing behavior, criminal conduct, general violence, and domestic violence. Detailed inquiry should be made about acting on threats that were previously made. In assessing a stalker's risk for violence, the evaluator should also look at the level of physical approach used in contacting the victim (James & Farnham, 2003; Palarea et al., 1999).

The psychosocial history may include reactions to authority figures, reactions to limit setting in the past, and the stalker's current social support system. Suicidality and a stalker's willingness to die to accomplish his goal should also be explored (Mullen et al., 2000) as part of the psychiatric history. Psychological testing can be helpful in sorting out personality style and may be useful to assess amenability to treatment.

ASSESSMENT OF THREATS BY STALKERS

A threat, oral or written, explicitly states a wish or intent to injure or kill the stalking victim. Threats may be expressive or instrumental. Expressive threats are used to regulate affect in the threatener. Instrumental threats are intended to control the behavior of the victim through aversive consequences (Meloy, 1999).

Threats by a stalker toward an intimate or former intimate partner may be an attempt to control and ultimately coerce her into returning to the relationship. If the threats are not successful in accomplishing that end, the stalker may use violence to exert control or to express his anger. Men whose partners have terminated relationships experience greater loss of control than men whose partners remain in the relationship. Therefore, one would expect a greater use of threats and violence in situations in which the wife or girlfriend has left the relationship (Brewster, 2000).

Some stalkers who make a threat do not pose a threat. Some stalkers who pose a threat do not make an explicit threat. Threats may be explicit or veiled, such as a picture of a tombstone. When a stalker expresses a threat, the clinician should consider the questions in Table 3.4 (Fein, Vossekuil, & Holden, 1997).

In Pathé and Mullen's (1997) research, two-thirds of the stalking victims had considered using violence to retaliate against the stalker. Many stalking victims

Table 3.4. Questions in Stalker Threat Assessment

1. What is the magnitude of the potential harm?
2. Why is the threat being made now?
3. What does the threatening stalker want?
4. How likely is the threat to induce a violent response by the stalking victim?
5. How serious is the intent behind the threat?
6. How developed is the plan for executing the violence?
7. Is the threat absolute and without alternative courses of action?
8. Is the threat based on likely or unlikely contingencies?
9. Does the threatener have a lethal weapon in mind?
10. How available is the weapon of choice?
11. How accessible is the potential stalking victim?
12. How soon is the stalker likely to carry out the threat?
13. Has the stalker already taken any steps to carry out the threat?
14. Has the stalker shown a recent decrease in his ability to control violent impulses?
15. Has the stalker been violent under similar circumstances in the past?
16. Has the stalker acted violently under similar stresses in the past?
17. Is the stalker likely to be disinhibited by substance abuse?
18. Does depression or paranoia distort the stalker's thinking?
19. Is the stalker willing to undergo the consequences of his violent act? For example, is the stalker planning suicide? Is going to prison acceptable?
20. Has the stalker been able to form a therapeutic alliance with a therapist?
21. Has the stalker approached his potential victim, either with or without weapons?
22. How acquainted is the stalker with the stalking victim's work, personal life, and daily comings and goings?
23. What thresholds have been crossed by the stalker? For example, has he violated restraining orders? Made a will? Given away personal items?
24. Does the stalker appear to be on a downward course? For example, has the stalker recently appeared to be giving up hope, becoming more desperate, or becoming suicidal?
25. Is the stalker organized enough to plan and execute a violent action against the stalking victim?
26. How concerned about safety is the stalking victim?

Source: Modified from Fein, Vossekuil, & Holden, 1997.

in Tjaden and Thoennes' (1998, 2000a) survey were provoked to take extreme actions such as getting a gun (17%), changing addresses (11%), or moving out of town (11%), to deter the stalker.

When a stalker makes a threat, the stalker must be evaluated for violence potential in general, not just evaluated for the likelihood of carrying out the threat toward the specified stalking victim. Threats should be only one element taken into account in the process of assessing the likelihood of dangerous be-havior. If threats are made in the context of long-standing delusional beliefs that have not been acted upon over several years, the danger may be quite low.

The more intimate the relationship between the stalker and the victim, the more likely the threat is to be carried out. A threat is more likely to be carried out if it is made face to face, rather than on the phone or in writing

Table 3.5. Risk Factors for Violence Among Stalkers After Threats

Intimate relationship
Threat made face to face
Specific threats
Signed threats
Threats introduced late

Sources: De Becker, 1997; Dietz, 1998.

(Dietz, 1998). The more specific the threat, the more likely it is to be carried out (Dietz, 1998). People who send threats anonymously are far less likely to pursue an encounter than those who sign their names. The threatener who provides his true name is not trying to avoid attention; he probably is seeking it. Threats that are introduced late in a controversy are more serious than those used early (De Becker, 1997), because threats used early are likely to represent an immediate emotional response as opposed to a considered decision to use violence (see Table 3.5).

Believing that others will react as we would is the single most dangerous myth of intervention. The issue must be viewed through the stalker's eyes. The clinician should not rely on an agreement by the threatening stalker that he will not now carry out a threat.

In concluding that a stalker who has made a threat no longer poses a risk, the evaluator should be able to (1) articulate why the stalker originally made the threat, (2) document changes in the stalkers' thinking and behavior that negate the original concerns, (3) describe why the stalker is unlikely to pose a future threat to the stalking victim (Fein & Vossekuil, 1998).

RESTRAINING (PROTECTION) ORDERS

Meloy, Cowett, Parker, Hofland, and Friedland (1997) concluded that approximately half of the studies have found restraining orders to be effective and one-third of the studies suggest mixed results. Harrell and Smith (1996) found that many victims are reluctant to seek a restraining order because they are afraid of the stalker. The primary reason that restraining orders are ineffective is that they are violated quite frequently. Given their potential to be violated, restraining orders are important to consider in any risk assessment of stalkers. In the National Institute of Justice study (1998), about 10% of men and 28% of women stalking victims reported filing for restraining orders . Unfortunately, 69% of female and 80% of male victims who obtained such an order reported its violation (Tjaden & Thoennes, 1998, 2000a). Previous studies have reported a violation rate ranging from 18% to 70% (Gill & Brockman, 1996; Harrell & Smith, 1996; Klein, 1996; Mechanic et al., 2000; Morrison, 2001; Mustaine & Tewksbury, 1999).

Häkkänen, Hagelstam, and Santtila (2003) made a major contribution to research in this area by reviewing court and police files of 240 Finnish stalking cases in which a restraining order had been issued. Restraining orders were violated in 35% of the cases. Of those who violated the restraining order, one-third did so within 2 weeks following the order issuance. In all seven cases in which the victim had voluntarily met with the stalker, a violation of the restraining order was reported.

Among the restraining order violators in this study, the proportion of stalkers using pursuit actions (e.g., making phone calls) did not decrease significantly following the restraining order. However, the proportion of stalkers who assaulted the victim before the restraining order compared to after the restraining order sharply decreased. None of those who had previously assaulted with a weapon before the restraining order repeated the behavior after the restraining order. Threats to kill the victim were reduced in half after the restraining order (Häkkänen et al., 2003).

The Häkkänen et al. (2003) study suggests that restraining orders can play a significant role in victim protection. It also suggests that restraining orders do not increase the risk of violence to the victim unless the victim does not behave in accordance with the restraining order intent by meeting with the stalker.

Failure to obey a past order, prior physical violence (Keilitz, Davis, Efkeman, Flango, & Hannaford, 1997), intense preoccupation with the victim, and poor enforcement all predict violations of a restraining order by stalkers (Meloy, 1999). Restraining orders that are obtained early carry less risk than those introduced after the stalker has made a significant emotional investment in stalking. Sometimes, mutual restraining orders for both the stalker and victim reduce the humiliation to the stalker and the likelihood of continued stalking. Meloy et al. (1997) found that arrests following the issuance of restraining orders were significantly lower among those with a mutual restraining order compared to those with a one-sided restraining order. Further discussion of the use of restraining orders for risk management purposes can be found in chapter 4.

CONCLUSION

Threats and violence are common in stalking. Although limited research is available, some risk factors for violence toward stalking victims are clear. A prior intimate relationship between the stalker and victim markedly increases the risk of violence. Prior criminal history, substance abuse, threats, and the absence of psychosis increase the risk of violence. Depression and suicidality in stalkers are also causes for concern. Evaluating the risk that a stalker will kill the victim may require examining risk factors different from those associated with general violence. For serious violence, the risk is increased by leaving threatening messages on the stalking victim's car and threats to harm the victim's children.

Effective strategies for ending stalking involve an appropriate combination of legal sanctions and therapy for the stalker (Mullen et al., 1999). In assessing stalking behavior, the clinician should consider the antecedents to the behavior, the behavior itself, and the behavior's consequences (Westrup & Fremouw, 1998). The next chapter explains how to manage violence risk in stalking situations.

REFERENCES

Adams, D. (1990). Identifying the assaultive husband in court: You be the judge. *Response, 13*, 13–16.

Bachman, R., & Saltzman, L. (1995). Violence against women: Estimates from the redesigned survey (Special Report No. NCJ-154348). Washington DC: Bureau of Justice Statistics, U.S. Department of Justice.

Bjerregaard, B. (2000). An empirical study of stalking victimization. *Violence and Victims, 15*, 389–406.

Borum, R. (1996). Improving the clinical practice of violence risk assessment: Technology, guidelines, and training. *American Psychologist, 51*, 945–956.

Brewster, M. P. (2000). Stalking by former intimates: Verbal threats and other predictors of physical violence. *Violence and Victims, 15*, 41–53.

Burgess, A. W., Baker, T., Greening, D., Hartman, Burgess, A. G., Douglas, J. E., & Halloran, R. (1997). Stalking behavior within domestic violence. *Journal of Family Violence, 12*, 389–403.

Campbell, J. C. (1995). Prediction of homicide of and by battered women. In J. C. Campbell (Ed.), *Assessing dangerousness: Violence by sexual offenders, batterers, and child abusers* (pp. 96–113). Thousand Oaks, CA: Sage.

Coleman, F. L. (1997). Stalking behavior and the cycle of domestic violence. *Journal of Interpersonal Violence, 12*, 420–432.

Davis, K. E., Ace, A., & Andra, M. (1999). [Stalking victimization data]. Unpublished raw data.

Davis, K. E., & Frieze, I. H. (2000). Research on stalking: What do we know and where do we go? *Violence and Victims, 15*, 473–487.

De Becker, G. (1997). *The gift of fear.* New York: Dell.

Dietz, P. (1994). *Stalking syndrome of pathological attachments.* Paper presented at the American Academy of Psychiatry and the Law Annual Meeting, Maui, Hawaii.

Dietz, P. (1998). *Assessment of violent threats.* Paper presented at the American Psychiatric Association Annual Meeting, Toronto, Canada.

Douglas, K. S., & Dutton, D. G. (2001). Assessing the link between stalking and domestic violence. *Aggression and Violent Behavior, 6*, 519–546.

Dutton, D., & Kropp, P. R. (2000). A review of domestic violence risk instruments. *Trauma, Violence, and Abuse, 1*, 171–181.

Edelson, J. L., Eiskovits, Z. C., Guttman, E., & Sela-Amit, M. (1991). Cognitive and interpersonal factors in woman abuse. *Journal of Family Violence, 6*, 167–182.

Eronen, M., Hakola, P., & Tiihonen, J. (1996). Mental disorders and homicidal behavior in Finland. *Archives of General Psychiatry, 53,* 497–504.

Farnham, F. R., James, D. V., & Cantrell, P. (2000). Association between violence, psychosis, and relationship to victim in stalkers, *Lancet, 355,* 199.

Fein, R. A., & Vossekuil, B. (1998). Preventing attacks on public officials and public figures: A secret service perspective. In J. R. Meloy (Ed.), *The psychology of stalking: Clinical and forensic perspectives* (pp. 176–194). San Diego, CA: Academic Press.

Fein, R. A., & Vossekuil, B. (1999). Assassination in the United States: An operational study of recent assassins, attackers, and near-lethal approachers. *Journal of Forensic Sciences, 44,* 321–333.

Fein, R. A., Vossekuil, B., & Holden, G. A. (1997): Assessing targeted violence. *Expert Opinion, 4*(4), 1, 3–7.

Gill, R., & Brockman, J. (1996). A review of section 264 (criminal harassment) of the criminal code of Canada (Working Document WD 1996–7e). Ottawa, Canada: Research, Statistics, and Evaluation Directorate, Department of Justice.

Häkkänen, H., Hagelstam, C., & Santtila, P. (2003). Stalking actions, prior offender-victim relationships and issuing of restraining orders in a Finnish sample of stalkers. *Legal and Criminological Psychology, 8,* 189–206.

Hall, D. M. (1998). The victims of stalking. In J. R. Meloy (Ed.), *The psychology of stalking* (pp. 113–137). San Diego, CA: Academic Press.

Harmon, R., Rosner, R., & Owens, H. (1998). Sex and violence in a forensic population of obsessional harassers. *Psychology, Public Policy, and Law, 4,* 236–249.

Harrell, A., & Smith, B. E. (1996). Effects of restraining orders on domestic violence victims. In E. S. Buzawa & C. G. Buzawa (Eds.), *Do arrest and restraining orders work?* (pp. 214–242). Thousand Oaks, CA: Sage.

James, D. V., & Farnham, F. R. (2003). Stalking and serious violence. *The Journal of the American Academy of Psychiatry and the Law, 31,* 432–439.

Keilitz, S. L., Davis, C., Efkeman, H. S., Flango, C., & Hannaford, P. L. (1997). Civil protection orders: Victims' views on effectiveness. *National Institute of Justice Journal, (233),* 23–24.

Kellerman, A. L., & Mercy, J. A. (1992). Men, women, and murder: Gender-specific differences in rates of fatal violence and victimization. *The Journal of Trauma, 33,* 1–5.

Kienlen, K. K., Birmingham, D. L., Solberg, K. B., O'Regan, J. T., & Meloy, J. R. (1997). A comparative study of psychotic and nonpsychotic stalking. *The Journal of the American Academy of Psychiatry and the Law, 25,* 317–334.

Klein, A. R. (1996). Re-abuse in a population of court-restrained male batterers. In E. S. Buzawa & C. G. Buzawa (Eds.), *Do arrest and restraining orders work?* (pp. 214–242). Thousand Oaks, CA: Sage.

Kropp, P. R., Hart, S. D., & Lyon, D. R. (2002). Risk assessment of stalkers: Some problems and possible solutions. *Criminal Justice and Behavior, 29,* 590–616.

Kropp, P. R., Hart, S. D., Webster, C. W., & Eaves, D. (1999). *Spousal assault risk assessment: User's guide.* Toronto, Canada: Multi-Health Systems.

Langhinrichsen-Rohling, J., Palarea, R. E., Cohen, J., & Rohling, M. L. (2000). Breaking up is hard to do: Unwanted pursuit behaviors following the dissolution of a romantic relationship. *Violence and Victims, 15,* 73–90.

Logan, T. K., Leukefeld, C., & Walker, B. (2000). Stalking as a variant of intimate violence: Implications from a young adult sample. *Violence and Victims, 15,* 91–111.

McFarlane, J., Campbell, J. C., & Watson, K. (2002). Intimate partner stalking and femicide: Urgent implications for women's safety. *Behavioral Sciences and the Law, 20,* 51–68.

Mechanic, M. B., Weaver, T. L., & Resick, P. A. (2000). Intimate partner violence and stalking behavior: Exploration of patterns and correlates in a sample of acutely battered women. *Violence and Victims, 15,* 55–72.

Meloy, J. R. (1996). Stalking (obsessional following): A review of some preliminary findings. *Aggression and Violent Behavior, 1,* 147–162.

Meloy, J. R. (1999). Stalking, an old behavior, a new crime. *Psychiatric Clinics of North America, 22,* 85–99.

Meloy, J. R. (2002). Stalking and violence. In J. Boon & L. Sheridan (Eds.), *Stalking and psychosexual obsession* (pp. 105–124). London: Wiley.

Meloy, J. R., & Boyd, C. (2003). Female stalkers and their victims. *The Journal of the American Academy of Psychiatry and the Law, 31,* 211–219.

Meloy, J. R., Davis, B., & Lovette, J. (2001). Risk factors for violence among stalkers. *Journal of Threat Assessment, 1,* 3–16.

Meloy, J. R., Cowett, P. Y., Parker, S., Hofland, B. & Friedland, A. (1997). Domestic protection orders and the prediction of subsequent criminality and violence toward protectees. *Psychotherapy, 34,* 447–458.

Meloy, J. R., Rivers, L., Siegel, L., Gothard, S., Naimark, D., & Nicolini, J. R. (2000). A replication study of obsessional followers and offenders with mental disorders. *Journal of Forensic Sciences, 45,* 189–194.

Menzies, R., Fedoroff, J. P., Green, C., & Isaacson, K. (1995). Prediction of dangerous behavior in male erotomania. *British Journal of Psychiatry, 166,* 529–536.

Morrison, K. A. (2001). Predicting violent behavior in stalkers: A preliminary investigation of Canadian cases in criminal harassment. *Journal of Forensic Sciences, 46,* 1403–1410.

Mowat, R. R. (1966). *Morbid jealousy and murder.* London: Tavistock.

Mullen, P. E., & Maack, L. H. (1985). Jealousy, pathological jealousy, and aggression. In D. P. Farrington & J. Gunn (Eds.), *Aggression and dangerousness* (pp. 103–126). New York: Wiley.

Mullen, P. E., Pathé, M., & Purcell, R. (2000). *Stalkers and their victims.* Cambridge, UK: Cambridge University Press.

Mullen, P., Pathé, M., Purcell, R., & Stuart, G. (1999). A study of stalkers. *American Journal of Psychiatry, 156,* 1244–1249.

Mustaine, E. E., & Tewksbury, R. (1999). A routine activities theory explanation for women's stalking victimization. *Violence Against Women, 5,* 43–62.

National Institute of Justice. (1998). *Stalking and domestic violence: The third annual report to Congress under the Violence Against Women Act.* Rockville,

MD: National Criminal Justice Reference Service. Retrieved May 15, 2006, from http://nij.ncjrs.org/publications/pub

Pagelow, M. D. (1992). Adult victims of domestic violence. *Journal of Interpersonal Violence, 7,* 87–120.

Palarea, R. E., Zona, M. A., Lane, J. C., & Langhinrichsen-Rohling, J. (1999). The dangerous nature of intimate relationship stalking: Threats, violence, and associated risk factors. *Behavioral Sciences and the Law, 17,* 269–283.

Pathé, M., & Mullen, P. E. (1997). The impact of stalkers on their victims. *British Journal of Psychiatry, 170,* 12–17.

Reiss, A. J., & Roth, J. A. (1993). *Understanding and preventing violence.* Washington: National Academy Press.

Rosenfeld, B. (2003, June). Recidivism in stalking and obsessional harassment. *Law and Human Behavior, 27*(3), 251–265.

Rosenfeld, B. (2004). Violence risk factors in stalking and obsessional harassment: A review and preliminary meta-analysis: *Criminal Justice and Behavior, 31,* 9–36.

Rosenfeld, B., & Harmon, R. (2002). Factors associated with violence in stalking and obsessional harassment cases. *Criminal Justice and Behavior, 29,* 671–691.

Rosenfeld, B., & Lewis, C. (2005). Assessing violence risk in stalking cases: A regression tree approach. *Law and Human Behavior, 29,* 343–357.

Sandberg, D. A., McNiel, D. E., & Binder, R. L. (1998). Characteristics of psychiatric inpatients who stalk, threaten, or harass hospital staff after discharge. *American Journal of Psychiatry, 155,* 1102–1105.

Schwartz-Watts, D., & Morgan, D. W. (1998) Violent versus non-violent stalkers. *The Journal of the American Academy of Psychiatry and the Law, 26,* 241–245.

Schwartz-Watts, D. M., & Rowell, C. N. (2003). Commentary: Update on assessing risk for violence among stalkers. *The Journal of the American Academy of Psychiatry and the Law, 31,* 440–443.

Shepherd, M. (1961). Morbid jealousy: Some clinical and social aspects of a psychiatric syndrome. *Journal of Mental Science, 107,* 687–704.

Sheridan, L., & Davies, G. M. (2001). Violence and the prior victim–stalker relationship. *Criminal Behavior and Mental Health, 11,* 102–116.

Silva, A. J., Ferrari, M. M., Leong, G. B., & Penny, G. (1998). The dangerousness of persons with delusional jealousy. *The Journal of the American Academy of Psychiatry and the Law, 26,* 607–623.

Soyka, M. (2000). Substance misuse, psychiatric disorder, and violent and disturbed behaviour. *British Journal of Psychiatry, 176,* 345–350.

Steadman, H. J., Mulvey, E. P., Monahan, J., Robbins, P. C., Appelbaum, P. S., Grisso, T., Roth, L. H., & Silver, E. (1998). Violence by people discharged from acute psychiatric inpatient facilities and by others in the same neighborhoods. *Archives of General Psychiatry, 55,* 393–401.

Tjaden, P., & Thoennes, N. (1998). *Stalking in America: Findings from the National Violence Against Women Survey* (Research in Brief Series, Publication NCJ 169592). Washington, DC: National Institute of Justice and Centers for Disease Control and Prevention.

Tjaden, P., & Thoennes, N. (2000a). *Full report of the prevalence, incidence, and consequences of violence against women: Findings from the National Violence Against Women Survey. Research Report.* Washington, DC: National Institute of Justice and the Centers for Disease Control and Prevention. Retrieved December 28, 2005, from http://www.ojp.usdoj.gov/nij

Tjaden, P., & Thoennes, N. (2000b). The role of stalking in domestic violence crime reports generated by the Colorado Springs Police Department. *Violence and Victims, 15,* 427–441.

Walker, L. E., & Meloy, J. R. (1998). Stalking and domestic violence. In Meloy, J. R. (Ed.), *The psychology of stalking: Clinical and forensic perspectives* (pp. 140–164). San Diego, CA: Academic Press.

Wallace, C., Mullen, P., Burgess, P., Palmer, S., Ruschena, D., & Browne, C. (1998). Serious criminal offending and mental disorder: Case linkage study. *British Journal of Psychiatry, 172,* 477–484.

Westrup, D., & Fremouw, W. J. (1998). Stalking behavior: A literature review and suggested functional analytic assessment technology. *Aggression and Violent Behavior, 3,* 255–274.

White, G. E., & Mullen, P. E. (1989). *Jealousy: Theory research and clinical strategies.* New York: Guilford Press.

White, S., & Caywood, J. (1998). Threat management of stalking cases. In Meloy, J. R.(Ed.), *The psychology of stalking: Clinical and forensic perspectives* (pp. 298–316). San Diego, CA: Academic Press.

Zona, M., Palarea, R., & Lane, J. (1998). Psychiatric diagnosis and the offender-victim typology of stalking. In J. R. Meloy (Ed.), *The psychology of stalking: Clinical and forensic perspectives* (pp. 69–84). San Diego: Academic Press.

Zona, M. A., Sharma, K. K., & Lane, J. (1993). A comparative study of erotomanic and obsessional subjects in a forensic sample. *Journal of Forensic Sciences, 38,* 894–903.

4   Risk Management of Stalking

James Knoll

This chapter will address the clinical, legal, and practical methods that may be used to manage the risk of stalking behaviors. Multiagency interventions and victim safety strategies are stressed. Practical security approaches and appropriate responses to stalkers' harassment are discussed. The special issue of managing the stalking of clinicians is addressed. Finally, psychiatric treatment of the stalker is discussed as a method of managing risk. The chapter concludes with a case example and discussion of practical methods of stalking risk management.

INTRODUCTION

The effective risk management of stalking is a dynamic process that requires skill and experience in many of the areas previously discussed. Understanding stalking from a medico-legal perspective (see chapter 7) as well as a risk assessment perspective (chapter 3) is necessary for an effective and comprehensive approach to risk management. This special knowledge is often necessary *in addition* to a skilled approach to psychiatric diagnosis and treatment due to the high rates of major mental illness observed in stalkers (Mohandie, Meloy, McGowan, & Williams, 2006). Because stalking can have a substantial impact upon victims, we have devoted a separate chapter to victim management and considerations (see chapter 5). This chapter will address the clinical, legal, and practical methods that may be used to manage the risk of stalking behaviors. Multiagency interventions and victim safety strategies are stressed. Finally, psychiatric treatment of the stalker is discussed as a method of managing risk.

GENERAL MANAGEMENT PHILOSOPHY

Any well-reasoned risk management approach to stalking behavior must first address the "intervention dilemma" (White & Cawood, 1998). The intervention dilemma involves the consideration that taking direct action toward the stalker to reduce stalking may actually increase the risk of violence, and in some cases, no direct action may be preferable. An active response by law enforcement or others may have three possible outcomes: (1) risk reduction, (2) risk enhancement, or (3) no effect.

In some cases, an active intervention may actually enflame the stalker by challenging or humiliating him or her. For this reason, there can be no single "best approach" to risk management. Rather, risk management approaches must consider the significance of individual-specific nuances and preferably involve the input of different disciplines.

Obtaining a protective order is one example of direct action, which may or may not be helpful. The majority of domestic violence research does indicate a positive protective effect for abused women who apply and qualify for a protective order (McFarlane et al., 2004). An area of overlap sometimes occurs between domestic violence and stalking in the rejected type of stalker. Although there are no conclusive studies of the effectiveness of protective orders specifically related to stalkers, it is generally accepted that a stalker's reaction to previous orders, if known, is the best guide in individual cases (Meloy, 1997).

If the decision is made to use a protective order, it is important for the victim to make a personal "commitment" to reporting all violations of the order. Failure to strictly enforce a protective order may send a message to the stalker that the order can be disregarded (Orion, 1997). The victim who obtains a protective order against an ex-intimate partner should guard against developing a false sense of security. This is because this type of rejected stalker is likely to have a great deal of emotional investment in the relationship that, in his perception, may outweigh potential criminal sanctions. Furthermore, in stalking cases involving psychotic individuals whose behavior is particularly irrational, criminal injunctions may be misperceived in a variety of ways and thus disregarded.

In rare cases, protective orders may actually escalate stalking and violence (Meloy, 1997). However, obtaining a protective order against a stalker can also be helpful in ways that go beyond preventing the stalking behavior. The protective order may serve as legal evidence of the course of stalking behavior, as well as documenting the legal necessity of a "fearful victim" for a criminal conviction. Restraining orders are covered in greater detail later in this chapter.

Another general risk management principle is the importance of remaining vigilant around "dramatic moments" during which violence risk may be especially heightened (Meloy, 1997). Certain events may result in the stalker experiencing intense shame or humiliation. Typical dramatic moments include legal

Table 4.1. Risk Enhancing Dramatic Moments

- Arrests
- Issuance of restraining orders
- Court hearings
- Custody hearings
- Anniversary dates
- Family-oriented holidays

Table 4.2. Courtroom Safety Precautions

- Sit as far away from the stalker as possible.
- Do not look at or talk to the stalker.
- Bring a friend or relative.
- Tell a bailiff or sheriff that you are afraid.
- Ask the judge or sheriff to allow you to leave before the stalker.
- Take your protection order wherever you go.
- Call police if the stalker follows you when you leave.

Adapted from ABA Commission on Domestic Violence.

intercessions such as when the stalker receives a protective order, is arrested, or appears in court. Table 4.1 provides a list of dramatic moments commonly observed by risk management experts.

The victim of stalking may be at the greatest risk of violence immediately after such events, primarily because the stalker is feeling the greatest humiliation, yet still maintains his freedom. Dramatic moments may also be less obvious, and involve events or dates that have symbolic meaning for the stalker, such as anniversaries, holidays, or other social events. Victims who are especially concerned about an impending dramatic moment should take steps to prepare, such as arranging to be out of town or notifying the court, law enforcement, and victim advocates. Because courtroom appearances are dramatic and sometimes dangerous situations, special precautions should be taken by stalking victims upon going to court (see Table 4.2).

MULTIAGENCY INTERVENTIONS

The stalker's risk of violence is managed most effectively by a multidisciplinary approach that accounts for the multiple facets of the stalker's social system. Agencies involved should typically include, when possible, law enforcement, criminal justice, mental health, attorneys, security specialists, victim advocates, the victim, and her social network. Victims should work to actively establish rapport with the senior police official and district attorney assigned to the case. This will increase the chances that the victim will be listened to and seen as a personal priority by officials (Orion, 1997; White & Cawood, 1998). In addition, the victim will be in a better position to learn the policies, laws, and resources available for managing risk in stalking cases.

An example of a well-established, comprehensive multidisciplinary approach is the San Diego Stalking Strike Force (Maxey, 2002). The Strike Force is a group of volunteer professionals from mental health, law enforcement, victim advocate and criminal justice agencies who manage stalking cases with a collaborative approach. They provide services such as training, education, victim support, and risk assessment of individual stalking cases. The Strike Force is in a unique position to promote the recognition of stalking cases, give legal updates, conduct investigations, and craft risk management strategies. They have produced educational materials such as training videos and victim support handbooks.

The Strike Force's Stalking Case Assessment Team meets every month to evaluate cases. Members also serve on an on-call basis, should an emergent situation arise. In addition to assessing risk and assisting with victim safety, the team frequently provides liaisons with state parole agencies. This can be critical in the postconviction stages when it is possible for the parole board to impose special conditions on the stalker. Continued supervision of the stalker is enhanced by the exchange of information between the case manager and the parole agent during the monthly meetings.

VICTIM SAFETY AND STRATEGIES

Most authorities emphasize the necessity that victims assertively take responsibility for their own personal safety (De Becker, 1997; McFarlane et al., 2004). This includes becoming familiar with local stalking laws, resources, and law enforcement policies. Certainly, these strategies should not be undertaken alone, but it is the victim who must take the lead in assuring that safety measures are in place. Table 4.3 provides a list of strategies that victims should consider in an effort to maximize their own safety.

In every case of unwanted contact, the victim should document and record each incident, resisting the urge to ignore or eliminate evidence that may evoke feelings of fear, shame, or disgust. Victims may find it helpful to keep an "incident log" or journal recording the times and dates of each unwanted contact. Such documentation helps establish a clear course of illegal conduct, and may prove valuable to police and prosecution efforts.

All evidence, including gifts, mementos, and other, perhaps bizarre, materials, must be preserved. Ideally, these items should be stored in a plastic bag and labeled with the date, time, and place they were received. Victims should avoid handling the evidence and should store it in a secure location. All forms

Table 4.3. Victim Strategies to Maximize Safety

- Document and record all evidence.
- Protect personal information.
- Convey one clear "stay away" message.
- Avoid all subsequent contact.
- Establish contact with a law enforcement liaison.
- Form a safety network.
- Seek counseling.
- Put in place security measures.

of unwanted contact, including vandalism, should be recorded in the incident log. Vandalism or damage to property by stalkers should be photographed and noted by date.

Voice messages left by the stalker should be preserved and dated. It is especially helpful if the victim's voicemail has a function that allows forwarding. If this is the case, the victim can simply forward the stalker's message to the police or prosecuting attorney's office. If the stalker calls or sends letters from a correctional facility, the victim should immediately inform the stalker's correctional case manager or warden (Abrams & Robinson, 1998). If the inmate's correctional case manager is not known, the victim could call the correctional facility in question and ask to speak to a corrections official who deals with victim services. Following up such notifications with a letter will increase the likelihood that the information will be communicated to the stalker's parole board.

It is also critical that victims take an active role in protecting personal information. Disclosing personal information should be a highly selective process, with only trusted persons receiving such information. Addresses, phone numbers, and e-mail addresses should be carefully guarded. Victims should consider establishing a post office box that will prevent the theft of mail containing personal information. Personal mail that is to be discarded should be destroyed instead of merely placed in the garbage.

In cases involving unwanted telephone contact, victims should consider obtaining a second, unlisted, phone line. The original number is preserved solely for the purpose of screening and recording unwanted contacts, whereas the second line is used for personal affairs (Mullen, Pathé, & Purcell, 2000). The stalker will hopefully remain unaware of the existence of the second line. The stalker's unwanted calls can then be recorded for evidence, and the problem of intermittent reinforcement is eliminated. De Becker (1997) recommends that the victim recruit a same-gender friend to record the answering message on the initial phone line to dissuade stalkers who call repeatedly for the purpose of listening to the victim's voice.

Victims should adhere to a policy of *no initiated contact* with the stalker. As soon as the unwanted pursuit is apparent, the victim should clearly and unequivocally state one time to the stalker that *no* relationship is wanted. The message should be firm, reasonable, and as clear as possible due to some stalkers' tendency to misinterpret such communications to their favor. For the same reason, the victim should not attempt to deliver the message gently by letting the stalker "down easy." This may be interpreted by the stalker to mean that the victim is ambivalent about the decision.

An example from the author's case files is the victim who responded to an incompetent type stalker by saying, "I'm sorry, I just don't have time for a relationship right now." This was subsequently interpreted by the stalker to mean that the victim might be available for a relationship with him in the future. Another example is the victim who told her rejected type stalker, "It's not you, it's me—I'm dealing with a lot of emotional baggage from my past and it wouldn't be fair to you." The rejected stalker interpreted this statement as a "call to arms" for him to increase his contact with her in an effort to help "heal" her past emotional wounds.

Mullen et al. (2000) suggest delivering this message "personally and directly" in a place where the victim feels safe, such as in public. It is important that the victim not entertain a stalker's attempts to negotiate, plead, or debate. Having delivered the message, the victim must not engage in any further discussion. From that point on, the victim should avoid all direct contact with the stalker so as to minimize the effects of "intermittent positive reinforcement" that will sustain or increase future approach behavior (Meloy, 1997).

Establishing contact with local law enforcement is an important safety strategy that may also serve to provide the victim with valuable resources such as victim advocate groups. Establishing contact generally entails going to local law enforcement department and speaking with a local police chief, who is usually in the best position to direct a victim to a particular officer or division within the department. Law enforcement will then be in a position to assist the victim in learning about the department's stalking risk management strategies. Victims should seek to establish rapport and have a frank discussion with law enforcement personnel about expectations for assistance.

The victim who establishes a good working relationship with law enforcement will be more likely to be heard and given personal priority (White & Cawood, 1998). Additionally, victims may wish to hire the services of a private investigator who is familiar with personal protection and stalking issues. However, public agency law enforcement officials should be contacted first so that at the very least, there will be documentation of the stalking behavior with the victim's local law enforcement agency. Private security consultants may be approached second, especially if it becomes clear that local law enforcement is unable to effectively manage risk (Meloy, 1997).

Forming a network of trusted social contacts will provide a "safety net" that victims can rely on to help manage risk. Victims should inform family, friends, coworkers, and neighbors about the stalking behavior and its potentially serious consequences. This may prove to be an effective preventive measure, especially in reducing the risk that personal information is inadvertently disclosed to the stalker by others (Mullen et al., 2000).

The victim may wish to distribute a photo of the stalker to the members of the safety network with instructions to call the victim if the stalker is spotted. Such a plan establishes a lookout strategy that provides an early warning system and greater sense of security to the victim (Meloy, 1997). It is common for stalking victims to experience emotional distress. Should emotional distress become disabling or progress to symptoms of mental illness, the victim should seek mental health counseling as discussed in chapter 5.

Stalking victims should consider having a home security check performed by local law enforcement or a private security company. Practical suggestions

Table 4.4. Home Security Measures for Victims

- Memorize emergency numbers.
- Keep a cell phone with you at all times.
- Plan an escape route.
- Have a packed bag ready in case you need to leave quickly.
- Block caller ID.

Adapted from ABA Commission on Domestic Violence (1999).

usually involve upgrading locks, installing security windows, and obtaining a home security system. Motion-sensitive lights may be installed outside. Windows and doors should be cleared of obstructions so as to prevent potential hiding areas (White & Cawood, 1998).

Some stalkers may establish an "observation area" that allows them to view the victim while remaining unseen. The observation area may be inside or outside of the victim's residence. One method of searching for an observation area is to stand at each window of the victim's house and survey the perimeter using binoculars. The interior of the victim's house, including attics, crawl spaces, and other concealed areas, should be inspected.

It is advisable for stalking victims to invest in a mobile phone that can be used in case of emergency. The American Bar Association (ABA) Commission on Domestic Violence (1999) has suggested a number of home security tips that are applicable to stalking victims (see Table 4.4).

Security experts often advise stalking victims not to adhere to their usual, predictable routines (Ramsey, 2000). This can be accomplished by taking different daily travel routes or being prepared to go out of town on weekends at short notice. Victims should also make contingency plans in the event that their social supports are unavailable in an emergency. Emergency contingency plans can be arranged by contacting victim advocacy agents who can give information about the services and locations of local "safe houses" or domestic violence shelters.

RISK MANAGEMENT IN THE WORKPLACE

Stalking behavior is often an integral part of domestic violence, and many stalking-related fatalities occur in the workplace. Approximately 5% of workplace homicides fall into the domestic violence category involving ex-intimate partners (University of Iowa Injury Prevention Research Center, 2001). Thus, it may be crucial for a victim to inform her employer and work colleagues of the stalking situation (Meloy, 1997; Mullen et al., 2000). This communication is essential not only for the safety of the victim, but also for the safety of coworkers.

Recently, workplace violence has become an issue of national concern. Most employers are seeking to reduce risk and liability by implementing workplace violence prevention programs. Some practical measures for reducing workplace violence include the following: requiring a check-in point for all nonemployees, isolating public access areas from employee areas, designating a "safe room" and alternate exits for emergencies, installing a security system, and hiring security guards (ABA Commission on Domestic Violence, 1999).

Employers should consider instituting security escorts and special parking for the victim. Coworkers can be instructed to screen the victim's calls and recognize the stalker if he appears at the workplace. Ideally, there should be some notification system and response protocol firmly in place to deal with appearances of the stalker (White & Cawood, 1998). Regrettably, in more serious cases, the victim may wish to consider temporary or permanent work relocation.

RISK MANAGEMENT FOR HEALTHCARE PROFESSIONALS AS STALKING VICTIMS

Health-care professionals constitute a unique, though understudied, group of stalking victims. In the mental health field, complex therapeutic transference issues can result in a patient misperceiving a clinician's empathy as a desire for a closer relationship (Lion & Herschler, 1998). Patients who suffer from severe personality disorders or erotomanic delusions may be vulnerable to developing such misperceptions. In addition, they are prone to hostile, retaliatory behavior in response to what they perceive as mistreatment (Sandberg, McNiel, & Binder, 2002). Major obstacles to stalking risk management for clinicians are denial of victimization and lack of firm doctor-patient boundaries (Galeazzi, Elkins, & Curci, 2005; Tsushima & Wong, 2003). The workplace violence safety measures described above apply equally to health-care professionals, who should consider alerting the hospital security department, if available, and coworkers to pertinent details of their situation.

Health-care professionals who adopt a detached stance or who minimize inappropriate patient communications toward them may inadvertently potentiate their own victimization. Professionals must first acknowledge the behavior in its early stages, and engage the patient in a frank discussion about appropriate boundaries. Depending on the severity of the inappropriate behavior, it may be necessary for the professional to transfer the patient's care and/or consider civil commitment if the patient meets state statutory requirements.

In a study of stalking and harassing behavior experienced by clinicians, the authors concluded that having a "repertoire of responses" permitted a necessary flexibility of risk management response. Potential responses included informing supervisors and coworkers, limit setting through direct confrontation, and involvement of law enforcement (Sandberg et al., 2002). Indeed, it would be prudent for clinicians and their professional organizations to develop action plans to raise awareness of the risks of stalking by clients, particularly in light of the fact that clinicians who are stalked may consider leaving the profession (Purcell, Powell, & Mullen, 2005).

When the patient's care must be transferred, the professional should consider informing the patient, by certified mail, of the termination of the relationship. In addition, the letter should provide contact information for a referral to another professional. The referral should be made in a thoughtful manner and with the consent and understanding of the receiving health-care professional. In situations in which it is not possible to secure a timely referral, the clinician may consider furnishing a list of community mental health providers for the patient to choose from. When possible, it may be desirable to have the letter come from a clinic or administrative director, as opposed to the victim (Meloy, 2002), particularly when the victim has already clearly communicated to the patient the intent to terminate treatment.

ADDITIONAL APPROACHES TO GENERAL STALKING RISK MANAGEMENT

In addition to more practical environmental safety measures, some authorities recommend that victims receive training in self-defense (Shrapnel, 1997). Self-defense training may have the effect of increasing victims' sense of power and security, as well as equipping victims with skills to protect their physical integrity. The option of a personal body alarm may be preferable to some victims. Central monitoring of the body alarm provides a more prompt police or security response (Mullen et al., 2000).

In some states, multiagency collaboration has resulted in such safety measures being provided by state government. For example, a prosecuting attorney's office in New Hampshire now provides stalking victims with cell phones programmed to dial 911 immediately, as well as personal body alarms (Roberts & Kurst-Swanger, 2002). A more recently developed technology is a part of the Juris Monitor Program, originally designed for domestic violence offenders (Archives of the Mayor's Press, 1999). The program requires the stalker to wear an electronic monitoring device. If the stalker comes within 500 feet of the victim, an alarm is set off that immediately notifies police and 911 operators. Each violation is automatically recorded in a computer system.

Restraining or Protective Orders

Research on restraining orders indicates that they are frequently violated (Gill & Brockman, 1996; Harrell & Smith, 1996; Klein, 1996; Mustaine & Tewksbury, 1999). Restraining order violations can have implications for the assessment of risk, and this topic is also discussed in chapter 3. With regard to risk management, although the majority of stalkers disobey court orders, obtaining a restraining order can still benefit the victim. Most importantly, a formal restraining order creates documentation that may be useful in later legal proceedings. In addition, police may be more likely to act faster and more decisively in cases with an active restraining order (Häkkänen, Hagelstam, & Santtila, 2003).

Restraining orders should not be sought reflexively, however; they should be carefully considered as a potential risk management option among other strategies (De Becker, 1997). Whether or not a restraining order is appropriate will depend on a variety of factors particular to the individual case. Table 4.5 lists a number of important factors to consider before obtaining a restraining order.

The primary danger is that a restraining order may provide a false sense of security to the stalking victim. In the interest of preventing a false sense of security, it is important to note that failure to obey a past order, prior physical violence, intense preoccupation with the victim, and poor enforcement of a protective order all predict violations of a restraining order by stalkers (Keilitz et al., 1997; Meloy, 1997).

Restraining orders are most effective on stalkers who have a limited emotional investment in the victim (De Becker, 1997). For example, a restraining order against a man who has only had several dates with the victim simply asks him to go about his life as it was before he met the victim. In contrast, a restraining order against an estranged husband asks him to abandon his emotional investment in many central features of his life (De Becker, 1997). For these reasons, it is desirable to obtain a restraining order in the early stage of the stalking, prior to the stalker developing significant emotional investment in the victim. Restraining orders are also more likely to be effective in the case of a naïve pursuer who does not recognize the inappropriateness of his behavior (De Becker, 1997). This type of individual would most likely correspond to the *incompetent* type stalker in the Mullen et al. (2000) classification.

Among domestic violence prevention advocates, the issue of the "mutual restraining order" is harshly critiqued. This is because in cases of spousal abuse, it is seen as potentially supportive of the perpetrator's distorted views about who is actually being victimized. In fact, some states have statutes banning the use of mutual restraining orders in cases of domestic violence. In general, mutual

Table 4.5. Restraining Order Considerations

- Stalker's response to past orders
- Stalker's prior physical violence
- Stalker's prior physical violence
- Capacity and responsiveness of local police
- Single versus mutual restraining order
- Current stage of stalking

restraining orders involve both stalker and victim obtaining a restraining order on each other.

For the stalker who does not have a history of domestic violence yet has accumulated a substantial degree of emotional investment in the victim, the mutual restraining order may be an option. Meloy (1997) found that there were fewer arrests of stalkers following the issuance of a mutual restraining order as compared to single restraining orders. In some select cases, the stalker's feelings of humiliation can act to fuel their continued pursuit, and a mutual restraining order may allow the stalker to abandon the pursuit by reducing the level of his humiliation.

COPING WITH INTIMIDATION

After their behavior has attracted the attention of the criminal justice system, some stalkers will use a variety of tactics to intimidate the victim. The stalker's motivation may be to frighten the victim into dropping charges, or simply to maintain some type of contact with the victim, no matter how aversive or unpleasant that contact might be. Victims are left feeling scared and as though they have no control over their circumstances. Table 4.6 lists common intimidation tactics used by stalkers.

Upon hearing that the victim is obtaining a protective order, some stalkers will file a "counter" protective order. This typically involves the stalker misinforming local law enforcement that he is being "stalked" or otherwise harassed by the victim. In doing so, he seeks to preempt the victim's claims of stalking by making his own. In some instances, the stalker may even rush to authorities in order to file for the protective order before the victim does. This serves to obfuscate the stalker's behavior, and causes law enforcement to view the situation as relationship dysfunction, rather than a course of harassing pursuit by the stalker. Further, it may provide stalkers with legal "evidence" to continue the obfuscation in court. For some stalkers, it serves to reinforce delusional beliefs that the victim desires a relationship. Stalkers may go as far as fabricating evidence that the victim has initiated contact with him. Such false claims of victimization include sending e-mails or letters to themselves and claiming that they were sent by the victim.

Table 4.6. Stalker's Intimidation Tactics

- Filing a "counter" protective order
- Approaching police before the victim
- Arriving first at the victim's usual destinations
- Threats to harm unless charges are dropped
- Threats during courtroom appearances

After a counterprotective order is filed, the stalker may then use the tactic of being the first party to engage police after he breaks a protective order. In this way, the stalker can continue to intimidate the victim, as well as initiate contact without fear of reprisal. In an attempt to exert control over multiple aspects of the victim's life, the stalker may attempt to arrive at some of the victim's favorite or preferred locations first, claiming that it was not his "fault" that the victim happened to show up.

Threats by the stalker to harm the victim if charges are pressed are usually made by rejected type stalkers with a history of domestic violence. Often, this results in charges being dropped due to the victim being too fearful to show up in court (Bennett, Goodman, & Dutton, 1999). Threats and intimidation can continue even into the courtroom itself. During courtroom appearances, stalker and victim are often required to park in the same lot, navigate the same passageways, and sit in the same hall while waiting for their case to be called. This affords the stalker plenty of opportunity to intimidate and threaten. An extreme example observed by an author (JK), was a rejected type stalker who filled the courtroom with members of his inner city gang. This created a frightening atmosphere and an unspoken threat of revenge.

Coping with such intimidation tactics is often extremely difficult for the victim to do alone. This is why the multiagency approach described above is the best approach. When the antistalking team is apprised of the situation in advance, steps may be taken to reduce the impact of the stalker's intimidation. For example, victim advocates can be used to inform prosecutors and judges about the serious nature of the stalking and the pattern of intimidation (Shepard & Pence, 1999).

Advocates can play a role in educating the judge about stalking behaviors to decrease the risk that they will be misperceived as "lovers' spats," or mere relationship dysfunction. In most cases, judges will be in a position to secure the safety of the victim in and around the courtroom (Ptacek, 1999). The antistalking team can facilitate communication with local law enforcement, clarifying any misperceptions caused by the stalker's counterprotective orders. In regions that lack advocates or antistalking services, it is important for the victim to mobilize resources and promote collaboration between professionals.

MENTAL HEALTH TREATMENT OF THE STALKER

Although stalking is a criminal behavior, mental illness often plays a role. It follows that failure to treat mentally ill stalkers may result in continued risk to the victim. For example, a stalker with erotomanic delusions who is confined without treatment will likely emerge from confinement with no significant reduction in risk. To date, there are no reliable outcome data on the treatment of stalkers, and mental health professionals must rely on empirically derived clinical data.

It is recommended that therapists involved in treating stalkers should have experience and/or receive some type of specialized training. Ideally, the therapist should have experience practicing in a forensic setting. At the very least, non–forensically trained therapists should receive training on the psychology of the stalker. One group has found it helpful to form a specialized "Stalkers' Clinic" that provides not only a center of clinical expertise, but also support and education for clinicians and the criminal justice system (Warren, MacKenzie, Mullen, & Ogloff, 2005).

Most stalkers have encountered a substantial amount of adverse life consequences as a result of their stalking behavior. Mullen et al. (2000) note that in order to obtain a stalker's investment in treatment, the distress experienced by the stalker "can potentially be used as a lever to alter the behavior and release the victims from continuing distress and disruption" (p. 279).

Although some stalkers may be willing to voluntarily engage in treatment, the majority will require some form of court mandate ordering them to comply with treatment. Therapists who are willing to treat stalkers must never collude with the stalker. However, it is helpful to view minor relapses of stalking behavior in the same way that therapists view substance use relapse. Specifically, that they are likely to occur, and should not result in automatic cessation of treatment. Rather, it is advisable to clearly communicate to the stalker that being in therapy will not provide any type of legal immunity from the consequences of reoffending.

Therapists working with stalkers should be familiar with their state's duty-to-protect statutes as well as relevant case law related to stalking, so that legal obligations can be discussed with the stalker from the outset of treatment. Local laws may be obtained by contacting a local prosecutor's office, and state statutes can usually be found on the Internet.

Prior to beginning treatment with the stalker, a therapist should perform a thorough assessment. The assessment should include review of past risk assessments, mental health records, criminal records, witness statements, and past management strategies. It is also helpful to gather collateral information from the stalker's family and friends, although often this is not possible due to the stalker's lack of a social support network. A thorough psychiatric evaluation should determine whether there are any current mental disorders that require treatment. The presence of substance abuse and personality disorders should also be identified and addressed. When an individual other than the therapist has been assigned the task of risk assessment, it is important that the therapist have access to the risk assessment information or reports. This is of particular importance to the treating therapist who needs to have a thorough understanding of the stalker's dynamic risk factors so that they can be implemented into a treatment and risk reduction plan. The notion of incorporating into treatment periodic risk assessments by an objective evaluator is discussed below. Further review related to the role of mental health professionals working with victims, stalkers, and risk assessment teams can be found in chapter 5.

Most stalkers will be difficult to engage in treatment, and arrive at the therapist's office only because they have been compelled by a court order. Initially, the therapist is likely to encounter the stalker's striking lack of insight into the nature and consequences of his behavior. The stalker may initially seek validation for his actions, while demonstrating little concern over ending his obsessions. Well-entrenched defenses of denial, rationalization, and minimization will usually become apparent. Nevertheless, as Mullen et al. (2000) note, "defining them as unchangeable makes them unchangeable" (p. 288). Table 4.7 gives a list of approaches that are helpful to consider when doing psychotherapy with a stalker.

From the outset, it is critical to establish rapport with the stalker by adopting a nonjudgmental approach. Inquiring about the stalker's motivations without judgment will elicit more helpful information than forcing the stalker to justify his actions. Once rapport has been established, the therapist can begin to reframe the stalker's motivations by shifting the focus from the unknowable feelings of the victim to the stalker's feelings for the victim. This begins to focus the stalker on his own feelings and judgments. His motivations are reframed as his own "hopes and desires." At the same time, the therapist should seek to clarify the extent of the stalker's loneliness and lack of relationships. This may allow the stalker to see his pursuit as a product of his situation and not the imagined feelings of the victim.

Continuing in an atmosphere of rapport building, the therapist may next help the stalker begin to identify the costs of his stalking behaviors. Here, all of the adverse consequences of the stalking behavior may be pointed out in an empathic manner. For example, legal consequences, emotional distress, and time and energy spent can all be discussed from a standpoint of personal loss. From the stalker's own losses, a transition can be made to the distress and losses of the victim. This is accomplished by reframing the actions of the stalker as disturbing and distressing to the victim. Techniques such as role-playing and encouraging empathy for the victim are useful.

Some therapists may wish to use videotaped interviews of stalking victims describing how the unwanted pursuit affected their lives. The therapist can then

Table 4.7. Helpful Psychotherapy Approaches

- Establish rapport.
- Reframe motivations.
- Identify costs and adverse consequences.
- Reframe actions.
- Allow stalker to abandon pursuit with "dignity."
- Develop social skills.

begin to challenge the stalker's distorted beliefs about how his behavior has affected the victim. All of these techniques are aimed at the goal of improving the accuracy of the stalker's processing of social information. Programs that have been successful in developing victim empathy in sex offenders may also be adapted for use with stalkers (Mullen, Pathé, & Purcell, 2001).

The next phase of therapy involves assisting the stalker to abandon his pursuit while affording him some dignity in the process. Avoiding humiliation will reduce the likelihood that the stalker will become enraged as a result of narcissistic injury. The therapist may wish to reframe the stalker's behavior as "understandable," given his particular vulnerabilities, but counterproductive and self-defeating. The stalker can then be encouraged to give up the behavior as an act of "generosity" and self-preservation.

After the stalker has made sufficient progress in psychotherapy, it is helpful to begin reconnecting the stalker to healthy, socially acceptable relationships. Some role-playing and constructive feedback may be required to teach and develop needed social skills. Because stalkers often have impoverished social networks, it is important to encourage their involvement in prosocial activities such as sports clubs or group activities.

By gradually increasing the level of socially acceptable pursuits, the stalker may overcome his social disabilities and acquire a satisfactory social network. In addition, stalking behavior usually consumes such a significant amount of time that stalkers are frequently under- or unemployed. A referral to a vocational rehabilitation program may be necessary to help integrate the stalker into the workforce.

Psychotropic medications should be used to treat specific mental disorders that are in need of psychopharmacologic intervention. Delusional disorders and other psychotic mental illnesses, for example, will require treatment with antipsychotic medications. For stalkers with psychotic mental illnesses who resist involvement in treatment, court-ordered involuntary treatment may be necessary.

When approaching the pharmacologic treatment of the stalker, it is prudent to conceptualize the stalking behavior and the mental disorder as overlapping, but distinct states (Badcock, 2002). The purpose of such a stance is to safeguard against the potentially false assumption that the stalking behavior is purely a function of the underlying mental disorder. Even in cases of intimacy-seeking and resentful stalkers, in which erotomanic or persecutory delusions heavily influence the stalker, behavioral reinforcers of the stalking may generate their own forces which should not be dismissed. Thus it is desirable to combine psychotherapy with well-targeted pharmacologic treatment if at all possible.

It is imperative that stalkers with underlying psychotic illnesses be treated with antipsychotic medications prior to attempting any in-depth psychotherapy. When a stalker with a psychotic illness must be treated with antipsychotic treatment, supportive psychotherapy and psychoeducational techniques such as those described above may be the most appropriate psychotherapeutic interventions. Insight-oriented psychotherapies may be contraindicated. In their study of over 1,000 stalkers, Mohandie and colleagues (2006) found that one in seven were psychotic at the time of the stalking offense. In terms of the Mullen et al. (2000) typology, intimacy-seeking, resentful, and incompetent type stalkers will have comparatively greater amounts of psychotic illness than other stalker types. For stalkers who suffer from chronic psychotic disorders, atypical antipsychotics are the medication of choice. The atypical antipsychotics, clozapine in particular, are thought to have specific antiaggressive effects (Glazer & Dickson, 1998). They may be particularly useful for individuals who have demonstrated persistent aggression and/or hostility (Buckley, Noffsinger, Smith, Hrouda, & Knoll, 2003). In particular, stalkers suffering from a chronic psychotic disorder who have failed adequate trials of other atypicals should be considered for treatment with clozapine. Clozapine has also been associated with reduced arrest rates in psychotic patients with past criminal histories (Frankle et al., 2001).

It is recommended that antipsychotic medication for the psychotic stalker take the form of monotherapy at first. If aggression persists despite adequate antipsychotic pharmacotherapy, the option of adjunctive medications may be considered. Adjunctive medication options include addition of a second atypical antipsychotic such as risperidone or mood stabilizers such as valproic acid or lithium. Carbamazepine may be considered but should not be used in combination with clozapine due to the increased risk of agranulocytosis.

Because many stalkers with psychotic disorders have limited insight leading to medication noncompliance, their long-term management may require the use of long-acting depot antipsychotics. Clinicians now have a long-acting atypical antipsychotic, risperidone, to consider in addition to typical depot antipsychotics. If the stalker fails to appear for an injection at the clinic, it should serve as a warning sign that stimulates notification of members of the risk management team.

Depressive disorders should not be overlooked. Selective serotonin reuptake inhibiters (SSRIs) are the agents of first choice, due to their favorable side effect profile, and especially when there are concerns about comorbid anxiety, obsessions, or sexual compulsivity. In addition, clinicians should remain vigilant around the issue of the stalker's suicide risk, and be knowledgeable about how to conduct a thorough suicide risk assessment (APA, 2003). Suicidal ideation or suicidal behaviors have been found to occur in approximately 25% of stalkers (Mohandie et al., 2006). Predatory type stalkers with paraphilias may require testosterone-lowering agents such as medroxyprogesterone acetate to help reduce deviant sexual drive and impulses (APA Task Force on Sexually Dangerous Offenders, 1999). Substance use disorders must be addressed before meaningful treatment can begin. It is often necessary to make regular urine drug screens and chemical addiction treatment a court-ordered condition of probation or parole.

As noted above, clinicians who elect to treat stalkers should be aware of what their individual jurisdiction's legal regulations are regarding stalking laws, as well as laws pertaining to the duty to protect third parties. Clinicians must be prepared for the reality that there will likely need to be an ongoing awareness of potential risk to victims. Many jurisdictions have case law requiring the clinician to take reasonable steps to protect the intended victim(s) of their patient. Some jurisdictions will have so-called *"Tarasoff*-limiting" statutes that articulate specific steps clinicians must carry out in order to discharge their duty. Other jurisdictions have remained silent on the issue; however, an argument could easily be made that the standard of care requires clinicians to take reasonable steps to protect third parties, given an explicit threat of violence against an identifiable target. Reasonable steps may include hospitalization or informing the potential victim, police, and stalking risk management team. It is possible, given the right clinical circumstances, that the clinician may protect third parties by undertaking a thoughtful and reasonable plan of outpatient treatment that includes steps designed to mitigate dynamic risk factors. In many cases involving danger to third parties, it is highly advisable to seek consultation from a colleague, both from an objectivity and liability reduction perspective (Buckley et al., 2003).

Finally, it is highly desirable for the stalker to undergo periodic risk assessments by a qualified forensic psychiatrist, when available. It is important that the forensic psychiatrist is not involved in the stalker's treatment so as to preserve the objectivity of the assessment. The periodic nature of the assessments is important due to the fact that the stalker's "dynamic" risk factors may change over time, and thus warrant a change of risk management strategies (Meloy, 1997). The details of risk assessment in stalking cases have been described in chapter 3. The results of the periodic assessments can be used to identify any weaknesses in the current risk management strategy, as well as to inform the therapist and stalking risk management team about any new concerns.

STALKING RISK MANAGEMENT: CASE EXAMPLE AND DISCUSSION

The following case example illustrates the stalking of a mental health professional by a patient, and a subsequent successful risk management approach.

CASE EXAMPLE 4.1: MS. KAYE

Ms. Kaye was a 28-year-old woman who began seeing a therapist for anxiety and depression stemming from childhood sexual abuse. Ms. Kaye had a history of suicide attempts, as well as self-mutilation to relieve her inner turmoil. Ms. Kaye quickly became enamored of her therapist, and felt that her therapy session was the only place she felt at ease. After several months of therapy, Ms. Kaye noticed a growing desire to be closer to her therapist. She began having fantasies that she and her therapist could become close friends, go to social functions together, and share each other's private concerns.

Ms. Kaye brought several gifts to her therapist to show her appreciation and desire to become more than "just a patient." Her therapist accepted the gifts; however, Ms. Kaye perceived that her therapist was not genuinely pleased by the gifts. Therefore, Ms. Kaye resolved to begin studying her therapist's likes and dislikes in order to get her a gift that better suited the therapist's personal tastes. Ms. Kaye used her therapy sessions to make mental notes of her therapist's office décor, dress style, and any comments she made that reflected her personal interests. Ms. Kaye diligently recorded all of her findings in a journal.

After a period of intense deliberation, Ms. Kaye purchased a small but expensive statue for her therapist. Ms. Kaye was troubled when her therapist accepted the statue with a look of hesitation. Ms. Kaye was further disturbed when her therapist indicated that she should not give her any more gifts. After leaving the session, Ms. Kaye became consumed with her therapist's reaction to her gift. She finally decided that she needed to see the inside of her therapist's house so she could satisfy herself that the statue was there, as well as get a better sense of her therapist's personal tastes.

Ms. Kaye went to her therapist's home during the daytime when the therapist was at work. She entered the house through an unlocked back door and proceeded to take a mental account of the interior décor. When she was unable to locate the statue, she decided to take a few small items that would help her feel "closer" to the therapist. The therapist's daughter entered the home and surprised Ms. Kaye, who immediately fled the scene. After involving the police, the therapist terminated care with Ms. Kaye and filed a restraining order against her.

Several months later, Ms. Kaye was distraught and overwhelmed by her need to see her therapist again. She again decided to enter her therapist's home, but this time she was met by the therapist's boyfriend who was now staying at the house. A physical altercation ensued during which Ms. Kaye stabbed the boyfriend with a knife she had been carrying. The boyfriend was ultimately able to subdue her and call the police. The therapist made it a priority to give her input at all the relevant sentencing and parole board hearings. After collecting evidence and discussing the matter with a victim advocate, she informed the court about all the details of her stalking victimization and requested that the judge require Ms. Kaye to submit to a forensic risk evaluation.

The therapist's attorney helped to coordinate a risk management team that included law enforcement, mental health, and a victim advocate. A risk management plan was crafted that required Ms. Kaye to have periodic risk assessments. After several parole board hearings, Ms. Kaye decided to move out of state. The risk management team made sure to transfer all of her relevant case information and court-mandated requirements with her to her new location.

This case example demonstrates the importance of the victim taking an active role in risk management. The therapist's efforts to establish a rapport with the court and law enforcement helped to ensure that her concerns would be taken seriously. In addition, coordinating the forensic risk assessment and risk management plan with a multidisciplinary team reduced the possibility that vital information would be omitted.

The forensic psychiatrist identified Ms. Kaye as an intimacy-seeking type of stalker. However, it was noted that due to the unique nature of the therapeutic relationship, Ms. Kaye also had some characteristics in common with the rejected type of stalker. When this was considered alongside her assaultive behavior and the fact that she had broken into the therapist's home twice, Ms. Kaye's risk of violence was estimated as high. The parole board strongly considered this finding in its decision to grant Ms. Kaye's parole as long as she agreed to move out of state.

It could be argued that the therapist might have intervened at an earlier stage by setting clear boundaries when the initial gifts were given. Health-care professionals who are uncertain about boundary violations in particular cases may wish to seek consultation from a colleague.

CONCLUSION

Stalking risk management is best approached with a multiagency stalking management team. The team should be comprised of professionals from different disciplines who regularly communicate about potential risk issues. Any risk management approach must carefully consider the intervention dilemma and individual-specific nuances of the case. Victims should play an active role in assuring their own safety. When mental illness plays a role in stalking behavior, risk management is best accomplished by monitoring the treatment of the stalker over time. Risk management plans that fail to consider psychiatric treatment of a mentally ill stalker will fail to address a major source of risk.

REFERENCES

Abrams, K., & Robinson, G. (1998). Stalking part II: Victim's problem's with the legal system and therapeutic considerations. *Canadian Journal of Psychiatry*, *43*, 477–481.

American Bar Association Commission on Domestic Violence. (1999). *A guide for employers: Domestic violence in the workplace.* Washington, DC: Author.

American Psychiatric Association. (2003). *Practice guideline for the assessment and treatment of patients with suicidal behaviors.* Washington, DC: Author.

American Psychiatric Association Task Force on Sexually Dangerous Offenders. (1999). *Dangerous sex offenders.* Washington, DC: Author.

Archives of the Mayor's Press. (1999, July 26). *Mayor Giuliani builds on successful domestic violence campaign with three innovative new programs.* Retrieved May 14, 2006, from http://www.nyc.gov/html/om/html/99a/pr295-99.html

Badcock, R. (2002). Psychopathology and treatment of stalking. In J. Boon & L. Sheridan (Eds.), *Stalking and psychosexual obsession: Psychological perspectives for prevention, policing and treatment* (pp. 125–163). Chichester, UK: Wiley.

Bennett, L., Goodman, L., & Dutton, M. (1999). Systemic obstacles to the criminal prosecution of a battering partner: A victim perspective. *Journal of Interpersonal Violence, 14*(7), 761–772.

Buckley, P., Noffsinger, S., Smith, D., Hrouda, D., & Knoll, J. (2003). Treatment of the psychotic patient who is violent. *Psychiatric Clinics of North America, 26,* 231–272.

De Becker, G. (1997). *The gift of fear: Survival signals that protect us from violence.* New York: Dell.

Frankle, W. G., Shera, D., Berger-Hershkowitz, H., Evins, A. E., Connoly, C., Goff, D. C., & Henderson, D. C. (2001). Clozapine-associated reduction in arrest rates of psychotic patients with criminal histories. *The American Journal of Psychiatry,158,* 270–274.

Galeazzi, G. M., Elkins, K., & Curci, P. (2005). The stalking of mental health professionals by patients. *Psychiatric Services, 56*(2), 137–138.

Gill, R., & Brockman, J. (1996). A review of section 264 (criminal harassment) of the criminal code of Canada (Working Document WD 1996–7e). Ottawa, Canada: Research, Statistics, and Evaluation Directorate, Department of Justice.

Glazer, W., & Dickson, R. (1998). Clozapine reduces violence and persistent aggression in patients with schizophrenia. *Journal of Clinical Psychiatry 59,* 8–14.

Häkkänen, H., Hagelstam, C., & Santtila, P. (2003). Stalking actions, prior offender-victim relationships and issuing of restraining orders in a Finnish sample of stalkers. *Legal and Criminological Psychology, 8,* 189–206.

Harrell, A., & Smith, B. E. (1996). Effects of restraining orders on domestic violence victims. In E. S. Buzawa & C. G. Buzawa (Eds.), *Do arrest and restraining orders work?* (pp. 214–242). Thousand Oaks, CA: Sage.

Keilitz, S. L., Davis, C., Efkeman, H. S., Flango, C., & Hannaford, P. L. (1997). Civil protection orders: Victims' views on effectiveness. *National Institute of Justice Journal, 233.*

Klein, A. R. (1996). Re-abuse in a population of court-restrained male batterers. In E. S. Buzawa & C. G. Buzawa (Eds.), *Do arrest and restraining orders work?* (pp. 214–242). Thousand Oaks, CA: Sage.

Lion, J., & Herschler, J. (1998). The stalking of clinicians by their patients. In J. R. Meloy (Ed.), *The psychology of stalking: Clinical and forensic perspectives* (pp. 165–175). San Diego: Academic Press.

Maxey, W. (2002). The San Diego Stalking Strike Force: A multi-disciplinary approach to assessing and managing stalking and threat cases. *Journal of Threat Assessment, 2*(1), 43–53.

McFarlane, J., Malecha, A., Gist, J., Watson, M., Batten, E., Hall, I., & Smith, S. (2004). Protection orders and intimate partner violence: An 18-month study of 150 Black, Hispanic, and White women. *American Journal of Public Health, 94*(4), 613–618.

Meloy, J. R. (1997). The clinical risk management of stalking: "Someone is watching over me. . . ." *The American Journal of Psychotherapy, 51*(2), 174–184.

Meloy, J. R. (2002). Commentary: Stalking, threatening, and harassing behavior by patients—The risk-management response. *Journal of the American Academy of Psychiatry Law, 30,* 230–231.

Mohandie, K., Meloy, J. R., McGowan, M. G., & Williams, J. (2006). The RECON typology of stalking: Reliability and validity based upon a large sample of North American stalkers. *Journal of Forensic Sciences, 51,* 147–155.

Mullen, P. E., Pathé, M., & Purcell, R. (2000). *Stalkers and their victims.* Cambridge: Cambridge University Press.

Mullen, P. E., Pathé, M., & Purcell, R. (2001). The management of stalkers. *Advances in Psychiatric Treatment, 7,* 335–342.

Mustaine, E .E., & Tewksbury, R. (1999). A routine activities theory explanation for women's stalking victimization. *Violence Against Women, 5,* 43–62.

Orion, D. (1997). *I know you really love me: A psychiatrist's journal of erotomania, stalking, and obsessive love.* New York: Macmillan.

Ptacek, J. (1999). *Battered women in the courtroom: The power of judicial responses.* Boston: Northeastern University Press.

Purcell, R., Powell, M., & Mullen, P. (2005). Clients who stalk psychologists: Prevalence, methods, and motives. *Professional Psychology: Research and Practice, 36*(5), 537–543.

Ramsey, B. (2000). *Stop the stalker: A guide for targets.* Morrow, GA: Securus House.

Roberts, A., & Kurst-Swanger, K. (2002). Court responses to battered women and their children. In A. Roberts (Ed.), *Handbook of domestic violence intervention strategies* (pp. 127–146). New York: Oxford University Press.

Sandberg, D., McNiel, D., & Binder, R. (2002). Stalking, threatening, and harassing behavior by psychiatric patients toward clinicians. *Journal of the American Academy of Psychiatry and Law, 30,* 221–229.

Shepard, M., & Pence, E. (Eds.). (1999). *Coordinating community responses to domestic violence: Lessons from Duluth and beyond.* Thousand Oaks: Sage.

Shrapnel, R. (1997). *Personal protection at home and abroad.* Singapore: Times Books International.

Tsushima, W., & Wong, R. (2003). Stalking of doctors by patients: A case study of love obsessional stalking. *Journal of Threat Assessment, 2*(4), 35–47.

University of Iowa Injury Prevention Research Center. (2001, February). *Workplace violence: A report to the nation* (p. 12). Iowa City, IA: Author.

Warren, L. J., MacKenzie, R. N., Mullen, P. E., & Ogloff, J. R. P. (2005). The problem behavior model: The development of a stalkers clinic and a threateners clinic. *Behavioral Sciences and the Law, 23,* 387–397.

White, S. G., & Cawood, J. S. (1998). Threat management of stalking cases. In J .R. Meloy (Ed.), *The psychology of stalking: Clinical and forensic perspectives* (pp. 295–314). San Diego: Academic Press.

5 Stalking: Perspectives on Victims and Management

Alan W. Newman
Kenneth L. Appelbaum

The potential of being stalked is a frightening prospect, in part because of the widespread media attention to the phenomenon, principally highlighting cases in which significant harm toward the victim has occurred. Victims may have little knowledge of how to manage a stalking situation. Civil and criminal remedies may provide some relief, but ultimately victims must manage their own safety in a way that they see as best for their particular situation. In assisting and assessing victims, the issue of false victimization must also be considered. This chapter will explore issues related to the effects of being stalked and methods of management for victims.

INTRODUCTION

Although much of the attention to stalking seen in the legal, clinical, and research literature has been related to stalkers and the act of stalking, there has also been a burgeoning interest in examining stalking victims. This allows for a greater opportunity to understand stalking behaviors, and their effects on others, from a perspective vastly different from that of the perpetrator. Moreover, it has become increasingly recognized that stalking creates very negative psychological (and at times physical) harm to victims. Understanding the phenomenology of victimization and victimology can help clinicians work from a foundation when they are faced with treating a person who may be a victim of stalking. Furthermore, although risk assessment and risk management of stalkers are discussed elsewhere in this book (see chapters 3 and 4), it is imperative that there be a mechanism to manage risk from the perspective of the victim. Stalking represents a dyadic tension, and approaches to mitigating risk must be done with recognition of the impact of stalking on the victim.

As we discussed in our GAP Committee on Psychiatry and the Law, important questions typically posed by a stalking victim include queries into whether the stalking will cease and whether the victim will be harmed. More nuanced aspects of victim assessment and management include an examination of day-to-day approaches in dealing with stalking behavior. Clinicians and law enforcement may come and go, but a victim may receive hundreds of phone calls or other communications daily, and each intrusion raises more questions and often more distress as to how a particular situation should be managed. A review of victimization, victimology, psychiatric sequelae of being stalked, and approaches to treatment of victims is included here to help the reader gain a foundation related to understanding and managing stalking victims.

STALKING VICTIMIZATION AND VICTIMOLOGY

The term used to describe the study of a victim or victims is *victimology* (Turvey, 1999). Attention to the victim has been a method increasingly used by the criminal justice system to better understand and potentially solve crimes, particularly when an attacker is unknown (Douglas, Burgess, Burgess, & Ressler, 1992).

Much has been written about the typology of individual stalkers, but much less effort has been made to classify the victims of stalkers. Mullen, Pathé, and Purcell (2001) have developed a schema of classifying victims according to the examination of two components: the relationship, if any, between victim and stalker and the setting or context of the stalking. Mullen, Pathé, and Purcell (2000) classify victims into seven types: ex-intimates, casual acquaintances, professional contacts, workplace contacts, strangers, the famous, and unusual victims.

Ex-Intimates

As the majority of stalking victims are women pursued by a man with whom she had a former intimate relationship, ex-intimates comprise the largest category of stalking victims (Pathé & Mullen, 2002). This relationship can range from a brief dating situation to a former long-term/spousal relationship. Mullen et al. (2000) notes that in addition to the wide range of harassment methods that can be used on these victims, these relationships are further complicated by the fact that perpetrator and victim may share children or have property division issues that may force the victim to interact with the stalker in ways not encountered by other victims. In Hall's (1998) study of 120 stalking victims, 57% of victims reported a former relationship with their stalkers. Victims of this type of stalking may also face less support from friends, family, or the legal system than do other victims. In Fremouw, Westrup, and Pennypacker's (1997) survey of 593 university undergraduates, 80% of the students who reported being stalked knew their stalker, and 43% of the females reporting stalking (and 24% of the male respondents) had seriously dated their stalker.

Casual Acquaintances

Another type of stalking victim identified by Mullen et al. (2000) is the victim stalked by a casual acquaintance or friend. This type of victim may be pursued by a variety of stalker types (see chapter 2 for a review of stalker typologies). Resentful stalkers may target a neighbor with whom they have a dispute; rejected stalkers may target a former friend or casual acquaintance after the dissolution of their relationship. Intimacy-seeking or incompetent stalkers may pursue someone with whom they have had only a casual acquaintance. In Hall's (1998) study of 120 stalking victims, 35% of victims reported that they were acquainted with their stalkers, although Hall did not further divide that into the nature of the relationship (i.e., friends, neighbors, or workplace contacts).

Professional Contacts

A stalking victim may be someone whose relationship with the stalker arises in the context of a professional relationship. Teachers and clinicians are at risk of being stalked by students, clients, or patients. According to Mullen et al. (2000), intimacy seekers or incompetent stalkers may pursue a mental health or primary care provider, whereas resentful stalkers may pursue a clinician with whom they are angry regarding some aspect of their relationship or treatment.

Workplace Contacts

Stalkers may also target victims in their immediate workplace environment. A wide range of stalker types may target these victims. In addition to intimacy-seeking or incompetent stalkers, whose relationship with their victims arises in the context of the workplace, a stalker may be motivated by resentment. This resentment may be directed at a real or perceived behavior by the victim or may be directed toward the workplace organization itself (i.e., the victim may represent an aspect of the company with which the stalker has a grievance). In addition, stalking by an ex-intimate may involve harassment at the victim's workplace regardless of whether the stalker is a coworker of the victim (Pathé & Mullen, 2002).

Stranger Victims

Mullen et al. (2000) characterize stranger victims as those who are unaware of any prior contact with the stalker. In Hall's (1998) survey, 6% of victims were certain that their stalker was someone whom they did not know, whereas 2% did not know the identity of their stalkers and could therefore not postulate the nature of the relationship. Mullen et al. (2000) suppose that these victims are usually pursued by intimacy-seeking or incompetent stalkers, but may also be targeted by sexually predatory stalkers. Intimacy-seeking stalkers may select their victims on the basis of the person's elevated social status or prominence, whereas the victim of the incompetent stalker may have been selected due to their physical appearance or simply because they had the misfortune to encounter the potential stalker (Mullen et al., 2000). Unless the stalker is discovered, the recipient of the stalking behavior may be unaware that he or she is being pursued.

Sexually predatory stalkers, in addition to pursuing victims who are aware of them, may also target a stranger. Mullen et al. (2000) postulates that sexual predators who stalk strangers may engage in fewer pursuit behaviors prior to an attack compared with predatory stalkers who pursue victims who are known to them. Indeed, a stranger pursued by a sexually predatory stalker may be unaware that they are at risk and therefore are unaware that they should take precautions until they have been the victim of an assault or attempted assault.

Mullen et al. (2000) note that stranger victims may also be targeted by resentful stalkers. In this situation, some victims may be selected due to a specific grievance perceived by the stalker, whereas others may simply be selected because the stalker identifies them as a member of a group disliked by the stalker.

Famous Victims

Another victim classification type recognized by Mullen et al. (2000) are those victims selected because they are famous. Due to the attention such cases have received from the media, these victims have perhaps been better studied than other types of victims (Dietz, Matthews, Duyne, et al., 1991; Dietz, Matthews, Martel, et al., 1991). Mullen et al. (2000) note that although these victims have their celebrity status in common, a number of stalker typologies are recognized in these cases, including socially incompetent stalkers, resentful stalkers, and stalkers with erotomanias and morbid infatuations. This subject is discussed further in chapter 10, Celebrity and Presidential Targets.

Unusual Victims

Finally, Mullen et al. (2000) recognize that some victims may be unusual and not clearly fit the typical profile of victims listed above. Examples include former stalkers themselves who find themselves the object of an obsessive pursuit by their former victims. Although Mullen et al. (2000) includes notorious prisoners as unusual victims, the media attention and subsequent celebrity status

Table 5.1. Common Links Between Stalker Typologies and Victim Typologies

			Stalker Type			
Victim Type*	Rejected	Resentful	Predatory	Intimacy Seeking	Incompetent Suitors	Erotomania/ Infatuations
Ex-intimates	x					
Casual acquaintances	x	x		x	x	
Professional contacts		x		x	x	
Workplace contacts		x		x	x	
Strangers		x	x	x	x	
Famous		x			x	x

*Unusual victim types not included in this table.
Source: Mullen et al., 2000; Pathé & Mullen, 2002.

accorded to notorious criminals may simply make them a variant of other famous victims.

Table 5.1 summarizes the points above, illustrating the way in which Mullen et al.'s (2000) typology of stalkers overlaps with the types of victims selected by the stalker. *Ex-intimates* are often stalked by *rejected* stalkers. Victims who are *casual acquaintances* with the stalker are commonly stalked by the *rejected, resentful, intimacy seeking,* and *incompetent suitors* subtypes. Victims stalked by those with whom they have *professional* or *workplace contacts* are commonly stalked by perpetrators who fit the *resentful, intimacy seeking,* or *incompetent suitors* subtypes. Victims who are *strangers* to their stalker may be pursued by stalkers fitting a number of subtypes, including *resentful, predatory, intimacy seeking,* and *incompetent suitors. Famous* victims may be pursued by stalkers with *erotomania,* as well as those fitting the typologies *resentful* and *incompetent suitors.*

INCIDENCE, PREVALENCE, AND DEMOGRAPHICS

The best-studied aspect of stalking research involves examinations of the most common characteristics of victims. Early reports on the effects of stalking on victims were based on limited data, such as victim impact reports taken by the police or depositions of victims during legal actions against stalkers (Mullen & Pathé, 1994). Although early reports like these were useful in helping to identify the nature of the problem, studies based on legal records suffer a referral bias toward more serious offenses as they identified only the cases that led to legal action. A detailed review of the epidemiology of stalking can be found in chapter 1. Below is an overview of this data, as it pertains to victims.

Gender of Stalking Victims

The most comprehensive examination of stalking victims comes from the report *Stalking in America* by Tjaden and Thoennes (1998), based on data from the larger National Violence Against Women survey. In this study, 8% of women and 2% of men in the study had been stalked at some time. Furthermore, 78% of the victims were women, the majority of whom were between the ages of 18 and 29. Alternately, in surveys by Hall (1998) and Pathé and Mullen (1997), 83% of stalking victims were women.

A high prevalence of stalking behaviors experienced by university under-graduates has also been reported (Fremouw et al., 1997). This was discussed in chapter 1. Briefly, Fremouw et al. found that the rate of reported stalking victimization among females was nearly twice that of males in this study. Westrup and Fremouw (1998) studied the effect of stalking on (female) undergraduates without requiring the presence of a "credible threat" but nonetheless distinguishing "stalking" from mere "harassment" (see detailed discussion below). This study surveyed 232 women, categorizing 36 (6.4%) as stalked and an additional 43 (5.4%) as being harassed.

Racial and Ethnic Issues in Stalking Victims

It is unclear what role race plays in stalking victims. In the National Violence Against Women study, there was no significant difference in the lifetime prevalence of stalking between White and minority women (Tjaden & Thoennes, 1998). However, when specific racial or ethnic groupings were compared, there was a statistically significantly higher prevalence of being a stalking victim among American Indian/Alaska Native women. The meaning of this finding was not clear from this study due to the relatively small number of women in this ethnic group in the sample. The study also did not look at whether the increased prevalence could be explained by nonracial demographic or other factors. Because the study looked only at Native Americans and Alaska Natives as a single group, any tribal differences in the prevalence of stalking were not established.

Child Victims of Stalking

Children, too, can be stalking victims; their stalkers can be other children, adolescents, or adults (McCann, 2000). This subject is covered in detail in chapter 8.

Same-Gender Stalking

The issue of victims being stalked by members of the same gender has only recently been studied (Pathé, Mullen, & Purcell, 2000). Many early case reports of this phenomenon used the term *homoerotomania* to describe the behavior. This term, although descriptive in some cases, can be deceptive, as not all such cases could be accurately described as erotomanic attachments (see chapter 2 for further explanation of erotomania). Further, the term suggests a same-gender sexual preference, despite the fact that the victim, perpetrator, or both may be heterosexual.

Many early surveys of stalking noted the presence of same-gender stalking with little exploration of the prior relationship between victims and their same-gender stalkers (Tjaden & Thoennes, 1998). In Tjaden and Thoennes' landmark survey, of the 2% of male respondents who reported a past history of stalking, 60% were stalked by other men, a rate somewhat higher than the 24–44% noted in other surveys (Hall, 1998; Pathé & Mullen, 1997). The rates of same-gender stalking of female victims have also been different based on the survey. Tjaden and Thoennes (1998) noted that of the 8% of women who reported past stalking, only in 6% of the cases was the perpetrator of the same gender. In contrast, Pathé and Mullen (1997) noted that 12% of the 83 female subjects had been stalked by a woman.

A later study by Pathé and colleagues (2000) attempted to explore the demographics, behaviors, and relationships involved in cases of same-gender stalking. In this study of 163 stalkers, 18% targeted victims of the same gender. In the cases of same-gender stalking, the victim was more likely to be a work colleague and less likely to be an ex-intimate of their stalker when compared with victims stalked by those of the opposite sex. Significantly, in 28% of the cases, the victim was either the treating doctor or a teacher of the victim.

Immigrant Victims of Stalking

A new area of study concerns the unique problems experienced by immigrants who are victims of stalking. An immigrant, particularly one who resides in their host country illegally, may be less likely to report stalking due to a number of reasons, including language barriers, fear of deportation, and limited knowledge of resources available to victims ("Immigrant Stalking Victims Face Complex Challenges," 2003). A female victim may originate from a culture that does not encourage her to report victimization out of concern for her family's reputation. She may also be much less aware that the stalking behaviors are illegal and unacceptable in the new country. Further, an immigrant victim may be more sensitive to the consequences of quitting a job or school than a native citizen.

In 1994, the *Violence Against Women Act* was passed, allowing (among other provisions) a battered noncitizen spouse of a U.S. citizen or permanent resident to apply for legal status in the United States without the threat of deportation for reporting abuse or without requiring the cooperation of their spouse ("Legal Protections for Immigrant Stalking Victims," 2004). Although many stalking victims have not been assaulted physically by their stalker, the law also affects those who have experienced "extreme cruelty." The law falls short of protecting all potential immigrant victims of stalking, as it requires the victim to be married to the abuser at the time of the petition and that the abuser have legal immigration status. Unmarried illegal immigrants would not be protected, nor would the partners of illegal immigrants.

In 2000, a new *Violence Against Women Act* was passed that somewhat broadened the rights of immigrant women but continued to emphasize that they have been married to their abuser ("Legal Protections for Immigrant Stalking Victims," 2004). The new act does provide a new type of visa (called the U-Visa), which allows immigrant victims (with valid visas) who are not married to their abuser but "who have suffered substantial physical or mental abuse flowing from criminal activity" to obtain legal immigrant status, provided that they fully cooperate with the legal investigation or prosecution of the criminal activity. It remains to be seen how successful this program will be.

THE PSYCHOLOGICAL, SOCIAL, AND OCCUPATIONAL EFFECTS OF STALKING

Spitzberg and Cupach (2007) depict the sequelae of stalking as resulting in wide-ranging effects. Within relational effects, or those that relate to the personal and larger-scale disruption due to being stalked, first-order effects consist of those that are experienced by the victim. Second-order effects include alterations in social and institutional networks as a result of the stalking (e.g. adaptation efforts by friends, family, and co-workers of the victim). Third-order effects include the impact of stalking on third parties who may inadvertently become a potential victim of the stalker as well (e.g., a new boyfriend of the stalking victim). The social system effects can include the workplace, the legal system, and law enforcement resources. Focusing on the effects of stalking on the individual victim, a number of factors are often at play, including the behavior of the stalker, the awareness by the victim of the stalking behaviors, and the psychological characteristics that influence the reaction of the victim to traumatic stress. It is important to recognize therefore that victim responses are unique to the individual. Also, the data on the effects of stalking on victims is relatively recent, and there is more to be learned regarding both long-term and short-term sequelae.

Psychological Consequences of Stalking

Although violence by stalkers is rare, media depictions often focus on worst-case examples of murder by stalkers, undoubtedly increasing the amount of fear experienced by stalking victims (Dietz, Matthews, Duyne, et al., 1991; Pruitt, 1996). Some sources of advice for victims may also increase victim fear by not distinguishing cases in which violence is a serious risk from those cases in which the behaviors are simply annoying or inappropriate.

Prior studies examining psychiatric sequelae of stalking have identified depression, anxiety, and suicidal thoughts and behavior as prevalent among stalking victims seeking treatment (Kamphuis & Emmelkamp, 2001; Pathé & Mullen, 1997). There is little evidence supporting the treatment of depression or suicidality in stalking victims as substantially different from the treatment of depression and suicidality arising outside a stalking context. Much of the writing on the impact of stalking on victims uses the framework of posttraumatic stress disorder (PTSD). Although the degree of stress and trauma may vary greatly among victims and classes of victims, Mullen et al. (2001) noted that unlike most victims of traumatic events or crimes, "victims of persistent stalking develop stress-related symptoms very similar to the victims of other forms of chronic trauma, such as domestic violence" (p. 15). Emotional sequelae can result both directly and indirectly from being stalked. These difficulties can include both the fear and uncertainty created by the stalker's behavior, as well as the consequences of the disruptions to normal living created by dealing with the stalker's behavior. In addition, victims may have problems coping with the legal system (Abrams & Robinson, 1998).

Mullen et al. (2000) and others noted that only recently had research on the impact of stalking on victims been studied, and there had been as yet no studies of stalking victims within a random sample of a population. Still, a growing body of research shows the impact that stalking behaviors have on victims. In a study of battered women, Mechanic, Uhlmansiek, Weaver, and Resick (2000) found that those who were relentlessly stalked by their former partners had higher rates of depression and PTSD compared with those who were less frequently stalked. Of note, this study points also to the idea that the classical model of PTSD may not accurately depict the stalking experience, in large part because stalking involves multiple events, many of which do not involve physical violence but the anticipation of violence or a significant life-threatening encounter (see also Spitzberg & Cupach, 2007).

A study by Pathé and Mullen (1997) examined the toll of stalking on its victims by surveying 100 victims on issues concerning the nature of the stalking, motives, and the impact on the victim. In this survey, 58 cases involved overt threats to the victim, third parties, or both. Thirty-four of the subjects were assaulted, 7 of them sexually. Of the 34 who were assaulted, 26 had received previous threats. The victims of stalking in this survey, as expected, showed a large number of psychiatric symptoms. Symptoms experienced with the highest frequency included increased anxiety (83 cases), feelings of powerlessness (75 cases), and sleep disturbance (74 cases). Sixty-five reported having aggressive thoughts directed to the stalker. Suicidal ideation or attempts were reported in 24 cases. Appetite disturbance and weight fluctuation were symptoms acknowledged in half of the subjects. Other symptoms acknowledged by subjects included increased fatigue (55 cases), increased frequency or severity of headaches (47 cases), nausea (30 cases), and increased consumption of alcohol or cigarettes (23 cases).

As one would expect, many of these subjects displayed evidence of PTSD. Fifty-five of the subjects described experiencing "intrusive recall and vivid flashbacks." Thirty-eight reported feelings of numbness and a desire to avoid others, whereas 37 of the subjects met the full criteria for PTSD as defined by the *DSM-IV-TR* (American Psychiatric Association [APA], 2000). However, an additional 18 subjects met enough criteria to be diagnosed with PTSD with the exception of not meeting criterion A1 (i.e., "the person experienced, witnessed, or was confronted with an event or events that involved actual or threatened death or serious injury, or a threat to the physical integrity of self or others"; APA, 2000, p. 467).

The authors acknowledge that the high degree of distress in the sample is likely due to the selection of the subjects of the survey. The subjects were all individuals who either contacted the authors after becoming aware of their research or were individuals who had been referred to the authors' clinic, which specializes in stalking issues (Pathé & Mullen, 1997).

Another study that focused on support-seeking victims showed similar levels of distress (Kamphuis & Emmelkamp, 2001). This study of Dutch female stalking victims showed that 59% of subjects reported significant levels of psychomedical symptoms on the General Health Questionnaire. On the Impact of Event Scale, the trauma symptoms experienced by stalking victims was similar to those experiencing many types of trauma associated with PTSD, although less severe than those experiencing violence, traffic accidents, and acute bereavement.

As noted above, Westrup and colleagues studied the phenomenon of stalking in undergraduate university students. One study, restricted to females, attempted to distinguish stalking from "harassment," as well as to explore the psychological consequences of both (Westrup, Fremouw, Thompson, & Lewis, 1999). The subjects were asked two questions:

1. "Have you ever had someone intentionally and repeatedly follow, and/or harass, and/or threaten you?"
2. "Would you label the situation you were in as one in which you were being stalked by someone?" (p. 555)

Subjects endorsing both items were considered "stalked." Those endorsing the first question only were categorized as "harassed." Subjects, as well as those in a control group (of never-stalked women who had been in a > 6-monthlong relationship) were administered a number of standardized psychological measures examining symptoms of PTSD and psychiatric symptoms. On measures of PTSD, victims from the stalking group had a statistically significant higher number of symptoms and a higher symptom severity score when compared to either the control group or the harassed group. On a measure of general symptomatology, stalked subjects showed statistically higher scores on scales of obsessive-compulsive symptoms, interpersonal sensitivity, and depression when compared with control subjects. In contrast, these scores in subjects from the harassed group were intermediate to (but not statistically significantly different from) the scores of either the control or stalked groups. Likewise, total scores and scales looking at the severity and presence of psychiatric symptoms were significantly higher in the stalked group when compared to the control group.

In a more recent large Australian study examining a random community sample ($n = 1,844$), Purcell, Pathé, and Mullen (2005) sent surveys examining the experience of harassment and the respondent's mental health. Among those persons defined as victims of stalking compared with those defined as having only experienced short-term harassment, a significantly higher percentage of subjects (36% vs. 22%) experienced psychological symptoms that appeared to impact the respondent's quality of life and occur at a frequency that would generally be seen among those who sought help from mental health professionals. Victims of stalking had significantly increased scores on scales assessing severity of depression. Stalking victims were more likely to endorse having had recent suicidal ideas. Moreover, approximately 10% of victims of persistent stalking acknowledged recent suicidal ideation, with one in eight reporting they had seriously contemplated suicide in the month prior to the survey. Interestingly, rates of psychiatric morbidity among the victims of stalking were not associated with the methods of pursuit, the nature of the prior relationship with the stalker, or the experience of threats and violence.

One-third of the victims in the study by Purcell et al. (2005) reported ongoing high levels of anxiety and depression well after the stalking had ended, which the authors concluded emphasized the chronic course of impairment that can be seen in stalking victims. The authors suggested that anxiety symptoms such as hypervigilance, panic, and insomnia continue often because the victim has faced repeated intrusions over which they have felt little control, leading to the development of long-lasting concerns about the dangerousness of the world and the fragility of their safety. Although actual physical assaults did not seem to affect levels of posttraumatic stress disorder, victims who had been directly threatened showed significantly more posttraumatic type symptoms than those who had not been threatened. The authors concluded that this suggests that threats can be more emotionally damaging in many ways than actual assaults. Furthermore, depression was viewed as an outgrowth of a sense of a loss of individual autonomy and decreased quality of life due to the intrusive nature of the stalking.

Social and Occupational Consequences of Stalking

Given the range of psychiatric symptoms experienced by victims of stalking, it is not surprising that there are social and occupational consequences to the victims as well. In Pathé and Mullen's (1997) study of stalking victims referred to their clinic (discussed above), all of the victims perceived that the stalking experience had an impact on their functioning. Ninety-four of the 100 victims reported that the experience led them to make major lifestyle changes. Eighty-two victims reporting modifying their usual activities, 73 victims reported increasing their security measures, and 70 curtailed their usual social outings. The experience led 39 of the victims to relocate as a consequence of stalking. Many in this group also had disturbed occupational functioning as a result of the experience. Fifty-three of the victims decreased or stopped working or attending school. Thirty-seven victims reported that the experience led them to change their workplace, school, or chosen career. Likewise, Kamphuis and Emmelkamp's (2001) study of Dutch female victims showed that 71% of victims had been stalked for over 2 years, and that feelings of powerlessness and fear for one's life were very high. Coping mechanisms included seeking legal counsel (69%), avoiding leaving home (55%), and increased security measures (51%). As with the study by Pathé and Mullen (1997), many victims changed addresses (30%) and 23% quit work or school in response to stalking (Kamphuis & Emmelkamp, 2001).

As discussed above, studies requiring either a credible threat of harm or subjects referred to specialists in stalking may show evidence of greater psychopathological consequences of stalking compared with subjects in studies that do not require a credible threat or allow subjects to self-identify as stalking victims without meeting a legal definition of stalking. In Fremouw et al.'s (1997) study of 593 university undergraduates, the majority of the 24% who reported being stalked did not contact law enforcement. The two most common behaviors of both male and female victims were to either ignore the behavior or directly confront the stalker. Both male and female students frequently changed their schedules to avoid the stalker, although it was not clear in this study the extent of the life disruption caused by changing their schedules. Female respondents were more likely than males to carry a repellent spray, and male victims were more likely to reconcile with the stalker in cases of being stalked by an ex-intimate.

One hypothesis for the common behaviors reported in this study (i.e., not contacting the law, confronting the stalker, reconciling with the stalker) suggests that many of the students likely experienced behaviors far less frightening than those experienced in Kamphuis and Emmelkamp's (2001) or Pathé and Mullen's (1997) studies discussed above. It may also be that this group typically would strive for independence and may not want to admit their fear and seek help, or they may not have the wherewithal to recognize the risk of being stalked. Furthermore, other avenues (e.g., contacting parents or campus administration) may have been pursued but were not specifically explored in these studies.

Like victims of opposite-gender stalking, common behaviors by victims of same-gender stalking included changing usual activities, decreasing social activities, and disruptions in the ability to work in their chosen career (Pathé et al., 2000). In addition, Pathé et al. noted that when seeking assistance, many victims of same-gender stalking reported frustration that their complaints were not taken seriously. Although the majority of victims of same-gender stalking were heterosexual and most relationships with the stalker arose out of a professional context, many victims perceived their complaints as taken less seriously by law enforcement because of the same-sex aspect of the case.

THE MANAGEMENT OF STALKING VICTIMS

Overview

Although the impact of stalking on its victims is well described, most of the recommendations in the literature on the clinical management of stalking victims are based primarily on the experience of individual clinicians with such patients. The authors are unaware at the time of this writing of the presence of any randomized controlled trials specifically relating to the management of the victims of stalking.

Pathé, Mullen, and Purcell (2001) recommended a variety of clinical methods in managing stalking victims. These include providing an empathetic, nonjudgmental environment, education on stalking, monitoring of substance use, pharmacotherapy with selective serotonin reuptake inhibitors, and psychotherapies (group, family, and cognitive behavioral). Meloy (1997) recommends a team approach comprising not only the victim and the mental health professional, but also a number of others including a supportive companion, law enforcement, prosecutors, and possibly even a private attorney and security guard. Specialized forensic psychiatric consultation can also help in that it can allow for an objective clinical risk assessment approach to help the victim, and it separates the roles of the treatment providers and those needing to provide more objective consultation. Although this team approach would allow the clinician to have access to a wide range of collateral information, one can imagine the issues some victims might have with both the cost of such an approach (especially if the clinician is charging for both case management and therapy) and the implications that such a diverse team might have on the victim's confidentiality. Additionally, Meloy (1997) does not cite any evidence that a formal team approach coordinated by a mental health professional would lead to better outcomes for the victim.

Abrams and Robinson's (1998) approach, although admitting a lack of outcomes research to support it, recommends education, supportive therapy to increase the victim's self-esteem, assertiveness training, insight-oriented therapy to explore the victim's approach to relationships, and a focus on practical issues such as safety. Abrams and Robinson also speculate on the importance of clinician awareness of the countertransference issues that might arise during therapy. Female therapists, they feel, are at greater risk of either blaming the victim for her bad choices or are at risk for "overidentifying" with the female stalking victim. In contrast, male therapists may be at risk of being "overly protective" to rescue the victim or may experience feelings of guilt for failing to protect female victims against violence by men. Additionally, some male therapists may be at risk of identifying with aspects of the stalker's behavior based on their own past feelings of being rejected by women.

Meloy (1997) advises victims to accumulate evidence that would be useful for law enforcement in an eventual prosecution. He also urges victims to avoid direct contact with the perpetrator, stating that "each victim contact with the perpetrator is an intermittent positive reinforcement and predicts an increase in frequency of subsequent approach behavior" by the stalker (p. 177).

Although most victims of stalking likely find themselves in a situation not of their own making, little has been written concerning the possibility that some behaviors might, in some cases, make certain people more likely to become targets of stalking. Some writers have dismissed this even as a possibility. Abrams and Robinson's (1998) statement that even if a "victim's unconscious conflicts or past history of low self-esteem leave her vulnerable to choosing abusive partners, she does not consciously seek abuse or deserve to be abused" suggests that any other view would "revictimize" the victim (p. 479). Although this view may be reasonable in the context of providing supportive therapy, it does nothing to address the question of what role, if any, a victim's behavior may play in being selected by a stalker.

Beyond the psychiatric treatment of the stalking victim, the therapist may find herself or himself in the role of providing safety advice and other victim management strategies. There appears to be a paucity of solid research on the topic of victim management; rather, much of the writing is based on anecdotes of clinicians' experience with stalking victims (Meloy, 1997). However, there are a number of resources that can be found through the Internet related to stalking victimization. Pathé (2002) has published a book that victims of stalking may also find quite useful.

Evidence-Based Treatments Related to Anxiety Symptoms Resulting From Stalking

Although the treatment of all the various psychiatric symptoms that are seen among stalking victims is beyond the scope of this chapter, it appears that symptoms of anxiety and depression appear to predominate. This chapter focuses primarily on treatment of anxiety symptoms, although when stalking victims approach treatment providers, a full diagnostic assessment and treatment regimen for any identified impairing symptoms would be appropriate.

Until there are controlled trials of specific therapies directed at stalking victims, based on the discussions we held within the GAP Committee on Psychiatry and the Law, the authors believe that the most rational approach to managing the anxiety symptoms related to stalking victimization involves extrapolating from the much more advanced and growing body of knowledge about treatments for posttraumatic stress disorder and acute stress disorder (ASD). PTSD and ASD describe anxiety disorders due to severe psychological trauma. PTSD and ASD share the same core symptoms, but are distinguished by the length of the symptoms following the trauma (APA, 2000). ASD describes the condition shortly after the experience of the trauma; if the symptoms persist after 1 month, the victim may meet criteria for PTSD. Although not everyone exposed to psychological trauma will develop PTSD, 80% of those meeting criteria for ASD will meet criteria for PTSD after 6 months (Harvey & Bryant, 1998).

Many victims of stalking may not meet criteria for PTSD or ASD simply by virtue of the fact that they may not have been threatened with death or serious injury, necessary components required to make the diagnosis under the *Diagnostic and Statistical Manual of Mental Disorders* (*DSM-IV-TR*; APA, 2000). Others may experience psychological symptoms that do not meet the full diagnostic criteria for these disorders. Even without meeting the full criteria, many stalking victims will have some of the core symptoms of PTSD and ASD, particularly increased anxiety and avoidance of stimuli that reminds the victim of the stalking behaviors.

Pharmacological Approaches to PTSD

Serotonin Selective Reuptake Inhibitors

Although there are many case reports and open label trials of medications for PTSD, there are relatively few randomized controlled trials on these treatments (Cooper, Carty, & Creamer, 2005). The class of medications best studied in the pharmacotherapy of PTSD is the serotonin selective reuptake inhibitors (SSRIs;

Marshall, Beebe, Oldham, & Zaninelli, 2001). As noted, a full review of the use of these medications is beyond the scope of this chapter. However, many drug studies on treatments for PTSD focus on the reduction of symptoms in three primary clusters: (1) avoidance and reexperiencing of the trauma, (2) impairment in social and occupational functioning, and (3) depression (Davidson & Connor, 1999; Marshall et al., 2001; Schoenfeld, Marmar, & Neylan, 2004).

Marshall et al.'s (2001) 12-week, randomized, placebo-controlled trial showed that patients treated with 20 or 40 mg per day of the SSRI paroxetine statistically had improvement in three major PTSD symptom clusters. A randomized, controlled trial by Davidson and Connor (1999) showed that the SSRI sertraline was significantly superior to placebo in reducing symptoms of PTSD in patients with moderate to severe symptoms.

Antipsychotic Medications

One class of medications that does not appear to have much efficacy in the treatment of PTSD is neuroleptics or antipsychotics. Sernyak, Kosten, Fontana, & Rosenheck (2001) reviewed two outcome studies of combat-related PTSD in male veterans. Although commonly used, particularly in more psychiatrically ill patients, the use of neuroleptics was not shown to significantly affect outcome, although there may be utility in using some antipsychotics in patients with explosive behavior, psychosis, or sleep disturbance (Schoenfeld et al., 2004).

Additional Classes of Medications

A number of adrenergic-inhibiting agents (including propranolol, clonidine, and prazosin), anxiolytics (benzodiazepines and buspirone), and anticonvulsants (including valproate, carbamazepine, lamotrigine, gabapentin, and lithium) have shown promise in open label trials and case reports in the treatment of PTSD (Schoenfeld et al., 2004). However, the lack of randomized, controlled trials of these agents makes it difficult to assess the true efficacy of these treatments.

Other classes of medications studied include anticonvulsants (Davis, English, Ambrose, & Petty, 2001), benzodiazepines (Cooper et al., 2005), and other antidepressants such as tricyclics, monoamine oxidase inhibitors (Davidson & Connor, 1999; Schoenfeld et al., 2004) and mirtazapine (Schoenfeld et al., 2004).

Although SSRIs appear to be the most superior class of medications in treating PTSD, not all patients respond as well as others. Davidson and Connor (1999) noted that although the core symptoms of PTSD are well known, patients meeting criteria for PTSD may have a variable response to medications due to a number of factors, including the origin of the trauma, gender of the victim, and other factors (Davidson & Connor, 1999; Schoenfeld et al., 2004).

Unfortunately, none of the studies reviewed focused on PTSD specifically as a consequence of stalking, nor were there any studies that focused on the pharmacotherapy of stalking victims whose symptoms did not meet criteria for PTSD.

Psychotherapeutic Approaches to PTSD

Like pharmacotherapies, there are few if any controlled studies that examine the most evidence based approach to psychological symptoms experienced by victims of stalking. If the model of PTSD is used to suggest treatment strategies, there is a body of evidence suggesting which therapies might ultimately show the greatest efficacy in treating the anxiety symptoms experienced by victims of stalking.

A wide number of psychotherapies have been studied in the treatment of PTSD, and many of them are superior to no treatment. Bradley, Greene, Russ, Dutra, and Westen's (2005) meta-analysis of psychotherapeutic approaches for PTSD concluded that psychotherapy for PTSD is effective. The two most effective models were cognitive behavioral therapy (CBT) and eye movement desensitization reprocessing (EMDR), both discussed below. Bradley et al. (2005) concluded that there was no difference in the efficacy of CBT and EMDR, nor a significant difference in efficacy of different types of CBT treatments. There is, however, evidence that some treatments may actually be more harmful than helpful (Rose, Bisson, Churchill, & Wessely, 2002). A review of these various treatments is discussed below.

Critical Incident Stress Debriefing (Psychological Debriefing)

One type of intervention intended to prevent the development of PTSD is known as critical incident stress debriefing, or psychological debriefing (Raphael & Wooding, 2004). Although taking various forms, this is a psychological modality that involves a single session interview given to victims, usually within a few days of the trauma (Foa, Zoellner, & Feeny, 2006). The treatment encourages victims to discuss the traumatic event and encourages them to recall and process the event. Although this model has been promoted to be helpful in preventing PTSD due to trauma, its utility has been increasingly questioned (Raphael & Wooding, 2004). Although initially developed as a technique used to address combat trauma and reactions to disaster, proponents have advocated its use in a wide range of distressing health situations such as childbirth, diagnoses of HIV and cancer, and even treatment of grief reactions, despite limited evidence supporting these uses (Raphael & Wooding, 2004). Kenardy (2000) categorized debriefing as a "grassroots intervention that is popular among many health and allied practitioners" (p. 1033) and predicted its continued use despite evidence that it is ineffective.

A Cochrane evidence-based review of 15 trials concluded that psychological debriefing was not useful in preventing PTSD (Rose et al., 2002). Other studies applying psychological debriefing to traffic accident victims (Mayou, Ehlers, & Hobbs, 2000) and burn victims (Bisson, Jenkins, Alexander, & Bannister, 1997) suggest that the technique may in fact be more harmful than helpful. Bisson et al. demonstrated that psychological debriefing actually worsened psychological symptoms in burn victims compared with those who did not receive debriefing. In Mayou et al.'s 3-year follow-up study of victims of automobile accidents, those receiving debriefing shortly after the accident had significantly worse symptoms than the unbriefed control group.

Eye Movement Desensitization and Reprocessing (EMDR)

Eye movement desensitization and reprocessing (EMDR) is a technique applied to a variety of psychological disorders. Shapiro (1989) developed specific techniques for the use of EMDR in the treatment of PTSD. In treating PTSD, it involves a patient concentrating on a major aspect of the traumatic memories while engaging in specific lateral eye movements directed by the therapist (Shapiro, 1996). Although the mechanism of action is unclear, EMDR appears to have efficacy in treatment of PTSD. Stapleton, Taylor, and Asmundson (2006) reported that EMDR significantly reduced symptoms of anger and guilt in PTSD victims and was of equivalent efficacy to treatments that utilize either prolonged exposure (a form of CBT; see section below) or relaxation training.

Cognitive Behavioral Therapies (CBT)

Cognitive behavioral therapies are well established as efficacious treatments for a variety of mood and anxiety disorders, including PTSD (Ursano et al., 2004). Most forms of CBT involve training patients to recognize distorted thinking that contributes to psychological symptoms and teaching them how to modify the distorted cognitions through a variety of techniques. Although not well studied as a specific treatment in victims of stalking, Pathé et al. (2001, p. 404) advocated the use of CBT to help restructure "the victim's morbid perceptions of the world, in particular that the world is a malevolent place where nobody can be trusted." Concerning the treatment of PTSD, Hembree and Foa (2000) proposed that the most appropriate treatment for processing trauma required "emotional engagement with the trauma memory, organization of the trauma narrative, and correction of dysfunctional cognitions" (p. 33), processes well suited to cognitive behavioral approaches.

CBT for PTSD is called by a number of names based on the method applied by the clinician. Trauma-focused cognitive behavior therapy/exposure therapy

(TFCBT) describes CBT that typically involves a combination of *exposure* to the trauma, *cognitive restructuring*, and anxiety management (Bryant, Sackville, Dang, Moulds, & Guthrie, 1999). In the form advocated by Bryant et al., the *exposure* component involved the patient reexperiencing the traumatic event via focusing of the memories of the event and identifying their emotional responses. The *cognitive restructuring* component was designed to decrease anxiety and comprised training the patient to identify irrational or distorted thinking and promote the evaluation of these disturbed thoughts against evidence.

Bryant et al. (1999) compared the efficacy of CBT to supportive therapy in decreasing the rate of PTSD in patients meeting criteria for acute stress disorder. Using this approach in subjects recently exposed to trauma, Bryant et al. concluded that CBT was correlated with a much lower incidence of developing PTSD after 6 months, approximately 15%, compared with the development of PTSD in 67% of subjects receiving only supportive psychotherapy. Surprisingly, Bryant et al. found no additional benefit to adding anxiety management techniques to the treatment utilizing prolonged exposure and cognitive restructuring.

Foa, Hearst-Ikeda, and Perry (1995) studied the efficacy of brief cognitive behavioral therapy in preventing the development of chronic PTSD. The treatment involved four sessions of CBT applied to female assault victims. Compared to matched controls, 10% of those receiving brief CBT met criteria for PTSD, compared with 70% of controls. After nearly 6 months, the treated group also had significantly fewer symptoms of depression and reexperiencing of symptoms.

Evolving models of TFCBT continue to show promise in improving treatments of PTSD. Foa et al.'s (2006) recent study of female survivors of sexual and nonsexual assault compared three types of interventions. *Brief prevention (B-CBT)* was the term used to describe a TFCBT technique that involved four sessions of in vitro exposure to traumatic reminders of the assault, followed by cognitive restructuring. *Assessment condition* was a second type of treatment that involved four sessions of repeated assessments of the patient's reactions to the trauma without any direct processing of the trauma as in B-CBT. A third group received supportive therapy only. In this study, B-CBT was clearly superior to supportive therapy in reducing PTSD symptoms both immediately after the intervention and after 3 months. B-CBT was not shown to be superior to the assessment condition, in contrast to an earlier study by Foa et al. (1995), which showed clear superiority of B-CBT to assessment condition. After 9 months, none of the treatments in the 2006 study appeared significantly superior to the others, suggesting improvement with all three forms of treatment but earlier improvement in those receiving B-CBT or repeated assessments compared to supportive therapy.

According to a Cochrane review of randomized controlled trials of non-EMDR psychotherapies, individual trauma-focused CBT, group trauma-focused

CBT, and stress management were superior to other treatments, with evidence that the individual TFCBT was the most superior treatment (Bisson & Andrew, 2005).

Supportive Psychotherapy

Supportive psychotherapy is an atheoretical and commonly practiced psycho-therapy used in a wide range of treatment situations (Winston, Rosenthal, & Pinsker, 2004). Key elements include establishing a positive therapeutic alliance with the patient, understanding the patient's problems, and setting realistic goals with the patient. Foa et al. (2006) compared brief CBT and repeated assessments to supportive therapy. Although in the early stages of the study supportive therapy was not superior to the other modalities, after 9 months none of the other interventions appeared significantly superior to supportive therapy, all being associated with improvement in symptoms.

In a study by Bryant et al. (1999) comparing the efficacy of CBT with supportive psychotherapy in patients with acute stress disorder, supportive psychotherapy was associated with the development of PTSD in 67% of subjects, compared with an incidence of 80% in prospective studies of untreated PTSD. Although superior to no treatment, supportive psychotherapy alone was clearly inferior to CBT.

Summary

Although there are few specific data on treatment of victims of stalking, the literature on treatment of PTSD suggests that a number of those treatments may have value in victims of stalking, particularly those meeting criteria for PTSD or acute stress disorder. Pharmacotherapy with selective serotonin reuptake inhibitors and psychotherapy with trauma-focused cognitive behavioral therapy techniques are postulated by the authors as having the most theoretical efficacy in victims of stalking experiencing anxiety symptoms. Although not studied in stalking victims, eye movement desensitization and reprocessing may also be beneficial in stalking victims with symptoms of PTSD.

FALSE ACCUSATIONS OF STALKING

Introduction

Any discussion of false accusations of stalking must begin with a disclaimer: the incidence of false reports of victimization pales in comparison to the problem of inadequate resources and recourse for true victims of stalking. As detailed elsewhere in this book, individuals who have the misfortune to become targets of stalkers often encounter little support, misinformation, and ineffective legal remedies. Their concerns may be discounted. They may receive conflicting or inaccurate information and advice. They may obtain minimal assistance from law enforcement agencies in jurisdictions that lack adequate resources or criminal statutes. Feelings of helplessness and frustration can compound their legitimate fears for personal safety. A comprehensive overview of the phenomenon of stalking requires a review of cases of false accusations of victimization, but this should not detract attention from the very serious problem of true stalking.

Although false claims of stalking have been estimated to represent only about 2% of all reported stalking cases (Mohandie, Hatcher, & Raymond, 1998; Zona, Palarea, & Lane, 1998), they also create serious problems. These cases divert limited investigatory, therapeutic, and supportive resources away from legitimate cases. Both the accused and the accuser may suffer avoidable harm. The accused may face undeserved criminal and civil sanctions. Reputations, re-lationships, and careers can be ruined. The accuser, meanwhile, may suffer from an untreated mental disorder while the false claim remains undetected.

Appropriate management of stalking cases requires an understanding and recognition of the phenomenon of false accusations. Proper identification of the rare case of false accusations can help avoid mistaken diversion of limited clinical and law enforcement resources. Prevention and safety interventions can focus on legitimate cases while false cases also receive appropriate interventions. Descriptions of false stalking victims are sparse. A search of the psychiatric lit-erature revealed only one empirical study. In a 1999 report, Pathé, Mullen, and Purcell compared 12 cases of presumed false victims with 100 cases of true victims. The false victims consisted of five types:

1. Stalkers who accused their victims of being the stalker;
2. Persons with severe mental disorders that included delusions of being stalked;
3. Individuals who had been stalked in the past, leading them to misper-ceive innocent situations as a recurrence of stalking;
4. Factitious victims;
5. Malingerers.

In comparison to the true victims, false victims used more medical ser-vices, were more likely to be involved in legal action, and were less likely to be involved in a stable intimate relationship. Their accounts also differed from those of the true victims. They tended to report shorter durations of stalking (17.4 versus 40.5 months) before seeking help. Perhaps most significantly, their accounts typically lacked objective information. For example, they rarely com-plained of receiving letters from their alleged stalkers, and they typically did not report threats or attacks by their purported stalker against a third party.

Clinicians and criminal justice personnel require an understanding of the motives of false accusers and the techniques to identify them. This next portion of this chapter attempts to present a framework for understanding those motives and for detecting cases of false accusations.

Motives for False Accusations of Stalking

Underlying motives for false accusations can be divided into at least three categories: engagement with the falsely accused "stalker," engagement with others, and engagement with a distorted internal reality.

Engagement With the Falsely Accused Stalker

The motive for a false accusation of stalking may involve an agenda exclusive to the person accused. In such cases, the accuser clearly identifies the alleged perpetrator. The accuser selects the alleged stalker deliberately and with a victim-specific goal. The accuser might choose the target for the purpose of harassment or as a perverse type of stalking in reverse. Harassment may be associated with some secondary goal for engagement, but stalking in reverse has engagement as its primary goal.

> CASE EXAMPLE 5.1: HARASSMENT
> Mark and Linda were a divorced couple in a small town involved in an ongoing dispute over the support of their two children. Angry that Mark received partial custody of the children, Linda reported to her friends, lawyer, and local police that Mark had been pursuing her since the time of their separation, eventually escalating to threats to kill Linda if she dated other men. Following the initial report, Mark was arrested and briefly detained. Although the local police did not find much evidence to support her claims, a restraining order against Mark was granted. The local newspaper described the arrest, leading the local Boy Scout leaders to ask Mark to resign as the scoutmaster of his son's scout troop. Linda subsequently wrote letters to Mark's employer and to several women he was dating, telling them of his alleged behavior. Suspecting that his employer passed him over for promotion due to the accusations, and finding few women willing to date him, Mark relocated to another town, leading a local judge to grant Linda's request for full custody of their children.

False claims of victimization can result in adverse consequences for the accused. The alleged stalker is likely to become the subject of police investigation and attendant public embarrassment. Consequent disruptions can occur in social and occupational functioning. A mendacious accuser could be motivated merely by a desire to vex the accused. False rape allegations have been described in cases in which the accuser sought revenge against a rejecting suitor (Kanin, 1994). In other instances, the accuser may have an underlying goal. For example, in child custody disputes, an accusation of stalking could result in restraining orders and more favorable custody arrangements for the accuser.

CASE EXAMPLE 5.2: STALKING IN REVERSE

Mary K. was an inpatient under the care of Dr. Smith, a male psychiatric resident. After Mary was discharged from the unit, Dr. Smith began to suspect that he was being followed by Mary. He would encounter her at his regular coffeehouse, grocery store, and gym. He also began to receive anonymous love notes from a "secret admirer" that he feared was his former patient. At the urging of his wife, Dr. Smith called the local police department, where he was surprised to hear that Mary had complained to the police that Dr. Smith was pursuing her. The police informed him that Mary reported that she had a brief affair with Dr. Smith, but ended it, leading to the unwanted pursuit. The police officer suggested to Dr. Smith that he get an attorney, because sex with patients was a violation of the state criminal code. Within the next few weeks, Dr. Smith received calls from his residency director, department chairman, and an investigator from the state medical board, all reporting that a former patient of his had reported him for inappropriate sexual contact and ongoing stalking behavior. After a period of administrative leave with pay, Dr. Smith was exonerated of the accusations, but chose not to pursue further action against Mary out of fear that he would have to face her in court.

Appearances can be deceptive. A true stalker may turn the tables on a victim by falsely claiming that the victim is the stalker. The allegation obfuscates the situation and diverts resources away from aiding the actual victim. Faced with accusations and counteraccusations, the police may find it difficult to correctly identify perpetrator and victim. The victim also must devote time, energy, and resources to defend against the accusations. The true stalker also may benefit through mandatory legal contacts with the actual victim. In an attempt to present a defense to the false accusations, the victim may be compelled to confront the stalker during legal proceedings. The stalker thus gains access, which might otherwise be denied, to the victim.

Engagement With Others

For some false accusers, the identity of the victim appears to have less significance. In these cases, the accuser might or might not clearly identify the alleged perpetrator. Although a relationship may exist with the victim, this relationship does not primarily motivate the accuser. Instead, the accuser seeks a response or reaction from third parties. The victim serves merely as the means to this end. Examples of false accusations in the pursuit of engagement with others include malingering and factitious disorder.

CASE EXAMPLE 5.3: MALINGERING

Jason was an information technology worker at a publishing company who was engaged in a brief affair with his boss Susan. After the affair ended, Jason's work performance began to suffer and he was being considered for termination. Jason decided to claim financial compensation. Inspired by the movie *Fatal Attraction*, Jason created a story that would present his boss as an unstable predator. Hacking into Susan's computer and adjusting her computer's clock, Jason created a series of bizarre and threatening e-mails to complement genuine love letters Susan wrote him during their affair. He then poisoned his own dog and vandalized his car. Studying a copy of the *DSM-IV* from the local bookstore, he was able to expertly mimic the symptoms of posttraumatic stress disorder convincingly enough to fool the evaluator hired to assess his symptoms. Jason "graciously" agreed not to pursue legal action against Susan once he was granted his workers compensation claim.

People who falsely claim to be victims of stalking are engaging in deception. They are not, however, engaging in malingering unless they are also endorsing false or grossly exaggerated symptoms of psychiatric or other illness in order to obtain some external incentive. The malingerer typically seeks to obtain a desired reward such as money or drugs, or to avoid an unwanted situation such as military duty, work, or criminal prosecution. Some malingerers pursue such rewards by feigning victim status. In sexual harassment cases, for example, plaintiffs have exaggerated symptoms for monetary rewards or work-related reasons (Feldman-Schorrig & McDonald, 1992; Long, 1994). Although malingered claims of victimization by a stalker are likely to be rare, such claims could occur for any of the reasons usually associated with malingering. Some jurisdictions, for example, provide financial compensation for crime victims. Malingerers also might receive special accommodations at work because of alleged harassment by a stalker.

The presence of confirmed malingering in an alleged victim of stalking does not necessarily disprove that the stalking occurred. For example, a victim of real stalking who has few genuine psychiatric symptoms might claim to meet the full criteria of posttraumatic stress disorder in order to obtain drugs or financial compensation.

CASE EXAMPLE 5.4: FACTITIOUS DISORDER

Tina presented to an emergency room, covered with superficial abrasions. She described a terrifying tale of having been stalked by a stranger, who attempted to assault her. She described nightmares and flashbacks associated with a protracted period of death threats in calls and letters by the alleged stalker. Despite her lack of identification or insurance, she was admitted to a specialized inpatient unit for victims of posttraumatic stress disorder. Tina appeared to enjoy the program and was very resistant to leave or participate in discharge planning or attempts to obtain new identification. Although the staff was unable to obtain any collateral information, a visiting attending psychiatrist recognized Tina as "Suzanne," a patient who had spent the previous month in a day hospitalization program for patients with eating disorders.

Similar to malingering, factitious disorders also involve the intentional production of false or exaggerated symptoms. Unlike malingering, however, external incentives such as obtaining rewards or avoiding unwanted situations do not provide the motivation. Instead, the symptoms are produced with the goal of assuming the sick role. Gratification of a psychological need to take on the sick role in the absence of external incentives characterizes factitious disorders.

Differentiating malingering from factitious disorder can be difficult, especially when a person with a factitious disorder receives some external, or secondary, gain along with the primary gain derived from the sick role. For example, individuals with factitious disorders sometimes pursue litigation for monetary reward based on their falsified symptoms. In addition to malpractice lawsuits, cases have been described in which plaintiffs have sought financial damages from a manufacturer and from a luxury hotel based on claims of victimization from product tampering or from mugging (Eisendrath, 1996). In each of these cases, gratification of psychological needs seemed to provide the original motivation for the apparently self-inflicted injuries, which included permanent visual loss in one case. Malingerers typically do not self-inflict such serious injuries. In contrast with malingerers, persons with factitious disorders are more likely to produce substantial injuries in pursuit of their psychological needs.

In the case of a factitious disorder, a false complaint of stalking represents a desire to assume the role of victim. Cases of factitious rape and factitious sexual harassment motivated by a desire to obtain victim status have been described (Feldman, Ford, & Stone, 1994; Feldman-Schorrig, 1996). The purported victim may receive attention and support similar to that received by a sick person. As the victim of an alleged stalker, the accuser establishes and maintains contact with law enforcement officers, victims' advocates, therapists, and other supportive persons or authority figures. The accuser obtains psychological gratification from the response of third parties, and the falsely accused person serves merely as a means to this end.

Engagement With a Distorted Internal Reality

An accusation of stalking can be false despite the lack of a deceitful intent by the accuser. The accuser's perception of being stalked may simply be mistaken. Such honest mistakes can result from psychotic symptoms, such as paranoid delusions, or can arise in the absence of underlying psychopathology.

CASE EXAMPLE 5.5: PSYCHOSIS

Beth was admitted to an inpatient psychiatry service after developing symptoms of severe depression. On the initial evaluation, the treatment team noticed that the patient was staring at a male psychiatry resident and asked that he be sent out of the room. When asked why, the patient said, "There are people here claiming to be doctors who are not doctors." Although this was the first time the resident had seen the patient, she accused him of previously following her and spying on her at her workplace. A few days later, Beth saw the resident in the hallway and asked him his name. Beth stared at him suspiciously, saying, "That's not the name you gave me when I saw you at my office last month."

The symptoms of some psychotic disorders can include ideas of reference. The sufferer mistakenly assumes that casual events have a direct personal reference. If of sufficient intensity, the incorrect interpretations can reach delusional proportions. A delusion consists of an idiosyncratic false belief that is firmly held despite clear evidence to the contrary. The perception of being stalked can be delusional.

Although many types of psychotic disorders could present with delusions of being stalked, one type is especially noteworthy. In delusional disorder, the individual has a persistent, nonbizarre delusion. A nonbizarre delusion involves situations that can occur in real life, such as being loved from a distance or being stalked. Apart from the impact of the delusion, the person functions and behaves without marked impairment. Delusional disorders are generally divided into at least five specific subtypes (erotomanic, persecutory, grandiose, jealous, and somatic) (APA, 2000). The erotomanic type has been described in chapter 2 because of its association with actual stalking cases. The persecutory type, however, has the greatest relevance to false accusations of stalking. This subtype involves paranoid delusions, which may include the belief of being followed or spied upon. Individuals with persecutory delusions may become violent against those they believe are harassing them. Paradoxically, they might stalk those they believe are stalking them.

CASE EXAMPLE 5.6: NONPSYCHOTIC
MISPERCEPTIONS

Jennifer was a 21-year-old college student at Amtola State University. She was fearful of being stalked again after being the victim of a cyberstalker when she was in high school. To avoid being cyberstalked again, she used an e-mail address that would not suggest her actual name. One day she received an e-mail that said, "Why haven't you written back?" She did not recognize the address. The next day, she received a message that said, "I know you're home. I saw your car outside." Jennifer began to panic, convinced that she was being stalked again. She reported her fears to campus security and refused to leave her dorm for 2 days. Security tracked down the e-mailer and discovered a nonsinister explanation: the sender mistakenly sent Jennifer an e-mail intended for a friend. The intended recipient's e-mail address was oceanbleu@amtolastate.edu, nearly identical to Jennifer's e-mail address, oceanblue@amtolastate.edu.

Distorted perceptions of being stalked can arise for reasons unrelated to psychosis or psychopathology. Although honest mistakes can occur for many reasons, past stalking victims may be especially prone to incorrect beliefs. Stalking victims often suffer psychological distress, including hypervigilance. They may become extremely watchful and alert to potential danger. This hypervigilance can lead to misperceptions in which they mistakenly suspect a recurrence of stalking. Unlike delusional beliefs, however, such suspicions will likely resolve with reassuring evidence to the contrary.

Table 5.2. Clues to the Possibility of False Victimization

Account	Inconsistencies
	Changes in account when specifics are questioned
	Bizarre or psychotic accusations/evidence of delusional disorder
Corroborating details	Absence of supporting data
	No physical evidence
	No letters or answering machine messages
	No witnesses
Behavior	More concerned with attention than resolution of problem (factitious disorder)
	Resists attempts to resolve problem
History	Prior complaints
	History of attention-seeking behavior
	Fabrication or exaggeration of other life events
	History of factitious disorder/unusual, unexplained symptoms especially as coping mechanism in response to stressors
	Symptoms of many disorders without objective findings
	Lack of expected response to treatment
	Seeks invasive procedures
	Physician shopping, especially in response to physician's skepticism
	Evidence of antisocial or borderline personality
Alternative motives	Other areas of conflict with the falsely accused stalker
	Custody dispute
	Rejecting suitor

Identifying Cases of False Accusations of Stalking

All claims of stalking warrant response and review by law enforcement and clinical professionals. Experience suggests that most such claims represent true cases of stalking. Techniques designed to tease out the rare false claim should not replace an appropriate investigation of the complaint. In those cases, however, in which a reasonable investigation suggests that the complaint lacks credibility, some details may help to confirm or refute suspicions about the veracity of the accusation.

CONCLUSION

Research on stalking victims is a relatively new enterprise, and much of the data available suffer from numerous problems, including flawed methodology, problems defining what it means to be stalked, limited sample sizes, and skewed populations subjected to study. Furthermore, much of the research on management of stalking victims is based on anecdotal experience rather than any controlled studies (Meloy, 2002).

Standard definitions of stalking often exclude behaviors such as nonmalicious inappropriate actions, unreciprocated "crushes," or inappropriate attempts at seduction (such as the seduction of minors on the Internet). Recipients of such behaviors may nonetheless consider themselves to have been stalked. Other stalking victims may be completely unaware they are being stalked, due either to a lack of behaviors by the stalker that would alert the intended victim, or to a nonrecognition of behaviors that might clearly fit standard definitions of stalking.

REFERENCES

Abrams, K. M., & Robinson, G. E. (1998). Stalking. Part II: Victims' problems with the legal system and therapeutic considerations. *Canadian Journal of Psychiatry, 43*(5), 477–481.

American Psychiatric Association. (2000). *Diagnostic and statistical manual of mental disorders* (4th ed., Text Rev.). Washington, DC: Author.

Bisson, J. I., Jenkins, P. L., Alexander, J., & Bannister, C. (1997). Randomised controlled trial of psychological debriefing for victims of acute burn trauma. *British Journal of Psychiatry, 171*, 78–81.

Bradley, R., Greene, J., Russ, E., Dutra, L., & Westen, D. (2005). A multidimensional meta-analysis of psychotherapy for PTSD. *American Journal of Psychiatry, 162*(2), 214–227.

Bryant, R. A., Sackville, T., Dang, S. T., Moulds, M., & Guthrie, R. (1999). Treating acute stress disorder: An evaluation of cognitive behavior therapy and supportive counseling techniques. *American Journal of Psychiatry, 156*(11), 1780–1786.

Cooper, J., Carty, J., & Creamer, M. (2005). Pharmacotherapy for posttraumatic stress disorder: Empirical review and clinical recommendations. *Australian and New Zealand Journal of Psychiatry, 39*(8), 674–682.

Davidson, J. R., & Connor, K. M. (1999). Management of posttraumatic stress disorder: Diagnostic and therapeutic issues. *Journal of Clinical Psychiatry, 60*(Suppl. 18), 33–38.

Davis, L. L., English, B. A., Ambrose, S. M., & Petty, F. (2001). Pharmacotherapy for post-traumatic stress disorder: A comprehensive review. *Expert Opinion on Pharmacotherapy, 2*(10), 1583–1595.

Dietz, P., Matthews, D., Martel, D., Stewart, T., Hrouda, D., & Warren, J. (1991). Threatening and otherwise inappropriate letters to members of the United States Congress. *Journal of Forensic Science, 36,* 1445–1468.

Douglas, J. E., Burgess, A. W., Burgess, A. G., & Ressler, R. K. (1992). *Crime classification manual: A standard system for investigation and classifying violent crimes.* New York: Lexington Books.

Eisendrath, S. (1996). When Munchausen becomes malingering: Factitious disorders that penetrate the legal system. *Bulletin American Academy of Psychiatry and the Law, 24*(4), 195–203.

Feldman, M., Ford, C., & Stone, T. (1994). Deceiving others/deceiving oneself: Four cases of factitious rape. *Southern Medical Journal, 87*(7), 736–738.

Feldman-Schorrig, S. (1996). Factitious sexual harassment. *Bulletin of American Academy of Psychiatry and Law, 24*(3), 387–392.

Feldman-Schorrig, S., & McDonald, J. (1992). The role of forensic psychiatry in the defense of sexual harassment cases. *Journal of Psychiatry and Law, 20,* 5–33.

Foa, E. B., Hearst-Ikeda, D., & Perry, K. J. (1995). Evaluation of a brief cognitive-behavioral program for the prevention of chronic PTSD in recent assault victims. *Journal of Consulting and Clinical Psychology, 63*(6), 948–955.

Foa, E. B., Zoellner, L. A., & Feeny, N. C. (2006). An evaluation of three brief programs for facilitating recovery after assault. *Journal of Traumatic Stress, 19*(1), 29–43.

Fremouw, W. J., Westrup, D., & Pennypacker, J. (1997). Stalking on campus: The prevalence and strategies for coping with stalking. *Journal of Forensic Science, 42*(4), 666–669.

Hall, D. M. (1998). The victims of stalking. In J. R. Meloy (Ed.), *The psychology of stalking: Clinical and forensic perspectives* (pp. 113–137). San Diego: Academic Press.

Harvey, A. G., & Bryant, R. A. (1998). The relationship between acute stress disorder and posttraumatic stress disorder: A prospective evaluation of motor vehicle accident survivors. *Journal of Consulting and Clinical Psychology, 66*(3), 507–512.

Hembree, E. A., & Foa, E. B. (2000). Posttraumatic stress disorder: Psychological factors and psychosocial interventions. *Journal of Clinical Psychiatry, 61*(Suppl. 7), 33–39.

Immigrant stalking victims face complex challenges. (2003, Fall). *Stalking Resource Center Newsletter, 3,* 1–5.

Kamphuis, J. H., & Emmelkamp, P. M. (2001). Traumatic distress among support-seeking female victims of stalking. *American Journal of Psychiatry, 158*(5), 795–798.

Kanin, E. (1994). False rape allegations. *Archives of Sexual Behavior, 23*(1), 81–92.

Kenardy, J. (2000). The current status of psychological debriefing. *British Medical Journal, 321*(7268), 1032–1033.

Legal protections for immigrant stalking victims. (2004). *Stalking Resource Center Newsletter, 4,* 1–10.

Long, B. (1994). Psychiatric diagnosis in sexual harassment cases. *Bulletin of the American Academy of Psychiatry and Law, 22*(2), 195–203.

Marshall, R. D., Beebe, K. L., Oldham, M., & Zaninelli, R. (2001). Efficacy and safety of paroxetine treatment for chronic PTSD: A fixed-dose, placebo-controlled study. *American Journal of Psychiatry, 158*(12), 1982–1988.

Mayou, R. A., Ehlers, A., & Hobbs, M. (2000). Psychological debriefing for road traffic accident victims: Three-year follow-up of a randomised controlled trial. *British Journal of Psychiatry, 176,* 589–593.

McCann, J. T. (2000). A descriptive study of child and adolescent obsessional followers. *Journal of Forensic Science, 45*(1), 195–199.

Mechanic, M. B., Uhlmansiek, M. H., Weaver, T.L., & Resick, P. A. (2000). The impact of severe stalking experienced by acutely battered women: an examination of violence, psychological symptoms and strategic responding. *Violence and Victims, 15*(4), 443–458.

Meloy, J. (1997). The clinical risk management of stalking: "Someone is watching over me . . ." *American Journal of Psychotherapy, 51*(2), 174–184.

Meloy, J. R. (2002). Commentary: Stalking, threatening, and harassing behavior by patients—the risk-management response [Comment]. *Journal of the American Academy of Psychiatry & the Law, 30*(2), 230–231.

Mohandie, K., Hatcher, C., & Raymond, D. (1998). False victimization syndromes in stalking. In J. Meloy (Ed.), *The psychology of stalking: Clinical and forensic perspectives* (pp. 224–6). San Diego: Academic Press, Harcourt Brace.

Mullen, P. E., & Pathé, M. (1994). Stalking and the pathologies of love. *Australian & New Zealand Journal of Psychiatry, 28*(3), 469–477.

Mullen, P. E., Pathé, M., & Purcell, R. (2000). *Stalkers and their victims.* Cambridge, UK; New York: Cambridge University Press.

Mullen, P. E., Pathé, M., & Purcell, R. (2001). Stalking: New constructions of human behaviour. *Australian & New Zealand Journal of Psychiatry, 35*(1), 9–16.

Pathé, M. (2002). *Surviving stalking.* New York: Cambridge University Press.

Pathé, M., & Mullen, P. E. (1997). The impact of stalkers on their victims. *British Journal of Psychiatry, 170,* 12–17.

Pathé, M. T., & Mullen, P. E. (2002). The victim of stalking. In J. Boon & L. Sheridan (Eds.), *Stalking and psychosexual obsession: Psychological perspectives for prevention, policing and treatment* (pp. 1–22). Chichester, UK: Wiley.

Pathé, M., Mullen, P. E., & Purcell, R. (1999). Stalking: False claims of victimisation. *British Journal of Psychiatry, 174*, 170–172.

Pathé, M. T., Mullen, P. E., & Purcell, R. (2000). Same-gender stalking. *Journal of the American Academy of Psychiatry and Law, 28*(2), 191–197.

Pathé, M., Mullen, P. E., & Purcell, R. (2001). Management of victims of stalking. *Advances in Psychiatric Treatment, 7*, 399–406.

Pruitt, B. (Writer). (1996). Dark obsession: The stalking and murder of Rebecca Schaeffer [Television series episode]. In *The E! True Hollywood Story*. Los Angeles: E! Entertainment Television.

Purcell, R., Pathé, M., & Mullen, P. E. (2005). Association between stalking victimisation and psychiatric morbidity in a random community sample. *British Journal of Psychiatry, 187*, 416–420.

Raphael, B., & Wooding, S. (2004). Debriefing: Its evolution and current status. *Psychiatric Clinics of North America, 27*(3), 407–423.

Rose, S., Bisson, J., Churchill, R., & Wessely, S. (2002). Psychological debriefing for preventing post traumatic stress disorder (PTSD). *Cochrane Database Systematic Review* (2), CD000560.

Schoenfeld, F. B., Marmar, C. R., & Neylan, T. C. (2004). Current concepts in pharmacotherapy for posttraumatic stress disorder. *Psychiatric Services, 55*(5), 519–531.

Sernyak, M. J., Kosten, T. R., Fontana, A., & Rosenheck, R. (2001). Neuroleptic use in the treatment of post-traumatic stress disorder. *Psychiatric Quarterly, 72*(3), 197–213.

Shapiro, F. (1989). Eye movement desensitization: A new treatment for posttraumatic stress disorder. *Journal of Behavior Therapy and Experimental Psychiatry, 20*(3), 211–217.

Shapiro, F. (1996). Eye movement desensitization and reprocessing (EMDR): Evaluation of controlled PTSD research. *Journal of Behavior Therapy and Experimental Psychiatry, 27*(3), 209–218.

Spitzberg, B. H., Cupach, W. R. (2007). The state of the art of stalking: Taking stock of the emerging literature. *Aggression and Violent Behavior, 12*, 64–86.

Stapleton, J. A., Taylor, S., & Asmundson, G. J. (2006). Effects of three PTSD treatments on anger and guilt: Exposure therapy, eye movement desensitization and reprocessing, and relaxation training. *Journal of Traumatic Stress, 19*(1), 19–28.

Tjaden, P., & Thoennes, N. (1998). *Research in brief*. National Institute of Justice Centers for Disease Control and Prevention.

Turvey, B. E. (1999). *Criminal profiling: An introduction to behavioral evidence analysis*. London: Academic Press.

Ursano, R. J., Bell, C., Eth, S., Friedman, M., Norwood, A., Pfefferbaum, B., et al. (2004). Practice guideline for the treatment of patients with acute stress disorder and posttraumatic stress disorder. *American Journal of Psychiatry, 161*(11 Suppl.), 3–31.

Westrup, D., & Fremouw, W. J. (1998). Stalking behavior: A literature review and suggested functional analytic assessment technology. *Aggression and Violent Behavior, 3*(3), 255–274.

Westrup, D., Fremouw, W. J., Thompson, R. N., & Lewis, S. F. (1999). The psychological impact of stalking on female undergraduates. *Journal of Forensic Science, 44*(3), 554–557.

Winston, A., Rosenthal, R., & Pinsker, H. (Eds.). (2004). *Introduction to supportive psychotherapy.* Washington, DC: American Psychiatric Press.

Zona, M. A., Palarea, R. E., & Lane, J. C. (1998). Psychiatric diagnosis and the offender-victim typology of stalking. In J. R. Meloy (Ed.), *The psychology of stalking: Clinical and forensic perspectives* (pp. 69–84). San Diego: Academic Press.

PART III

Stalking and the Law

6   Trends in Antistalking Legislation

David J. Kapley
John R. Cooke

This chapter examines antistalking statutes in the United States and abroad. All state and the federal governments have adopted legal mechanisms to address stalking. These enactments attest to the growing awareness of stalking with its associated suffering and economic losses. The statutes are remarkable for both their innovation and their diversity, as different jurisdictions have chosen a wide variety of approaches. In the United States, this variety can be attributed in part to the division of lawmaking power inherent in federalism, as well as linked to the challenging nature of a problem whose characteristics and effects are just now coming into focus. International legal strategies also vary. In both U.S. and international statutes, criminal law is most often invoked, but civil remedies are increasing. The latter includes injunctions and protection orders, as well as civil rights of action, notice provisions, stalker surveillance, stalker registries, victim compensation, and mental health evaluations and treatment.

INTRODUCTION

The murder of the television actress Rebecca Schaeffer in 1989 drew a great deal of media attention to the problem of stalking; in 1990 California became the first state to adopt an antistalking law. The movement progressed rapidly: by 1996, all 50 state legislatures and the U.S. Congress had passed antistalking legislation.

There is considerable variation in the existing antistalking laws. Academic commentators have raised questions concerning the constitutionality of these laws under the state and federal constitutions. Early concerns were that limiting a stalker's contact with his victim might unreasonably intrude on the stalker's First Amendment rights of free speech and assembly. Statutes were criticized as being vague and overbroad in limiting these rights (Faulkner & Hsiao, 1993). In general, however, state courts have not been receptive to such claims (see, e.g., *Bouters v. State*, 1995). For example, the Supreme Court of Montana upheld the constitutionality of that state's antistalking statute against an argument that the law violated the defendant's free speech rights, finding that the law was not unconstitutionally vague since certain undefined terms had an accepted common usage (*State v. Martel*, 1995). In a separate case, the same court rejected another First Amendment attack, finding the statute did not reach constitutionally protected activity (*State v. Helfrich*, 1996). As a separate concern, Pathé, Mackenzie, and Mullen (2004) commented on the potential that certain aspects of stalking statutes could be manipulated by stalkers, placing the victim at greater risk. Nevertheless, stalking statutes have become prominent in the United States and elsewhere.

Antistalking laws can be arranged in three groups: (1) criminal statutes; (2) statutes containing criminal provisions with an added, but narrow, approach in the civil law; and (3) statutes with a comprehensive approach. The first group focuses on punishment of the stalker. The second adds the civil remedy of injunction. The third group provides remedies additional to injunction, imprisonment, and fines. The trend among the states has been toward comprehensively combining criminal and civil provisions. Specific interpretation of each statute is left to the individual state and federal governments.

Clinicians who work with stalkers or victims should be aware of the stalking laws of their own jurisdictions. The purpose of this chapter is to address the common themes in antistalking laws (also referred to as stalking laws), as well as to convey a sense of the range of variation. The chapter is not intended to be a complete catalog of current law, a task that would be outdated quickly in any event because laws can change rapidly. Rather, statutes will be cited to provide examples of the themes that are relevant to the chapter. The chapter is not a substitute for advice from a competent, licensed attorney. We recommend that the reader seek competent legal counsel if the reader has legal questions.

STATE CRIMINAL STATUTES

In this chapter, state statutes are referred to by the names of their respective states. Specific citations can be found in the reference section. A minority of states have exclusively criminal provisions. Criminal law remedies against stalking can be broken down into several common elements, handled differently in individual jurisdictions.

Elements of Stalking

Criminal statutes define stalking in a number of ways. Typical elements, listed in Table 6.1, include: (1) repeated proscribed acts ("course of conduct") by the stalker; (2) a certain mental state on the part of the stalker; (3) a threat, often defined as "credible," which some statutes say may be "either expressed or implied," or some other offensive behavior; and (4) a reaction of the victim, often with

Table 6.1. Typical Elements in State Stalking Statutes

- Repeated proscribed acts ("course of conduct") by the stalker
- Required mental state of the stalker
- Threats or other prohibited behavior
- Required mental state of the victim

the added requirement that the reaction be a "reasonable" fear, and sometimes a fear "of death or serious bodily harm."

Statutes commonly require repeated acts or a "course of conduct" by the stalker (see, e.g., Alabama, Arizona). In some statutes, a threshold must be reached, such as two or more acts (South Carolina), or three or more acts (Delaware). Some states require that the acts occur within a certain time period (South Carolina). In certain state statutes, the repeated acts of the stalker must be both within a certain period of time and separated by a different period of time (Arkansas).

Statutes vary in the mental state required of the stalker. Some provide that the stalker must act intentionally, willfully, or maliciously (see, e.g., Alabama, Connecticut, Florida). Accordingly, such laws do not necessarily reach the stalker who only wishes to reestablish an actual or fantasized relationship with the victim, wishes the victim no harm, and makes no threat, expressed or implied. Other states require only that the stalker act recklessly (Connecticut, Hawaii), knowingly, or even negligently (Washington). Connecticut statutes incorporate both requirements to distinguish varying degrees of stalking behavior. A statute may expressly state that it is no defense if the stalker did not intend to frighten, intimidate, or harass the victim (Washington). Still other statutes allow the mental state of the stalker to differ in the separate elements of the crime. For example, Alaska provides that stalking occurs if the stalker "knowingly engages in a course of conduct that recklessly places" the victim in certain fearful situations described in the statute. Thus, the stalker must know that he is committing the acts; but he is not required to know that the acts have resulted in reasonable fear in the victim, if he recklessly induces that fear.

Statutes typically define a variety of prohibited acts or threats. Some require acts that lead to fear of death or serious physical injury (see, e.g., Alabama, Alaska). Arkansas sets a higher level of intimidation and requires that the stalker "make . . . a terrorist threat" concerning "imminent fear of death or serious bodily injury" toward the victim or an immediate family member.

Not all states require that the victim or a family member of the victim be in fear of death or serious physical injury. Some states proscribe the infliction of substantial emotional distress upon the victim if a reasonable person would suffer such distress (see, e.g., Colorado). In Idaho, a defendant who knowingly and maliciously "engages in a course of conduct that seriously alarms, annoys, or harasses the victim and is such as would cause a reasonable person substantial emotional distress" is guilty of stalking. Other states have used this broader concept of stalking to prohibit repeated behavior that would induce in the victim reasonable fears that could thereby lead to emotional distress (Utah).

It is common for statutes to require that the reaction of the victim be reasonable (see, e.g., Arizona, Idaho). Sometimes statutes mandate that a victim demonstrate a subjective and an objective reaction. In other words, the victim must in fact have the fears required by the statute, whereas a reasonable victim would have had the fears required by the statute as well (Arizona).

At the time of this writing, Hawaii appears to be the state that requires the least effect on the victim. The stalker must act "with intent to harass, annoy or alarm another person, or in reckless disregard of the risk." There must be "a course of conduct involving pursuit, surveillance, or nonconsensual contact" "on more than one occasion without legitimate purpose." Nonconsensual contact is broadly defined without any requirement of threat by the stalker or injury to the victim. Instead, it means contact "without that individual's consent or in disregard of that person's express desire that the contact be avoided or discontinued." Thus, the Hawaii statute appears to make criminal certain repeated, impolite, and annoying conversation once the victim has requested no further contact. A court might construe the statute as consistent with the First Amendment because it requires that the acts of the defendant serve no legitimate purpose.

Some states have statutes that combine harassment with stalking (see, e.g., Texas). Hawaii combines the two to create the crimes of harassment by stalking, a misdemeanor, and aggravated harassment by stalking, a felony. Other states use terms such as harassing in the definition of stalking (Georgia).

Degrees of Stalking

States often divide stalking into misdemeanor and felony offenses (see, e.g., Alaska, Connecticut, Hawaii), and, sometimes, into differing levels of felony offenses (Delaware). Felonies or more serious levels of felonies occur under differing circumstances, such as threat of death or serious physical injury (Delaware), "reasonable" fear of death or bodily injury to the victim or certain persons related to the victim (Florida), possession of a deadly weapon (Delaware, Idaho), violation of a court order (Delaware, Idaho), prior conviction for stalking (Delaware, Idaho, Massachusetts), violation of probation or parole (Alaska, Idaho), and age of the victim less than 16 (Florida, Idaho). The fines and imprisonment for stalking vary considerably among the states.

Some states use different levels of the defendant's mental state to distinguish different crimes of stalking. In Florida, for example, cyberstalking includes a course of conduct through electronic media that is directed against a specific person, that causes substantial distress to the person, and that does not have a legitimate purpose; such behavior is a misdemeanor when the defendant willfully, maliciously or repeatedly cyberstalks, whereas it constitutes the felony of aggravated stalking when the defendant cyberstalks and makes a credible threat with the intent to place the victim or certain family members of the victim in reasonable fear of death or bodily injury. More information related to cyberstalking can be found in chapter 9.

Arizona defines two felonies of stalking according to the fear induced in the victim. The less serious felony occurs when the stalker causes the victim to reasonably fear for the safety of the victim or an immediate family member. The more serious felony occurs when the stalker causes the victim to reasonably fear for death of the victim or an immediate family member.

Other states consider prior offenses against the same victim not resulting in stalking to increase the seriousness of stalking and its punishment. In Idaho, a more serious form of stalking occurs when the defendant has been previously convicted of other serious offenses involving the same victim, such as poisoning, forcible sexual penetration with a foreign object, malicious harassment, or act of terrorism. In Georgia, each conviction for stalking after a prior conviction is a felony punishable by between 1 and 10 years in prison, but the more serious crime of aggravated stalking occurs when the defendant stalks after violating various court orders or conditions of release.

Burden of Proof and Prima Facie Evidence

States have adopted a variety of evidentiary rules in stalking cases. In Oklahoma, repeated contact after the victim requests no further contact creates a rebuttable presumption that the victim felt "terrorized, frightened, intimidated, threatened, harassed, or molested." The statute further specifies an extensive list of activities that constitute "unconsented contact."

The state of Washington specifies that there is prima facie (adequate without further proof) evidence that the defendant intends to frighten, intimidate, or harass if the defendant continues to have contact with the victim after notice that the victim does not want contact. In addition, the defendant violates the statute when the defendant knows or should know that the victim would be frightened—even if the defendant does not intend that result.

Peek v. State (2002), which affirmed the conviction of a stalker, illustrates evidentiary problems that can occur in stalking cases. In *Peek* the appeals court ruled that the jury was entitled to disbelieve the victim's sworn testimony at trial that she had wrongfully attacked the stalker, her boyfriend, when at the scene she had told a police officer that her boyfriend had been angry, dragged her from a car, kicked her, and punched her in the face. The court noted that at the scene the victim was tearful, upset, had facial bruises, and a large cut on her ankle.

Peek illustrates how facts can be sharply in dispute in stalking cases. Rules concerning burden of proof and prima facie evidence can help to determine the outcome in cases in which there are conflicting versions of what happened, especially when in court a victim recants prior allegations.

Law Enforcement Powers and Responsibilities

Various states use technology in prosecuting stalking. In Delaware, stalking is one of the crimes that justify electronic surveillance. Other states participate in electronic databases that track stalkers. For example, Georgia has adopted the Georgia Protective Order Registry, which provides a centralized database of protective orders in domestic violence and stalking cases. Police, prosecuting attorneys, and the courts have full access to the database, and it is linked to the National Crime Information Center Network.

The states differ considerably on whether a police officer may arrest a suspect for misdemeanor stalking not committed in the presence of that officer. Some states, such as Florida, give broad powers to the police, permitting an arrest without a warrant for misdemeanor and felony stalking if the police have probable cause to believe that a violation has occurred. In Idaho, the officer may arrest without a warrant for misdemeanor and felony stalking when the officer has probable cause "upon immediate response" to the report of a crime. In Mississippi, a law enforcement officer is entitled to arrest without a warrant for misdemeanor stalking only if the victim and the defendant are family or household members under the domestic violence statute.

Restrictions on the Release of the Defendant

Statutes address the issue of release of the defendant in criminal stalking cases at three stages of the proceeding: before conviction, after conviction, and after completion of sentence. In some states, courts have the power to jail the defendant before trial. In Georgia, only the superior court can set bail for serious offenses such as aggravated stalking; appeal bonds are not allowed after the defendant has been convicted. In Illinois, the court has the power to deny bail when "necessary to prevent fulfillment" of a real and present threat to the physical safety of the alleged victim."

An important concern in the forensic behavioral sciences is the defendant who is legally incompetent to stand trial, and who harms others after being released from custody. (See chapter 7 for an in-depth review of forensic evaluations related to competence to stand trial and criminal responsibility of stalkers.) Georgia provides that certain offenses, including aggravated stalking, trigger a statutory obligation for the criminal court to retain custody over the defendant who is likely to remain incompetent to stand trial. The statute calls for a hearing to determine whether the incompetent defendant meets criteria for involuntary civil commitment. The court may obtain independent forensic evaluation from a psychiatrist or a psychologist to assist with the determination. Even if the defendant does not meet criteria for involuntary commitment, the court may impose bond or other conditions before discharging the defendant.

Several states have placed limits on the ability to parole, find an alternative disposition for, or work release the convicted stalker. In Delaware, defendants guilty of stalking are not eligible for placement in boot camp and are not eligible for work release until 6 months before release from custody.

DOMESTIC VIOLENCE AND STALKING STATUTES

As discussed elsewhere in this chapter, there is a common connection between stalking and domestic violence. Studies have suggested that statutes related to domestic violence and stalking have been helpful in accomplishing ultimate prosecution (Logan, Nigoff, Walker, & Jordon 2002), but also may have some potential unintended consequences for victims (Romkens, 2006) warranting ongoing consideration for new interventions. Certain stalking legislative provisions appear to be grafted onto the definition of domestic violence. States accomplish this through a definition of domestic violence that includes stalking of a family or household member or stalking in other domestic situations. In some states, the victim of stalking involving domestic violence may enjoy more legal protection than the victim of stalking not involving domestic violence (see, e.g., Florida, Georgia). In such jurisdictions, injunctions authorized in domestic violence cases could be applied to some stalking behaviors. Georgia also provides for merger of violations during sentencing when the defendant's course of conduct is simultaneously a violation of the domestic violence and stalking law.

STALKING AND TECHNOLOGY

States are working to keep pace with use of technology by stalkers. Some states, such as Georgia, have defined crimes of cyberstalking. Numerous statutes proscribe the use of computers or electronic devices to stalk (see, e.g., Florida, Georgia, Idaho, Ohio). An uncommon statute in Idaho defines stalking to include allowing the telephone to ring repeatedly without having a conversation. As noted above, chapter 9 addresses cyberstalking in more detail.

STATES WITH CIVIL AND CRIMINAL
STATUTES ON STALKING

Some states have crafted more comprehensive remedies in stalking cases with the combination of criminal and civil law. Table 6.2 lists potential remedies that can be found in integrated stalking statutes. Injunctions can be available in criminal and civil cases.

Table 6.2. Remedies Seen in State Stalking Statutes

Common Remedies
- Criminal punishment of the stalker
- Injunctive relief (ex parte, temporary, permanent)

Less Common Remedies
- Victim's right to damages against the stalker
- Various other benefits to the victim
- Loss of other rights by the stalker

South Carolina is a prominent example of a state that provides comprehensive criminal and civil remedies. Mental health evaluations may be ordered after criminal conviction but before sentencing, or as a condition of bail. South Carolina has an extensive procedure for obtaining a temporary restraining order, even without notice to the defendant, for "good cause shown" if the plaintiff offers proof by a preponderance of the evidence, that is, "[a] prima facie showing of present danger of bodily injury, verified by supporting affidavits." Law enforcement officers shall arrest for violations of a restraining order after service and notice of the order, even if there is no arrest warrant. The statute establishes an important public policy: "The primary responsibility of a law enforcement officer when responding to . . . [a] stalking incident is to enforce the law and protect the alleged victim." South Carolina also provides limited immunity for a person who reports alleged stalking, files a criminal complaint, files a complaint for restraining order, or participates in a stalking case.

As in South Carolina, other states use injunctions and protective orders to bolster criminal and civil provisions. Such laws can contain unique provisions, such as:

- providing authority for injunctions of up to 10 years (California);
- requiring that notices on forms for obtaining restraining orders be printed in English and Spanish (California);
- specifying short time periods within which law enforcement agencies must act on protection orders (Georgia);
- awarding costs and attorneys fees (Michigan);
- requiring that the victim notify the court if the stalker is licensed to and required by occupation to carry a concealed weapon (Michigan);
- empowering a peace officer to arrest without warrant if the defendant does not immediately comply with the protection order or if there is reason to believe the defendant has violated a protection order (Michigan);
- establishing a plan for ordering and reviewing ex parte orders against the defendant (Ohio).

Montana and California are two other states that provide comprehensive remedies. In Montana, a court may issue a permanent order of protection in certain cases based on the history of violence of the stalker, the severity of the offense, and the evidence. The attorney general in Montana is obligated to provide forms for protective orders, which are required to conspicuously state the punishment for violating the order. The order must further state that the respondent must not violate the order "even if invited by" the alleged victim or another person. The court in California may base the restraining order "upon the seriousness of the facts before the court, the probability of future violations, and the safety of the victim and his or her immediate family."

Mental Health Evaluations

As stated in various sections of this book, evaluation and treatment of both stalker and victim can help decrease the incidence of stalking as well as symptoms in the stalker and victim. The GAP Committee on Psychiatry and the Law recommends a flexible system that provides the court with the power to order mental health and substance abuse evaluations and, when appropriate, treatment of the defendant. In our opinion, it is important to provide the flexibility to the court to order such evaluation and treatment at different stages of both civil and criminal proceedings: at the time of issuance of a temporary protective order and injunction; as a condition for bail; after conviction, as part of parole, probation, work release, and other disposition; and before release into the community, even after the sentence has been served. We further recommend that the court have the power to order mental health and substance abuse evaluations along with treatment of the victim if needed, as these types of mental health interventions, along with legal remedies, can decrease the recurrence of stalking and reduce symptoms in the victim.

As an adjunct to criminal remedies, a number of states authorize mental health evaluations of the defendant, typically permitting a judge to order the evaluation before sentencing (see, e.g., Georgia, South Carolina). Statutes can authorize psychological treatment as part of sentence, probation, or other disposition. Georgia authorizes the court to order a mental health evaluation as part of a protective order; South Carolina, as a condition of bail. Georgia further empowers the court to order mental health treatment for both stalker and victim.

Ohio has a descriptive statute for obtaining mental health evaluations in domestic violence and stalking cases. The statute organizes a framework to assess the risk of harm, violence, and threats posed by the stalker. The statute outlines the contents of the forensic report:

> [T]he findings of the examiner; the facts in reasonable detail on which the findings are based; the opinion of the examiner as to the mental condition of the defendant; the opinion of the examiner as to whether the

defendant represents a substantial risk of physical harm to other persons as manifested by evidence of recent homicidal or other violent behavior, evidence of recent threats that placed other persons in reasonable fear of violent behavior and serious physical harm, or evidence of present dangerousness; and the opinion of the examiner as to the types of treatment or counseling that the defendant needs. [Ohio Rev. Code Ann. §2919.271(D)]

Injunctive relief is not the only civil remedy that states have used in an attempt to curtail stalking. Other novel civil remedies include actions, claims, and other benefits for the victim; loss of the stalker's right to have a firearm; and loss of other civil liberties of the stalker.

Actions, Claims, and Other Benefits for the Victim

The usual approach in civil stalking laws has been to use protection orders and injunctions. Occasionally the victim has been granted a statutory right of damages against the stalker (Michigan). Damages in Michigan can include those that result from the stalking, exemplary (punitive) damages, costs of the action, and reasonable attorney fees. The civil action can exist even if the stalker was never charged in a criminal case.

In New York, victims of stalking can receive payments from a state crime victim board. Payments can be awarded even when the victim has not been physically injured, and can include compensation for lost earnings, destroyed essential personal property, security devices, transportation expenses to court, unreimbursed counseling, and expenses for occupational training.

In certain situations Montana grants unemployment benefits to an employee who is a victim or whose child is a victim of stalking. The employer's account is not to be charged under the statute, however. Montana also protects stalking victims from exclusion or discrimination by an insurance company or a health maintenance organization. The statute also covers family members, household members, or intimate partners of stalkers.

In some states the victim of stalking can receive official help to conceal her location from the stalker. For example, Montana has a program to provide the victim with a substitute address to be used for "official purposes," such as receiving service of process and mail. The statute includes other protections, including that the victim may change his or her address for registering to vote, is entitled to a substitute address card, and can request that his or her residential address not be placed on the list of registered voters. There is even a limited confidential privilege between advocate and victim, such as between an employee or volunteer at a domestic shelter and a victim of stalking by a partner or family member.

Notification to the Victim of the Stalker's Release From Custody

A thoughtful but seldom recognized right is notification to the victim of the stalker's release from custody. Some statutes mandate that the victim (and others, such as witnesses) be notified verbally and in writing when the stalker is released from custody. The Georgia statute provides that notification shall be on a landline telephone, not a pocket pager or a cell phone, and describes in detail when and how many attempts will be made to contact the victim by telephone. The statutes commonly state that violation of the notice requirement does not confer civil liability on the custodian of the stalker for damages suffered by the victim. The Georgia statute, however, does provide that the custodian who fails to warn the victim "shall be subject to appropriate disciplinary action, including termination for such failure."

Washington State has a detailed plan for notification of the release of a juvenile stalker requiring that notice must be given to the victim, the chief of police, the sheriff, and the school board. Under the law the victim shall receive notice if the victim makes a request for notification.

Loss of Stalker's Right to Have a Firearm

Several states deny a stalker access to a firearm. In Oklahoma, a prior misdemeanor conviction under the stalking law prevents the stalker from having the right to a handgun license. Other states specify different violations of the stalking laws that lead to revocation of the right to have a firearm (see, e.g., New York, Washington).

In Georgia, loss of the right to bear a firearm occurs after conviction for a "forcible felony," a term defined in the statute to include aggravated stalking, which occurs when the defendant stalks in violation of various court orders, injunctions, bonds, or conditions or release. The first-offense stalker does not automatically lose the right to bear a firearm unless he uses the threat of physical force or violence or commits one of the other violent offenses listed as a "forcible felony."

Loss of Other Civil Liberties of the Stalker

A few states have imposed other restrictions on the civil liberties of stalkers. In Minnesota, a stalking conviction can require that the stalker prove he or she is entitled to custody in a child custody dispute involving the stalker, and that a guardian be appointed to protect the interests of the child. There is a requirement in the statute for the transfer of custody rights if the stalker is convicted of certain forms of felony stalking. A Missouri law prevents a parent who is otherwise entitled to custody of a child from obtaining custody if the parent has a history of stalking within the previous 5 years.

In New Jersey, a convicted stalker is forbidden from working in a wide variety of occupations, including teacher, school physician, school nurse, and other workers at school. There is a complicated provision requiring that bureaucrats in the education system make certain background checks of applicants for those positions.

An uncommon provision is the requirement for publication of second and subsequent convictions of stalking as a legal notice (see, e.g., Georgia). The law requires publication of name, address, and photograph of the stalker, as well as date, place, and time of arrest. The publisher of the notice has a limited immunity for errors made in good faith.

FEDERAL STATUTES

The federal interstate stalking statute was first passed in 1996, during the administration of President Bill Clinton. On January 5, 2006, President George W. Bush signed into law the *Violence Against Women and Department of Justice Reauthorization Act of 2005*, which greatly expanded the power of the federal government to prosecute stalking. The law passed with overwhelming approval in Congress. This act contains provisions to combat stalking, cyberstalking, violence against women, domestic violence, and date violence. It also provides funding for various government endeavors, such as annual grants of three million dollars from 2007 through 2011 to fund the national stalking database. The largest expansion of federal power concerning stalking was in the amendment of the interstate stalking statute, 18 U.S.C. § 2261A.

Section 2261A has two primary stalking provisions. The first applies to the defendant who travels in interstate commerce or certain other locations within federal jurisdiction. The second applies to the defendant whose victim is in a different state or a different location within federal jurisdiction when that defendant makes use of certain entities, such as the mail, the Internet, or any facility of interstate or foreign commerce. Section 2261A(1) addresses interstate travel:

> Whoever—
> (1) travels in interstate or foreign commerce or within the special maritime and territorial jurisdiction of the United States, or enters or leaves Indian country, with the intent to kill, injure, harass, or place under surveillance with intent to kill, injure, harass, or intimidate another person, and in the course of, or as a result of, such travel places that person in reasonable fear of the death of, or serious bodily injury to, or causes substantial emotional distress to that person, a member of the immediate family (as defined in

section 115 [18 U.S.C. § 115]) of that person, or the spouse or intimate partner of that person . . . shall be punished as provided in section 2261(b) of this title [18 U.S.C. § 2261(b)].

The 1996 federal statute against interstate stalking was narrower in scope. Under the 1996 version of the statute it was necessary that the victim be in reasonable fear of death or serious bodily injury to the victim or a member of the victim's immediate family. In 2000, the statute was expanded. Under the 2000 version and the current version of the statute, a defendant commits interstate stalking when the defendant travels interstate, in foreign commerce, or within certain other federal locations; has an intent to kill, injure, harass, or intimidate another person; and, in the course of, or as a result of, that travel, places in reasonable fear of death or serious bodily injury that person or the close relation of that person as defined by the statute.

One major change in the current law of Section 2261A(1) is to make criminal the infliction of "substantial emotional distress" in the victim or close relation. According to the office of Senator Domenici (2005), a cosponsor of the law, the language regarding substantial emotional distress was borrowed from state stalking laws. Another change in the current law is the prohibition against surveillance of the victim, which the senator's office further noted was designed to make illegal stalking through the use of technology such as global positioning systems.

Section 2261A(2) addresses the defendant who does not travel interstate:

(2) [Whoever] with the intent—

   (A) to kill, injure, harass, or place under surveillance with intent to kill, injure, harass, or intimidate, or cause substantial emotional distress to a person in another State or tribal jurisdiction or within the special maritime and territorial jurisdiction of the United States; or

   (B) to place a person in another State or tribal jurisdiction, or within the special maritime and territorial jurisdiction of the United States, in reasonable fear of the death of, or serious bodily injury to-

    (i) that person;

    (ii) a member of the immediate family (as defined in section 115 [18 U.S.C. § 115] of that person; or

    (iii) a spouse or intimate partner of that person;

    uses the mail, any interactive computer service, or any facility of interstate or foreign commerce to engage in a course of conduct that causes substantial emotional distress to that person or places that person in reasonable fear of the death of, or serious bodily injury to, any of the persons described in clauses (i) through (iii) of subparagraph (B); shall be punished as provided in section 2261(b) of this title [18 U.S.C. § 2261(b)].

Criminal liability under this subsection is imposed on a defendant who acts with either of two criminal intents when the defendant uses the mail, any interactive computer service, or any facility of interstate or foreign commerce and engages in "a course of conduct" that causes substantial emotional distress to, or reasonable fear of death of, or serious bodily injury to, the victim or the victim's close relation, and the victim is in another state or in certain federal locations. The first illegal mental state is the intent "to kill, injure, harass, or place under surveillance with intent to kill, injure, harass, or intimidate, or cause substantial emotional distress" to the victim. The second illegal mental state is the intent to place the victim or the close relation "in reasonable fear" of death or serious bodily injury.

Intent to kill is not required to violate Section 2261A(2). For example, the defendant, intending to "harass," need only use the mail or the Internet "to engage in a course of conduct that causes substantial emotional distress" for the victim. This is a broad increase of federal power, which, to our knowledge, has yet to be fully tested in the federal courts.

A related and substantial addition to federal power under the 2005 *Violence Against Women Act* was an amendment to criminalize the use of the Internet in interstate or foreign communications when the defendant acts anonymously, even if there has been no actual communication, if the defendant intends "to annoy, abuse, threaten, or harass" the victim (47 U.S.C. § 223(a)(1)(C)). This law, which resembles some of the state harassment statutes, shows the overlapping interests between antiharassment and stalking legislation in both the federal and state law.

Federal Punishment and Restitution

The federal prohibition against interstate stalking is parallel with the federal prohibition against interstate domestic violence. The criminal penalties are fines and a multitiered system of imprisonment based upon factors including the victim's death, differing levels of injury to the victim, or the use of a dangerous weapon by the defendant. Prison terms vary from 5 years to life (18 U.S.C. § 2261(b)). A prior domestic violence or stalking conviction doubles the maximum sentence allowed under federal law (18 U.S.C. § 2265A). The 2005 *Violence Against Women Act* further amended the sentencing statute to increase to 1 year the minimum punishment for violating a protective order in a stalking case (18 U.S.C. § 2261(b)). A pattern of stalking (two or more separate incidents), in addition, increases the term of imprisonment under federal sentencing guidelines (18 U.S.C. § 2A6.2). There is another independent crime of interstate violation of a protection order, which occurs when the defendant travels into certain locations within federal jurisdiction while violating a domestic violence or stalking protection order (18 U.S.C. § 2262).

Victims of interstate domestic violence or interstate stalking have a mandatory right to restitution from the defendant in addition to other civil and criminal remedies. The statute contains a long list of victim losses that the defendant must pay, including, but not limited to, "medical services relating to physical, psychiatric, or psychological care" (18 U.S.C. § 2264(b)(3)(A)).

Federal Procedure

In a federal case of interstate stalking, the court may not release a defendant before trial without providing to the alleged victim "an opportunity to be heard regarding the danger posed by the defendant" (18 U.S.C. § 2263). Federal law maps out in detail a procedure whereby protection orders from one state, tribal, or territorial court shall be enforced in another state, tribal, or territorial court (18 U.S.C. § 2265). This statutory approach helps to ensure that valid state protection orders against stalking will have full faith and credit in the courts of another state, as required by the U.S. Constitution. Federal law prohibits state, tribal, and territorial courts from publishing protection orders on the Internet if the publication "would be likely to publicly reveal the identity or location" of the person to be protected (18 U.S.C. § 2265).

Other Federal Laws Concerning Stalking

Not all federal laws are limited to the prohibition against interstate stalking. There are numerous federal programs to help address the problem of stalking even if such stalking is not interstate in scope, such as: legal assistance for victims of stalking (42 U.S.C. § 3796gg-6); grants to state and local governments concerning the recording of stalking data in a national system (42 U.S.C. § 14031); and grants to combat violent crimes against women on campuses, including stalking (42 U.S.C. § 14045b).

In some limited circumstances, a seller of firearms is prohibited from selling to stalkers. For example, a gun dealer may not sell a firearm to a stalker if there is a type of state protection order that forbids stalking of an intimate partner or a child of an intimate partner of the stalker (18 U.S.C. § 922(d)). The seller may be forbidden to sell to other stalkers, such as those convicted of misdemeanor domestic violence or of crimes punishable by imprisonment for more than 1 year.

FOREIGN STATUTES

Stalking laws are not unique to the United States. As an example of their development around the world, we turn now to consider selected statutes in the common law jurisdictions of the United Kingdom, Canada, and Australia. In the United Kingdom, the relevant enactment is the *Protection From Harassment Act 1997*. (For further review of this statute, see also Infield & Platford, 2002.) In Canada, it is Chapter 264 of the Canadian Criminal Code. All states of Australia have passed stalking laws; in this chapter we, however, will look to the most comprehensive of those laws, Chapter 33A of the Queensland Criminal Code 1899.

Elements

United Kingdom: The Protection From Harassment Act 1997

England and Wales, on the one hand, and Scotland, on the other, offer diverging solutions for the problem of stalking. (In this chapter England also refers to Wales because both England and Wales adopt the same sections in the act.) The act uses concepts such as harassment and fear of violence instead of defining stalking as in the statutes of the states and the federal government in the United States.

England and Scotland have important similarities and differences in their statutes. England and Scotland adopt a similarly defined civil action of harassment. England, but not Scotland, creates a crime of harassment, and a crime related to putting people in fear of violence. England further makes criminal the violation of protection orders against harassment and putting people in fear of violence. In Scotland there is a similar offense of breach of non-harassment order, which has different standards from the English crimes.

Scotland has an unusual position on account of the Scottish refusal to make a crime of harassment. As this chapter demonstrates, a common pattern in statutes is the creation of crimes against stalking, with some jurisdictions adding civil remedies onto the criminal law. In Scotland, however, it is the reverse; there is a basic civil remedy against stalking, which is the civil action of harassment. The criminal law in Scotland is invoked only after the defendant breaches a non-harassment order. An apparent philosophy, as expressed in the Scottish statute, is that harassment is first an issue for the civil, not the criminal, law.

In England, harassment is generally described as a course of conduct that amounts to harassment, which the defendant knows or ought to know amounts to harassment. The reference for culpability is whether a reasonable person in possession of the same information would think that the course of conduct would amount to harassment of another. In contrast to the English definition of harassment, the civil action of harassment in Scotland occurs only when the defendant intended the harassment.

In England and Scotland harassment is not fully defined, but instead includes causing "alarm" or "distress." The statutes that apply to England and Scotland have similar references to conduct, as including "speech," and course of conduct as requiring at least "two occasions."

In England the offense of putting people in fear of violence occurs when the defendant shows a course of conduct that causes someone else to fear on at least two occasions that violence will be used against that person if on each of those two occasions the defendant knew or ought to have to have known that his course of conduct would have caused the fear. Again, the reference is whether a reasonable person in possession of the same information would think that the course of conduct would cause the other to so fear on that occasion.

Canada

Under Chapter 264 of the Canadian Criminal Code, "No person shall, without lawful authority and knowing that another person is harassed or recklessly [*sic*] as to whether the other person is harassed, engage in conduct" that causes the other person "reasonably, in all the circumstances," to fear for his or her safety or the safety of anyone known to him or her. The prohibited conduct consists of:

a. repeatedly following from place to place the other person or anyone known to them;
b. repeatedly communicating with, either directly or indirectly, the other person or anyone known to them;
c. besetting or watching the dwelling-house, or place where the other person, or anyone known to them, resides, works, carries on business or happens to be; or
d. engaging in threatening conduct directed at the other person or any member of their family.

Australia

Under the Chapter 33A of the Queensland Criminal Code, "[u]nlawful stalking" is "conduct" directed at "the stalked person" engaged in on more than one occasion (or one occasion if the conduct is "protracted") consisting of one or more acts (or "similar" acts) of the following types:

i. following, loitering near, watching or approaching a person;
ii. contacting a person in any way, including, for example, by telephone, mail, fax, e-mail or through the use of any technology;

    iii. loitering near, watching, approaching or entering a place where a person lives, works or visits;

    iv. leaving offensive material where it will be found by, given to or brought to the attention of, a person;

    v. giving offensive material to a person, directly or indirectly;

    vi. an intimidating, harassing or threatening act against a person, whether or not involving violence or a threat of violence;

    vii. an act of violence, or threat of violence, against, or against property of, anyone, including the defendant.

It is also required that the conduct:

    i. would cause the stalked person apprehension or fear, reasonably arising in all the circumstances, of violence to, or against property of, the stalked person or another person; or

    ii. causes detriment, reasonably arising in all the circumstances, to the stalked person or another person.

The act broadly defines "circumstances" and "property." "Violence" also has an expansive definition, but does not include "any force or impact" within the limits of what is acceptable as "incidental to social interaction or to life in the community."

"Detriment" to the stalked person includes the following:

    a. apprehension or fear of violence to, or against property of, the stalked person or another person;

    b. serious mental, psychological or emotional harm;

    c. prevention or hindrance from doing an act a person is lawfully entitled to do; compulsion to do an act a person is lawfully entitled to abstain from doing.

The following examples of detriment are provided (emphasis deleted):

A person no longer walks outside the person's place of residence or employment.

A person significantly changes the route or form of transport the person would ordinarily use to travel to work or other places . . .

A person sells property the person would not otherwise sell.

Notwithstanding the ostensible requirement of specific intent, the act states that it is immaterial whether the defendant "intends that the stalked person be aware that the conduct is directed" at the victim, is "mistaken about the identity" of the victim, or intends "to cause apprehension or fear, or the detriment." In fact, it is immaterial "whether the apprehension or fear, or the violence" is "actually caused." In addition, it is immaterial whether "the conduct directed at the stalked person consists of conduct carried out in relation to another person or property of another person" or whether the proscribed course of conduct, protracted or otherwise, "consists of the same or different acts."

Defenses

United Kingdom

For all defenses in England and Scotland the burden of proof lies with the defendant. The first two defenses in England under the harassment and fear-of-violence provisions are the same:

  a. that [the course of conduct] was pursued for the purpose of preventing or detecting crime, [or]
  b. that [the course of conduct] was pursued under any enactment or rule of law or to comply with any condition or requirement imposed by any person under any enactment. . . .

England further allows a defense under the harassment provision that in the particular circumstances the course of conduct was reasonable. Scotland has essentially adopted these three defenses in the Scottish civil action of harassment. The English fear-of-violence section has a similar defense that the course of conduct was reasonable for the protection of the defendant or another or the protection of the defendant's or another's property. England allows a defense of reasonable excuse for not following a protection order. The Scottish section, however, does not expressly allow reasonable excuse for breach of a non-harassment order.

A related issue is the provision for a certificate from the secretary of state, which applies in England and Scotland. A person's conduct described in the certificate is "conclusive evidence" that there is no violation of the act, if the actions of the person related to: "(a) national security, (b) the economic well-being of the United Kingdom, (c) the prevention or detection of serious crime. . . ."

Canada

The Canadian act has no express defenses.

Australia

It is not stalking under Chapter 33A of the Queensland Criminal Code to engage in "reasonable conduct" for a lawful trade, business or occupation, or "reasonable conduct" by a person to obtain or give information in which that person has a legitimate interest. Under the Australian act, unlawful stalking does not include the following:

    a. acts done in the execution of a law or administration of an Act or for a purpose authorised by an Act;

    b. acts done for the purposes of a genuine industrial dispute;

    c. acts done for the purposes of a genuine political or other genuine public dispute or issue carried on in the public interest.

Punishment

United Kingdom

In England a conviction under the harassment section is punishable by up to 6 months imprisonment and/or a fine. The punishment on conviction of indictment for the English fear-of-violence provision is imprisonment up to 5 years and/or a fine. Punishment for a breach of a protective order in England is also 5 years and/or a fine. The court may also issue a restraining order.

The Scottish statute initially defines harassment as only creating a civil action of harassment, in which the court may award damages as well as a "non-harassment order," which functions as an injunction. If the defendant violates the non-harassment order, then such a crime may be punished by conviction on indictment by imprisonment up to 5 years and/or a fine.

Canada

A conviction under the act is punishable by imprisonment of up to 10 years. Aggravating factors that must be considered by the court are whether the defendant's behavior contravened an order issued under a separate provision prohibiting his contact with children under the age of 14 or contravened another provision regarding orders of protection.

Australia

The maximum sentence under the Queensland act for a conviction is 5 years but can be extended to 7 years if the defendant threatens to use violence, illegally possesses a weapon, or violates or threatens to violate a court order. The court has broad powers under the act to issue a restraining order against the accused "whether he is found guilty or not guilty or the prosecution ends in another way."

A person who knowingly contravenes a restraining order can be imprisoned for up to 1 year.

Civil Remedies

United Kingdom

Under the English harassment section of the act, an "actual or apprehended" breach of the act confers a civil right of action on the person "who is or may be the victim of the course of conduct in question." Recovery can include, among other things, damages for "anxiety" and financial losses. The trial court may issue an injunction in support of the action and, if the victim concludes that the defendant has violated that order, he or she may seek an arrest warrant for the stalker. In England the fear-of-violence section confers no express civil cause of action.

As mentioned earlier, a similar civil action of harassment exists in the Scottish section of the act, with a major difference being that there is no Scottish crime of harassment, but instead, only a crime of violation of a non-harassment order. Damages under the Scottish action of harassment are for resulting anxiety and any financial loss.

Canada

The act has no express provision for a civil remedy.

Australia

The Queensland act has no express provision for a civil remedy.

CONCLUSION

The state and federal jurisdictions differ considerably on the definition and prosecution of stalking, as well as on the associated civil remedies available to the victim and related persons. In the United States a long-embraced tradition of federalism influences the creativity of the state statutes. In 2005, the U.S. federal government borrowed from the states during an amendment that increased the power of the federal government to punish and prevent interstate antistalking. Foreign nations have also enacted divergent stalking laws. A parallel process existed in the United States and the United Kingdom: lawmakers fashioned both similar and different antistalking remedies in connected political entities—the states and the federal government in the United States, and England and Scotland in the United Kingdom. We believe this reflects the nascent character of this jurisprudence.

In the opinion of our Committee on Psychiatry and the Law, an integrated approach is to be preferred. A statutory scheme that is comprehensive, with roots in the criminal and civil law, allows important flexibility. The prosecutor can select criminal or civil solutions, whereas a victim of stalking can directly assert rights in civil court. Mental health evaluations and treatment of both the stalker and victim can play an important role at different stages in criminal and civil proceedings. This approach can also attend to the protection of constitutional rights of the defendant in both civil and criminal court.

ACKNOWLEDGMENT

Dr. Kapley is grateful to his wife, Trudy Nelson Kapley, JD, and their daughter, Sarah, for assistance in preparing the manuscript.

REFERENCES

Ala. Code §§ 13-A6–90, 13-A6–92(a) (LexisNexis 2005).
Alaska Stat. §§ 11.41.260(a)(2)(3), 11.41.270(a) (LexisNexis 2006).
Ariz. Rev. Stat. § 13–2923.A, B, C.1 (LexisNexis 2006).
Ark. Code Ann. § 5–71–229(a)(1),(d)(1)(A) (LexisNexis 2006).
Bouters v. State, 659 So.2d 235 (Fla. 1995), *cert. denied* 516 U.S. 894 (1995).
Cal. [Pen.] Code §§ 15–646.9(f),(k), 646.91 (LexisNexis 2006).
Canada Criminal Code, R.S.C., ch. C-46, § 264 (LexisNexis 2006).
Colo. Rev. Stat. § 18–9-111 (LexisNexis 2005).
Conn. Gen. Stat. § 53a-181d, -181e (LexisNexis 2004).
Criminal Code (Stalking) Amendment Act, 1999, ch. 33A (Queensl. Cons. Acts). Retrieved February 7, 2007 from http://www.legislation.qld.gov.au/ LEGISLTN/ACTS/1999/99AC018.pdf
Del. Code Ann. tit.11, §§ 1312A(e)(f), 2402(c)(3), 2405(1), 6533(d), 6705(b)(3) (LexisNexis 2005).
Domenici, P., Office of. (2005). *Congress votes to extend* Violence Against Women Act *through 2011*. Washington: States News Service.
Faulkner, R. P., & Hsiao, D. H. (1993). And where you go I'll follow: The constitutionality of antistalking laws and proposed model legislation. *Harvard Journal on Legislation, 31*, 1–62.
Fla. Stat. Ann. §§ 741.28, 741.30, 784.048(1–7) (LexisNexis 2005).
Ga. Code Ann. §§ 16–3-1740, -1760, -1800, -1810(A), -1820, -1840, 16–5-90(a)(1),(c)(d), 16–5-91(a), 16–5-93(b),(c)(2),(i), 16–5-94(d)(3)(4),

16–5-95(c), 16–5-96, 16–11–131(e), 17–6-1(a)(12),(g), 17–7-130(e)(2)(A)(x), 19–13–1(2), 19–13–52(a)(d) (LexisNexis 2005).

Haw. Rev. Stat. Ann. §§ 711–1106.4, -1106.5 (LexisNexis 2005).

Idaho Code Ann. §§ 18–7905, -7906, 19–603.6 (LexisNexis 2006).

725 Ill. Comp. Stat. Ann. § 5/110–4(a) (LexisNexis 2005).

Infield, P., & Platford, G. (2002). Stalking and the law. In J. Boon & L. Sheridan (Eds.), *Stalking and psychosexual obsession: Psychological perspectives for prevention, policing and treatment* (pp. 221–235). West Sussex, UK: Wiley.

Logan, T. K., Nigoff, A., Walker, R., & Jordon, C. (2002). Stalker profiles with and without protective orders: Reoffending or criminal justice processing? *Violence and Victims, 17,* 541–553.

Mass. Ann. Laws ch. 265, §43 (LexisNexis 2005).

Mich. Comp. Laws Serv. §§ 600.2950(2),(22), 600.2954 (LexisNexis 2005).

Minn. Stat. Ann. §§ 211.037(3), 518.179, 609.749, 631.152–1,-2 (15) (LexisNexis 2005).

Miss. Code Ann. §§ 97–3-107, 99–3-7(5) (LexisNexis 2005).

Mo. Rev. Stat. § 211.037(3) (LexisNexis 2006).

Mont. Code Ann. §§ 33–18–216(1)(3)(6), 39–51–2111, 45–5-220 (LexisNexis 2005).

N.J. Stat. Ann. §§2C:12–10, 18A6–7.1 (LexisNexis 2005).

N.Y. [Exec.] Law § 631; [Fam. Ct. Act] §842-a (LexisNexis 2005).

Ohio Rev. Code Ann. §§ 2903.211, 2919.26(D)(2), 2919.271(D) (LexisNexis 2006).

Okla. Stat. tit. 21, §§ 1173.E,F4, 1290.10.5c (LexisNexis 2005).

Pathé, M., Mackenzie, R., & Mullen, P. E. (2004). Stalking by law: Damaging victims and rewarding offenders. *Journal of Law and Medicine, 12,* 103–111.

Peek v. State, 259 Ga. App. 13, 576 S.E. 2d 31 (2002).

Protection from Harassment Act, 1997, ch. 40 (Eng.). Retrieved February 7, 2007, from http://www.opsi.gov.uk/acts/acts1997/1997040.htm

Romkens, R. (2006). Protecting prosecution: Exploring the powers of law in an intervention program for domestic violence. *Violence Against Women, 12,* 160–186.

S.C. Code Ann. §§ 16–3-1700(b), (D), 1720, 1740, 1840 (LexisNexis 2004).

State v. Helfrich, 277 Mont. 452, 922 P.2d 1159 (1996).

State v. Martel, 273 Mont. 143, 902 P2d 14 (1995).

Tex. [Penal] Code Ann. §§ 42.07, 42.072(b) (LexisNexis 2005).

18 U.S.C. §§ 2A6.2, 115, 922(d), 2261, 2261A, 2261(b), 2262, 2263, 2264(b)(3)(A), 2265, 2265A (LexisNexis 2006).

42 U.S.C. §§ 3796 gg-6, 14031, 14045b (LexisNexis 2006).

47 U.S.C. § 223(a)(1)(C) (LexisNexis 2006).

Utah Code Ann. §76–5-106.5 (LexisNexis 2005).

Violence Against Women and Department of Justice Reauthorization Act of 2005, Pub. L. No. 109–62 (2006).

Wash. Rev. Code Ann. §§ 9A.46.110(2)(d), 9.41.040(1)(b),13.40.215 (LexisNexis 2005).

7   Stalking, Competence to Stand Trial, and Criminal Responsibility

Douglas Mossman

In the 1990s, stalking emerged as a new category of criminal offense and a distinct type of disordered behavior. A substantial fraction of stalkers suffer from delusional disorders or other severe mental illnesses, and many persons charged criminally with stalking adduce irrational beliefs to explain and justify their conduct. Such beliefs pose special challenges for mental health professionals who assess or help restore an accused stalker's competence to stand trial, or who evaluate an accused stalker's criminal responsibility. This chapter explores the clinical and forensic problems that arise when severe psychiatric symptoms—in particular, disruptions in reality testing (e.g., erotomanic delusions)—affect legal determinations concerning competence to stand trial, *mens rea*, and insanity.

INTRODUCTION

The term "stalking" unites under a single rubric behavioral patterns that until recently might have been regarded variously as manifestations of erotomanic delusions (Esquirol, 1845/1976), harassment (Jason, Reicher, Easton, Neal, & Wilson, 1984), or quaint expressions of courtly love (Singer, 1987). Beginning in the early 1990s, a confluence of social trends and news events—including heightened fears of stranger violence, increasing fragility of interpersonal relationships, and the stalking and murder of actress Rebecca Shaeffer—led the English-speaking world to construe stalking as a major mental health problem and a new category of criminal offense (Mullen, Pathé, & Purcell, 2001a). In turn, the existence of stalking as a distinct offense led to increased public recognition of the problem and, in some jurisdictions, to the filing of an unexpectedly large number of criminal stalking charges (Nadkarni & Grubin, 2000).

The acts that constitute stalking bear a superficial similarity to common (if annoying) behaviors in which "normal" people engage and that may have roots in human evolution (Brüne, 2003). Familiar examples include awkward attempts to start a dating relationship, persistent and insistent requests for attention or services, and unwanted pursuit by a former lover who hopes to rekindle a relationship (Mullen, Pathé, Purcell, & Stuart, 1999; Mullen et al., 2001a). By contrast, the types of persistent stalking toward which antistalking laws are directed involve approaches and intrusions repeated over weeks, months, or even years, in which the victim reasonably experiences fear and psychological distress. (For further information regarding stalking statutes, see chapter 6.) In many cases, the stalkers' extreme behavior, and their reasons for it, raise questions about whether their acts are motivated by serious psychopathology. When a stalker's actions lead to criminal charges, the possible presence of mental illness may generate concerns about whether the defendant's thinking is so compromised as to impair his capacity to grasp the criminality of his behavior or to understand the legal proceedings against him.

Research suggests that a substantial fraction of stalkers suffer from delusional disorders or other severe mental illnesses (a topic discussed further in chapters 1 and 2 of this volume), and many defendants charged with stalking adduce irrational beliefs to explain and justify their behavior. Such beliefs pose special challenges for mental health professionals who assess or help restore an accused stalker's competence to stand trial, or who evaluate an accused stalker's criminal responsibility. This chapter explores the clinical and forensic problems that arise when severe psychiatric symptoms—in particular, disruptions in reality testing (e.g., erotomanic delusions)—affect legal determinations concerning competence to stand trial, *mens rea*, and insanity.

STALKING AND PSYCHOPATHOLOGY

Clinicians who evaluate or treat defendants charged with stalking should recognize that such individuals often suffer from one or more forms of diagnosable mental disorders. Research suggests that one-third to one-half of stalkers referred to forensic psychiatry clinics have personality disorders, the most common types being paranoid, dependent, narcissistic, or antisocial (Mullen, Pathé, & Purcell, 2001b; Rosenfeld, 2003). In Mullen and colleagues' (1999) series, one-quarter of the stalkers had substance abuse disorders. More significant for our present purposes, however, is Mullen and colleagues' (1999) diagnosis of psychotic disorders in more than 40% of the stalkers whom they evaluated; a comparable proportion of the stalkers in Rosenfeld's (2003) series also suffered from psychoses. Defendants with psychoses constitute the subgroup of accused stalkers who are most likely to be compromised in their ability to understand the trial process or in their capacity to perceive why their alleged actions might give rise to criminal charges.

Among the several types of psychotic symptoms that are associated with stalking, erotomanic delusions are frequently encountered (Mullen et al., 2001b; Rosenfeld, 2003; Zona, Sharma, & Lane, 1993). In such cases, the stalker firmly believes that his persistent (but, in reality, unwanted) gestures, messages, or actions are directed toward someone who either is somehow responding affectionately to his behavior or will one day come to do so (Goldstein, 1978, 1987; Harmon, Rosner, & Owens, 1995; Leong, 1994; Mullen & Pathé, 1994; see also chapter 2 of this volume). Often, the erotomanic stalker's pursuit of and preoccupation with his imagined loved one become the near-exclusive foci of his mental life. Although any condition that gives rise to delusions can give rise to erotomanic beliefs, Mullen and colleagues' (1999) series suggests that delusional disorder is the most common diagnosis among those stalkers with psychotic disorders. Other conditions that sometimes produce erotomanic delusions include schizophrenia and bipolar disorder. Besides erotomanic delusions, stalkers may have psychotic motivations that reflect persecutory delusions, delusions of jealousy, delusions of perceived mistreatment, and misidentification syndromes (i.e., delusional beliefs that a person is someone other than whom he really is; see Odom-White, de Leon, Stanilla, Cloud, & Simpson, 1995).

Stalking sometimes is a manifestation of the energy, intrusiveness, and disinhibition that may occur during manic episodes. Although mania typically is characterized by distractibility rather than persistence, a few manic individuals may repeatedly harass individuals toward whom they feel especial affection, anger, or resentment.

Stalkers' preoccupation with their victims and the persistent, repetitive quality of their behavior makes it natural to wonder whether some stalking is a manifestation of obsessive compulsive disorder (OCD). The diagnostic criteria for OCD include the individual's recognition, at some point during the illness, "that the obsessions or compulsions are excessive or unreasonable" (American Psychiatric Association, 2000, p. 457). OCD sufferers also attempt to ignore the obsessions and resist compulsions, which are a source of great distress to them. Occasionally, a stalker recognizes that his preoccupations are irrational and tries to counteract his ruminations and behavior. "Such cases are, however, the exception rather than the rule," note Mullen and colleagues (2001b, p. 337). In fact, it is much more common for stalkers to completely lack insight into their behavior, and this phenomenon may generate questions about a stalker's ability to understand why his actions are wrong and why (once he is charged with a criminal offense) those actions are grounds for prosecution.

STALKING, COMPETENCE TO STAND TRIAL, AND COMPETENCE RESTORATION

By the time that Hale and Blackstone wrote their famous commentaries (Blackstone, 1765–1769; Hale, 1736), English common law had firmly established a prohibition against trying a criminal defendant who was incompetent. One of the earliest and most cited English formulations of criteria for judging competence to stand trial appears in *King v. Pritchard* (1836), in which the court instructed a jury to consider whether a defendant was "mute of malice or not; secondly, whether he can plead to the indictment or not; thirdly, whether he is of sufficient intellect to comprehend the course of proceedings on the trial."

Canada followed *Pritchard* until 1992, when its Criminal Code formally defined incompetence (or "unfitness") to stand trial as being

> unable on account of mental disorder to conduct a defence at any stage of the proceedings before a verdict is rendered or to instruct counsel to do so, and, in particular, unable on account of mental disorder to (a) understand the nature or object of the proceedings, (b) understand the possible consequences of the proceedings, or (c) communicate with counsel. (Criminal Code of Canada, [1992] R.S.C., Ch. C-46)

Australian law continues to acknowledge the fitness criteria of *Pritchard*, further specifying that a defendant must have

> the ability (1) to understand the nature of the charge; (2) to plead to the charge and to exercise the right of challenge; (3) to understand the nature of the proceedings, namely, that it is an inquiry as to whether the accused committed the offence charged; (4) to follow the course of the proceedings; (5) to understand the substantial effect of any evidence that may be given in support of the prosecution; and (6) to make a defence or answer the charge. (*Kesavarajah v. R*, 1994, p. 243)

The 1960 *Dusky* decision established the minimal constitutional standard for fitness to stand trial in the United States, holding that when the question of competence is raised, trial courts must determine whether a defendant "has sufficient present ability to consult with his lawyer with a reasonable degree of rational understanding, and whether he has a rational as well as factual understanding of the proceedings against him" (*Dusky v. United States*, 1960, p. 402). Fifteen years later, *Drope v. Missouri* (1975) supplemented the *Dusky* test with the additional requirement that the defendant be able to "assist in preparing his defense" (p. 171). The *Drope* court noted that several possible circumstances, including "evidence of a defendant's irrational behavior," might be sufficient to raise the issue of a defendant's competence to stand trial, a matter that "is often a difficult one in which a wide range of manifestations and subtle nuances are implicated" (p. 180).

Defendants charged with stalking frequently display (to use the language in *Drope*) "a wide range of manifestations" of mental disorders and "subtle nuances" in their conditions that can make competence assessment and restoration difficult (*Drope v. Missouri*, 1975). One reason for this is that, in some cases, stalkers "happily indulge in their harassment and the associated fantasies," and do not recognize "that the behaviour is in any way remarkable, let alone damaging and criminal" (Mullen et al., 2001b, p. 337). Even when accused stalkers clearly suffer from psychotic disorders, their lack of insight makes it difficult for them to conceive of themselves as lacking trial competence or as needing treatment.

But in many cases, it may be difficult for evaluators to tell whether a stalker's extreme ideas and actions are signs of a mental illness that impairs reality testing, or simply reflect nonpsychotic emotions such as anger or disgust. The following case history, prepared (with names changed) from a published criminal appeal, illustrates this ambiguity.

CASE EXAMPLE 7.1: MR. APPLE

Mr. Apple's criminal charges stemmed from his alleged behavior toward Judge Angela Rudd, who had presided over a landlord-tenant case involving Mr. Apple and one of his tenants. Mr. Apple failed to appear for the trial, and Judge Rudd awarded Mr. Apple's tenant compensatory and punitive damages totaling several thousand dollars.

Shortly after the ruling, Mr. Apple phoned Judge Rudd's chambers, referring to her as "Judge Bimbo . . . a cockroach . . . a gangster, a mobster." Mr. Apple demanded his money back from the judge, insisting that she had "stolen" it. Despite being told that his proper recourse was to appeal the decision, Mr. Apple continued to phone the Judge's chambers demanding repayment and using derogatory language. The calls occurred at least twice a week for several months. In and around the county courthouse, Mr. Apple distributed leaflets that denounced the judicial system in general and that accused Judge Rudd of robbing him.

During telephone calls to the judge's office (some of which were taped), Mr. Apple made these ominous-sounding statements:

- "This is her last week to straighten this mess up."
- "Tell that stinkin' bitch I will collect."
- "She's getting a taste of it now. I'd say I'm doing a pretty good job of that. . . . Tell that cockroach . . . that I've just begun."

Asked whether he knew that his calls might frighten the judge, Mr. Apple replied, "I would hope so, I work hard enough at it." The calls alarmed both the judge and the judge's secretary, who was intimidated by Mr. Apple's saying things such as "Wait and see what's going to happen next."

Judge Rudd took several measures to protect herself. She starting carrying a gun (even into her courtroom); a peephole was installed in the door entering into the chambers; new locks were installed in the judge's office; the judge stopped taking lunchtime walks. City police watched the judge's home, and her home phone was equipped to register all calls. Because the judge had heard testimony in the landlord-tenant case about Mr. Apple's volatile behavior, she believed Mr. Apple was "a potentially very dangerous man."

Mr. Apple was eventually charged with making threats and other improper influences in official and political matters, retaliation for past official action, harassment, stalking, and obstructing or impeding the administration of justice by picketing. At his trial, jurors found him guilty as charged, and he received a prison sentence of 17–23 months.

The published appellate record does not say whether Mr. Apple's competence to stand trial was ever questioned or whether he suffered from mental illness. Had the issue of trial competence been raised, however, evaluators might well have had difficulty deciding whether Mr. Apple's behavior reflected a mental disorder or merely his idiosyncratic perspective on legal matters. The ambiguity here is only heightened by the claims made at Mr. Apple's trial. There, defense counsel maintained that Mr. Apple sought only to achieve a political goal and was doing nothing beyond exercising his constitutional right of free speech. His counsel claimed that Mr. Apple's leaflet distribution, courthouse picketing, and phone calls were efforts to change how rent was escrowed in landlord-tenant proceedings, and that Mr. Apple had expended no energy toward threatening, annoying, or alarming Judge Rudd.

The *Dusky* test does not require that a defendant suffer from a particular type of psychiatric syndrome to be found incompetent to stand trial. Thus, if a psychiatrist can show that a defendant's poor understanding of criminal proceedings or lack of cooperation with defense counsel reflects a genuine mental incapacity—and not merely the defendant's unwillingness to understand or to cooperate—that incapacity may justify a finding of trial incompetence, even if the incapacity stems only from the defendant's characterological problems. This "nonrequirement" of a specific clinical syndrome may be important in cases in which specific functional impairments may be present but precise diagnosis is difficult. In Mr. Apple's case, if both the defendant and his attorney agreed to and could collaboratively plan a criminal defense that characterized Mr. Apple's prearrest behavior as political (and constitutionally protected) action, Mr. Apple might well meet the *Dusky* criteria for competence, irrespective of any mental problems. Also, Mr. Apple's willingness to defend his acts as constitutionally protected speech reflects an ability to share the perspective and legal assumptions of the general public. If, however, Mr. Apple made persistent, blanket denials of any possible evidence against him, or if his anger and irritability repeatedly kept him from reaching any agreement with counsel about a defense, an evaluator might conclude that he lacked competence, even if the evaluator thought Mr. Apple's problems stemmed only from personality characteristics.

Another conundrum for forensic evaluators arises from the fact that, even when it is clear that an accused stalker suffers from a mental illness, many aspects of the defendant's mental functioning remain relatively unaffected. Individuals with erotomania, for example, may exhibit little or no thought disorganization, mood lability, or other signs of severe mental illness. Despite holding delusional beliefs or having other clear signs of mental illness, many stalkers articulate an understanding of the legal system, recognize that they face criminal charges, and realize that they face prison terms if convicted. The problem for forensic examiners and courts is that some of these individuals also believe that their prosecution is just another feature of (what they delusionally believe is) a real, if difficult, love relationship. The following two cases illustrate the puzzles examiners can face in rendering opinions about whether defendants are competent to stand trial, even when defendants' beliefs clearly indicate they are suffering from serious mental illness. (All names are pseudonyms, and several case facts are altered for illustrative purposes and to preserve confidentiality.)

CASE EXAMPLE 7.2: MS. BONCE

Ms. Bonce developed the delusional belief that George Stench, the state's governor, was responsible for the breakup of Ms. Bonce's relationship with her boyfriend 5 years earlier. For years, psychiatrists had treated Ms. Bonce for schizoaffective disorder, and since the breakup, doctors had documented Ms. Bonce's chronic paranoid delusions about the governor. Ms. Bonce was charged with stalking after she sent many letters to Governor Stench and made several telephone calls during which she expressed anger about the breakup and threatened to "seek revenge."

Ms. Bonce went to a psychiatric hospital for evaluation of her competence to stand trial. There, she displayed marked irritability, agitation, and disorganized thoughts. Almost every utterance digressed into incoherent, delusional rantings about how Governor Stench was controlling other people in Ms. Bonce's life. After being found incompetent, Ms. Bonce remained at the hospital for restoration. She thought her treating psychiatrist was controlled by Governor Stench, and at one point, she vowed to "get even" with the governor for having convinced the trial court to order the hospitalization.

After several months of treatment with an antipsychotic and mood-stabilizing medication, however, Ms. Bonce was no longer agitated or irritable. She did not talk spontaneously about the governor, and she coherently acknowledged that she faced serious criminal charges. This apparent stability led to a reassessment of Ms. Bonce's competence to stand trial.

Ms. Bonce's reevaluation took place over 2 days. The first day, Ms. Bonce described the specific allegations she faced, the potential verdicts, and their associated penalties. She accurately explained the purpose of a trial and basic trial proceedings. She acknowledged writing letters to Governor Stench and knew that others had construed the letters as threatening. She was pleasant and cooperative, and even thanked the evaluator for his patience in answering her questions.

When the evaluator returned the next day to complete the evaluation, he asked Ms. Bonce about where things stood with her and the governor. In response, Ms. Bonce described her intense concerns about the governor's ability to influence her upcoming trial. Ms. Bonce said she could tell whether the governor was controlling the judge by watching when the judge sighed or took notes during courtroom proceedings. Ms. Bonce also said that if the judge gave a ruling that was inaccurate, she would know for certain that the governor was influencing the judge. Ms. Bonce was convinced that the police officers who investigated the case were manipulated or heavily influenced by Governor Stench because she had heard them chuckling to themselves at the time of her arrest. Ms. Bonce also referred obliquely to "a significant monetary transfer" involving the judge and the governor. Although certain potential witnesses had seemed kind, Ms. Bonce could not be certain that they were not also influenced by the governor.

Ms. Bonce had fired a previous attorney because she believed that lawyer had been working with the governor. Ms. Bonce liked her current attorney because she thought he was a "shrewd, clever" guy who could "outfox" Governor Stench. Yet Ms. Bonce wondered whether her new lawyer's recent delays in returning phone calls was evidence that he, too, was now being influenced by Governor Stench and was likely beginning to work against her.

To be competent to stand trial under the *Dusky* definition, a defendant must have "a rational as well as factual understanding of the proceedings against him" (*Dusky v. United States*, 1960, p. 402). *Dusky* also requires that a defendant have the capacity to consult with an attorney with "a reasonable degree of rational understanding." Ms. Bonce's case exemplifies situations in which stalking defendants remain irrational about key features of their own legal proceedings, despite having a good grasp of how the criminal justice system works and the facts of their own case. Ms. Bonce's persisting belief that her arrest and upcoming trial reflected Governor Stench's control over legal authorities clearly was irrational. The fact that Ms. Bonce began to wonder whether her new attorney might be under Governor Stench's influence suggests an additional impairment in collaborative capacities that has its basis in persisting mental symptoms. In our view, therefore, Ms. Bonce remained incompetent to stand trial, despite her substantial recovery during treatment.

CASE EXAMPLE 7.3: MR. CRUMB

As a young man, Mr. Crumb began frequenting a restaurant where he encountered a married waitress, Mrs. Uxor. To Mr. Crumb, Mrs. Uxor certainly was in love with him because (as he perceived it) she filled his drinks fuller than she did the drinks of other customers. Also, Mr. Crumb thought Mrs. Uxor signaled her affection by the special way she leaned when she served his food. Mr. Crumb began writing Mrs. Uxor letters—eventually, they came daily—declaring his reciprocated love for her and his understanding that Mrs. Uxor could not respond openly because doing so would upset her husband.

When Mrs. Uxor told Mr. Crumb that she did not love him, Mr. Crumb took this to mean that Mrs. Uxor certainly was in love with him, but had to say she was not for fear that her husband would become jealous. Mr. Crumb continued to frequent the restaurant and leave love letters for Mrs. Uxor. Several times, Mrs. Uxor asked him to leave the restaurant. As she did so, the tone in the letters became ominous, escalating to the point where Mr. Crumb threatened to come after Mrs. Uxor if she did not finally acknowledge what he knew to be her true feelings for him. Mrs. Uxor obtained a restraining order against Mr. Crumb, but he continued to contact her and was charged criminally with stalking.

At an evaluation of competence to stand trial that took place soon after his arrest, Mr. Crumb's thinking was disorganized, and he uttered a variety of grandiose delusions about religious issues and his relationships with famous historical figures. Mr. Crumb spent several months undergoing inpatient psychiatric treatment, during which time his thinking became coherent and his grandiose ideas waned. He then underwent another competence evaluation at which he was occasionally tearful, but calm. Mr. Crumb knew he was charged with stalking and understood this was a criminal charge that could lead to punishment. He also knew his lawyer's job was to defend him, and that the judge would play a neutral role in the proceedings.

Yet Mr. Crumb insisted that the stalking charge really was Mrs. Uxor's way of saying that she loved Mr. Crumb so much that she could not control her feelings. He thought that filing criminal charges had been Mrs. Uxor's last-ditch effort to stop herself from leaving her husband and joining Mr. Crumb. Mr. Crumb believed that once Mrs. Uxor appeared on the witness stand, she would break down and finally confess that she loved Mr. Crumb as he knew she did. In discussions with his attorney, Mr. Crumb insisted on testifying so that he could state his version of the story, and he insisted that his attorney question Mrs. Uxor about her true love of him. Mr. Crumb stated he would represent himself if his attorney refused to question her in this way.

Mr. Crumb's case illustrates another issue for evaluators to consider: whether the stalking defendant's beliefs prevent him from considering a defense strategy that rationally protects his self-interest. Though Mr. Crumb held delusional beliefs that his stalking charge was really Mrs. Uxor's expression of love and that she would confess her love during her testimony, these beliefs might not, by themselves, affect his relationship with his attorney. But Mr. Crumb's insistence on cross-examining Mrs. Uxor about her love for him represents an irrationality-based impairment in collaborative capacity that, in our view, justifies a conclusion that he is unfit to stand trial. His inability to consider the possibility that his views are wrong might also prevent him from giving proper consideration to a lawyer's recommendations about an insanity defense (a topic discussed later in this chapter).

Treatment to Restore Competence

To our knowledge, scientific publications contain no rigorous, double-blind study of the treatment of delusional stalkers, let alone studies of stalkers in need of competence restoration. However, psychotropic medication usually is a key element in treating incompetent defendants whose impairments stem from serious mental illnesses (Leong & Silva, 1988; Pinals, 2005).

As was noted earlier, erotomania is the type of delusional pattern most commonly found in psychotic stalkers. The delusion may occur in schizophrenia or stand alone in an erotomanic delusional disorder. Several authors (Gillett, Eminson, & Hassanyeh, 1990; Leong, 1994; Segal, 1989) suggest that erotomanic delusions respond poorly to treatment. Mullen and colleagues (2001b) disagree, however, and note that when an individual's primary diagnosis is schizophrenia or an affective psychosis, the erotomanic delusions often abate, along with other symptoms, as the underlying thought or mood disorder is treated. Reviewing available literature on the treatment of delusions and obsessive fixations, Rosenfeld (2000) also concludes that antipsychotic medications, mood stabilizers, and electroconvulsive therapy often can diminish delusional symptoms in persons with mood disorders, schizophrenia, and organic psychoses.

Clinical lore suggests that delusional disorders respond poorly to any form of treatment. Yet a few publications report that antipsychotic drugs yield some benefit and that psychotherapy may help reduce delusional beliefs that do not respond to medication. Two older reports (published before atypical antipsychotics were in widespread use) suggest that pimozide is an especially useful agent, achieving more success that other standard neuroleptics (Gillett et al., 1990; Munro & Mok, 1995). Rosenfeld's (2003) finding of lower recidivism by stalkers with delusional disorders weighs in favor of expecting some medication responsiveness in these individuals. Psychotherapy has been recommended as an adjunct to pharmacotherapeutic interventions. For example, Chadwick and Lowe (1990, 1994) describe how cognitive therapy and psychoeducational treatments produced reductions in—and occasional remissions of—delusions in persons with schizophrenia.

Mullen and colleagues (2001b) recommend a combination of novel antipsychotic agents (dosed judiciously to minimize side effects) and individual psychotherapy for treatment of stalkers who suffer from delusional disorders. These authors note that for many stalkers, pursuit of the victim is not merely the focus of the patient's mental life; stalking also becomes "the organising principle around which the patient's current existence and future hopes revolve" (p. 337). These stalkers misinterpret refusals and distort repeated rejections. As is the case with most delusional patients, pointing out the factual inaccuracy of a stalker's beliefs is ineffectual and may antagonize the stalker. However, stalkers pay a great price—in time, money, and disappointment—to pursue the targets of their delusions; once they are arrested, the price also includes the prospect of prosecution and punishment. Because of this, Mullen and colleagues (2001b) believe that "repeatedly drawing attention to the personal costs of continuing the pursuit and gently urging the patients to consider the likely implications of rebuffs and rejections can, over time, produce benefit" (p. 337). Other types of delusions that lead to stalking can be addressed with similar types of psychotherapeutic interventions.

Many of the just-discussed points concerning the treatment of delusional stalkers in nonforensic contexts might be adopted for individuals who are receiving treatment to restore their competence to stand trial. In the authors' experience, antipsychotic medications (and, for individuals with affective psychoses, mood stabilizers) help many delusional forensic patients to act and think more rationally, even when these drugs leave unchanged the delusional beliefs that underlie the patients' criminal charges. In many cases, the delusions, though persistent, occupy a smaller space in the patients' consciousness, allowing the patient to devote more mental energy to discussing (and presumably thinking about) reality-based matters. Although patients' delusional interpretations of past (e.g., prearrest) experiences often remain unchanged, medications often halt the accretion of new, delusionally tainted memories. Being confined in a jail or (during competence restoration) a psychiatric hospital reduces or eliminates contact between stalkers and victims, and removes patients from environments associated with their delusional pursuits. Pharmacotherapy, psychotherapy, and placement in a different environment allow patients to accumulate experiences and attitudes that are minimally influenced by delusional ideas. Patients can then use this set of nondelusional conceptualizations and recollections to address their legal situations more realistically and flexibly than they could before their arrest, when their thinking and behavior were dominated by delusional beliefs.

Warren, MacKenzie, Mullen, and Ogloff (2005) have developed a "problem behavior model" for conceptualizing the evaluation and treatment of stalkers and individuals who make threats. Although their "Stalker's Clinic" and "Threatener's Clinic" serve already adjudicated individuals, the principles underlying their care model may translate well to the treatment of incompetent stalking defendants who have not yet undergone adjudication. In addition to medication, Warren and colleagues (2005) offer individuals referred to their clinic a comprehensive psychological assessment, a "functional analysis" that examines motives and needs that sustain clients' problem behaviors, and individualized cognitive-behavioral treatment aimed at countering clients' distortions and self-deceptions.

As the cases of Ms. Bonce and Mr. Crumb suggest, however, even treatment that succeeds in greatly reducing clinical symptoms and problematic patterns of interaction may not be sufficient to render a defendant fit to stand trial.

In the United States, administering pharmacological treatment to restore an accused stalker's competence to stand trial may be complicated by the legal requirements in *Sell v. United States*, a 2003 Supreme Court decision concerning a mentally ill dentist. After Dr. Sell was found incompetent to stand trial, he refused to accept medication that psychiatrists thought would alleviate symptoms of a delusional disorder and restore his competence to stand trial. The U.S. Supreme Court held that criminal defendants who were not dangerous might be forced to take competence-restoring medication, but only when "*important* governmental interests are at stake" the medication will "*significantly further* . . . those interests . . . involuntary medication is *necessary* to further those interests" and administration of the drugs is "*medically appropriate, i.e.,* in the patient's best medical interest in light of his medical condition" (*Sell v. United States*, 2003, p. 181; italics in original). *Sell* (2003) also held that, when assessing whether prosecuting a defendant is an "important" government interest, trial courts must consider the consequences of not providing pharmacological treatment, which "may mean lengthy confinement in an institution for the mentally ill—and that would diminish the risks that ordinarily attach to freeing without punishment one who has committed a serious crime" (p. 180). Given the protection that such confinement would offer a stalker's victim and the limited success medications may enjoy in reducing erotomanic delusions, courts may well find that the government's interest in prosecuting an accused stalker would not be strong enough to overcome a stalker's wish to avoid medication. How U.S. courts will weigh these matters will become clearer over the next few years as jurisdictions adopt procedures and develop case law related to the *Sell* ruling.

STALKING AND *MENS REA*

In the United States, Canada, Australia, and other jurisdictions where legal principles derive from English common law, criminal liability traditionally is conceptualized as requiring the co-occurrence of an *actus reus* (Latin for "bad act") and *mens rea* ("guilty mind").

Actus Reus

The term *actus reus* refers to the behavioral features of a criminal act and typically points to some voluntary act that has caused social harm. In this context, an act refers just to a criminal's physical behavior, distinct from any inferred mental activity (e.g., planning or desiring a result) in which the criminal engaged. Traditionally, conduct is deemed voluntary if it is the kind of behavior to which one could ascribe a conscious volition, as opposed to spasms, seizures, and other body movements that occur without a person's conscious awareness. Examples of nonvoluntary body movements include reflexes, convulsions, behavior performed while unconscious or under hypnosis, and any behavior that "is not a product of the effort or determination of the defendant, either conscious or habitual" (*Model Penal Code*, American Law Institute, 1962, § 2.01(2)(d)).

The social harm caused by an *actus reus* is defined by common law principles or by statute. Some offenses (e.g., speeding or carrying a concealed weapon) designate certain behaviors as wrong even if they do not harm others. Other offenses (e.g., robbery or murder) require a prohibited result, and lead to criminal charges irrespective of the specific means (e.g., a firearm) that the defendant used to carry out the criminal act. As stalking is typically defined in U.S. statutes, it has both "conduct" and "result" requirements, because it requires repeated following or approaching behaviors that cause the victim to experience mental distress or fear of physical harm.

Mens Rea

Mens rea refers to the mental state required to regard conduct as being criminal. Although at common law it was once sufficient to show that a defendant acted with a generally culpable state of mind, the more prevalent practice in the United States is to make a particular, required mental state an element of an offense by including it in the offense's statutory definition.

Common law contains several (sometimes confusing) designations for mental states, so that conviction for some crimes requires that an act be done "with malice aforethought" (as opposed to actions done "in the heat of passion") or "willfully" (referring to an act done "with a bad purpose," "an evil motive," or "a purpose to disobey the law"). A still-important common law distinction (as subsequent portions of this chapter will show) is between crimes requiring "specific intent" and "general intent."

Specific intent crimes require (usually in the statutory definition of the offense) that the illegal action have some aim, purpose, or motive beyond simply accomplishing what the action itself achieves. General intent crimes, by contrast, contain in their definition just the mental state that relates to the *actus reus* itself. Iowa's jury instructions, which explain the practical distinction between specific and general intent, appear in Table 7.1.

Statutes in many U.S. jurisdictions have eschewed traditional common law designations of *mens rea* and instead refer to the mental states defined in the *Model Penal Code* (MPC; American Law Institute, 1962). Guilt is established only when the prosecution has shown that the accused committed each

Table 7.1. Examples of Instructions on General and Specific Intent From Iowa Criminal Jury Instructions

Instruction 200.1

To commit a crime a person must intend to do an act which is against the law. While it is not necessary that a person knows the act is against the law, it is necessary that the person was aware [he] was doing the act and [he] did it voluntarily, not by mistake or accident. You may, but are not required to, conclude a person intends the natural results of [his] acts.

Instruction 200.2

"Specific intent" means not only being aware of doing an act and doing it voluntarily, but in addition, doing it with a specific purpose in mind.

   Because determining the defendant's specific intent requires you to decide what [he] was thinking when an act was done, it is seldom capable of direct proof. Therefore, you should consider the facts and circumstances surrounding the act to determine the defendant's specific intent. You may, but are not required to, conclude a person intends the natural results of [his] acts.

Source: Iowa State Bar Association, Special Committee on Uniform Court Instructions (1988–2004).

element of the offense with the requisite state of mind as established by statute. The MPC limits culpable mental states to actions done "purposely," "knowingly," "recklessly," or "negligently." An example of a state's adopting MPC mental states appears in Table 7.2, which quotes text from New Hampshire's criminal code.

The Drafting and Interpretation of Stalking Statutes

As Mullen and colleagues (2001a) have noted, the designation of stalking as a crime has been a phenomenon largely restricted to English-speaking jurisdictions. In all U.S. states (U.S. Department of Justice, 2002), Canada, England, Wales, and Australia, lawmakers have passed laws that criminalize stalking, either as a form harassment (e.g., *Protection From Harassment Act* in England and Wales) or as a distinctly defined criminal offense. (For a detailed description of stalking statutes, see chapter 6.)

   In U.S. jurisdictions, the crime of stalking is typically defined as repeatedly contacting or approaching another individual person in ways that would cause a reasonable person to experience fear and that in fact have caused the victim to fear for his safety. The antistalking statutes first passed by U.S. state legislatures made stalking a specific intent offense. For example, New Jersey's original antistalking law required that the accused have acted with "the intent of annoying or placing the other person in reasonable fear of death or bodily injury." Similarly, the antistalking statute in New South Wales (*Crimes Act 1900*, §562AB(1))

Table 7.2. General Requirements of Culpability

II. The following are culpable mental states:

(a) "Purposely." A person acts purposely with respect to a material element of an offense when his conscious object is to cause the result or engage in the conduct that comprises the element.

(b) "Knowingly." A person acts knowingly with respect to conduct or to a circumstance that is a material element of an offense when he is aware that his conduct is of such nature or that such circumstances exist.

(c) "Recklessly." A person acts recklessly . . . when he is aware of and consciously disregards a substantial and unjustifiable risk that . . . exists or will result from his conduct. The risk must be of such a nature and degree that, considering the circumstances known to him, its disregard constitutes a gross deviation from the conduct that a law-abiding person would observe in the situation. ...

(d) "Negligently." A person acts negligently . . . when he fails to become aware of a substantial and unjustifiable risk that . . . exists or will result from his conduct. The risk must be of such a nature and degree that his failure to become aware of it consti-tutes a gross deviation from the conduct that a reasonable person would observe in the situation.

Source: Criminal Code of New Hampshire, Title LXII, Section 626:2.

provides for the potential prosecution and punishment of a "person who stalks or intimidates another person with the intention of causing the other person to fear physical or mental harm."

The problem with specific intent formulations, however, is summarized succinctly in the Colorado legislature's explanation of its amendment to that state's antiharassment law:

> A stalker will often maintain strong, unshakable, and irrational emotional feelings for his or her victim, and may likewise believe that the victim either returns these feelings of affection or will do so if the stalker is persistent enough. Further, the stalker often maintains this belief, despite a trivial or nonexistent basis for it and despite rejection, lack of reciprocation, efforts to restrict or avoid the stalker, and other facts that conflict with this belief. (Colo. Rev. Stat. 18–9-111(4)(a))

In clinical terms, stalkers often have erotomanic delusions such as those expe-rienced by Mr. Crumb: they believe that their victims love them and—despite causing their victims intense distress—may intend only to establish or continue relationships with them.

Recognizing this, drafters of the National Criminal Justice Association's (NCJA; 1993) Model Antistalking Code recommended that legislatures define stalking as a general intent offense. Under this scheme, a person acts illegally if he "purposefully" commits the actions that constitute stalking and "has knowledge or should have knowledge" that because of his acts, the victim "will be placed in reasonable fear." Several states responded by amending their statutes in line with the NCJA's model code. For example, in 1996, New Jersey redefined a stalker as someone who "[p]urposefully engages in a course of conduct directed at a specific person that would cause a reasonable person to fear" harm to himself or a family member, and who "[k]nowingly, recklessly or negligently places the specific person in reasonable fear" of such harm (New Jersey Stat. Annot. 2C:12–10(b)).

Despite suffering from delusions, stalkers with erotomania know that they are contacting or following their victims. Thus, in states with general intent antistalking statutes, a defendant accused of stalking will have difficulty obtaining a "not guilty" verdict by invoking his sincere-but-delusional belief that his attentions were desired by the victim and were not intended to cause fear. The clearest statement of this reasoning appears in *State v. Neuzil* (1999), an Iowa Supreme Court decision holding that making stalking a general intent crime represented a "sound public policy" decision by the legislature. Rightfully, the *Neuzil* court stated, Iowa's antistalking "statute's focus is not on the defendant's [specific] mental state but on the result the defendant's purposeful acts cause in a reasonable person" (p. 711). Were the statute to have a specific intent requirement, the Court continued,

> an accused stalker [could] avoid conviction by asserting an emotional inability to form the requisite specific intent. Here, for example, Neuzil [the defendant] sought to convince the jury that his conduct stemmed from his love for Sheetz [the complainant], and the hundreds of phone calls placed to her home were either the product of his depression or attempts to contact his children. To excuse his harassing conduct on these grounds would effectively negate the purpose of the antistalking statute—to enable law enforcement to get involved in a harassing situation before physical confrontation results. (*State v. Neuzil*, 1999, p. 712)

The New York Court of Appeals offered similar reasoning in interpreting its state's antistalking statute:

> The Legislature's decision to require intent as to a particular course of conduct—as opposed to a specific result—was purposeful. . . . [T]he Legislature enacted Penal Law § 120.45 recognizing that many stalkers are mentally or emotionally disturbed and that trying to discern their specific motivations would prove difficult, if not impossible. The statute thus focuses on what the offenders do, not what they mean by it or what they intend as their ultimate goal. . . . If the Legislature had required that the stalker intend to frighten or harm the victim, the statute would be debilitated and a great many victims endangered. Stalkers would be free to continue as long as they

harbored the notion that they stood to win, rather than harm, their prey. We cannot tell how many stalkers intend no harm. The Legislature did not want to give them license. (*People v. Stuart*, 2003, p. 427)

Even in states where the statutes appear to require specific intent to cause distress or frighten, interpretations courts actually give to those statutes may prevent defendants from avoiding punishment by claiming that their actions had benign motives. For example, Pennsylvania formerly defined the crime of harassment (in a statute that also covered behavior that constitutes stalking) as occurring "when, with intent to harass, annoy or alarm another, the person . . . follows the other person in or about a public place or places, . . . communicates repeatedly in an anonymous manner, . . . communicates repeatedly at extremely inconvenient hours . . ." (former 18 Pa.C.S. § 2709). In a decision that rejected a convicted man's claim that this law was unconstitutionally vague and placed a bar on protected free speech, a Pennsylvania appellate court noted that the law "requires the fact-finder to infer a specific intent on the part of the accused" (*Commonwealth v. Duncan*, 1976, p. 549). Note, however, the following description of actions for which the defendant was found guilty and the *Duncan* majority's reasoning about how the defendant's intent should be judged:

> Testimony of the prosecutrix, Miss Deborah Hartman, established that appellant approached her as she dozed on a couch in a dormitory lounge area. With his face in close proximity to hers, appellant made repeated requests that Miss Hartman permit him to engage in [oral sex] with her. Although Miss Hartman asked appellant to leave, he persisted in his requests. Not until he had made three or four requests [and was] asked to leave three or four times did appellant finally desist. Miss Hartman made it clear from the beginning that she wanted to be left alone. . . . Miss Hartman's replies made it clear, *or should have made it clear to a reasonable person* [emphasis in original], that continued entreaties would be offensive to her. The lower court was justified in finding that appellant had engaged in a course of conduct which alarmed or seriously annoyed another person. Appellant argues that no evidence was presented to show that he possessed the requisite intent to harass. Our courts have often found that a defendant's intent to commit a criminal act may be inferred from his words or actions when viewed in the light of all the attendant circumstances. (pp. 543–544)

STALKING AND THE INSANITY DEFENSE

Psychiatric physicians once used the term "insanity" to refer to a broad range of mental infirmities. Now, however, mental health professionals restrict use of the term to a single forensic context: being excused, by virtue of a mental disorder, from criminal responsibility for a particular offense. English-speaking jurisdictions have many different ways of defining legal insanity and specifying the required relationship between legal insanity and mental illness. To simplify matters, our discussion here will focus on psychiatric impairment of two mental capacities addressed in insanity standards: the defendant's capacity to recognize the wrongfulness of his alleged action, and his ability to control or "conform" his conduct to meet the requirements of the law.

Stalking and the Recognition of Wrongfulness

The most famous (and a still frequently used) formulation of the connections linking mental illness, knowledge of wrongfulness, and criminal responsibility comes from the so-called "M'Naghten rules" promulgated by the House of Lords in 1843:

> [T]he jurors ought to be told in all cases that every man is presumed to be sane, and to possess a sufficient degree of reason to be responsible for his crimes, until the contrary be proved to their satisfaction; and that to establish a defence on the ground of insanity, it must be clearly proved that, at the time of the committing of the act, the party accused was labouring under such a defect of reason, from disease of the mind, as not to know the nature and quality of the act he was doing, or, if he did know it, that he did not know what he was doing was wrong. (*M'Naghten's Case*, 1843).

The M'Naghten rules provide two potential ways for a defendant to be excused on grounds of insanity. First, a defendant's mental illness may preclude having the requisite *mens rea* for the offense. It is rare, however, to encounter individuals accused of serious crimes who, at the time of their alleged offenses, genuinely lacked knowledge of the nature and quality of their actions. Although persons suffering from severe psychotic disorganization may not realize that they are loitering, jaywalking, or engaged in disorderly conduct, defendants who commit actions that lead to serious charges usually know what they have done, despite suffering from severe mental illnesses. If stalking is defined as a general intent offense—knowingly engaging in a "pattern" of repeated, goal-directed behavior related to a specific individual—then it is hard to conceive of a defendant's following, phoning, or writing to a victim (i.e., carrying out the actions needed to generate a stalking charge) without knowing that he has done those things.

Though the idea that mental illness could negate a stalker's *mens rea* seems farfetched, the notion that hallucinations or delusions might provide psychotic justifications for stalking is quite plausible. Thus, the second potential ground for exculpation under *M'Naghten*—lack of knowledge of wrongfulness—is a likely focus of evaluation for accused stalkers who raise the insanity defense.

Borrowing from ideas formulated by Slobogin (2000), one might anticipate that having a mental disorder could impair a stalker's apprehension of wrongfulness in one of two potential ways. First, the stalker's mental disorder might create a false belief about circumstances such that, if the world really were as the stalker believed, those circumstances would provide a legal justification for the stalker's actions. Individuals who might fall into this first category include some of the stalkers classified as "resentful" by Mullen and colleagues (1999). These authors briefly describe a man who "stalked a medical practitioner who he believed had failed to diagnose his wife's cervical cancer" (p. 1247). Suppose that the stalker was mentally ill and that the source of his belief was a delusion (as opposed to a real failure by the doctor); suppose further that the stalker's goal was to get the doctor to admit his error, because the stalker held the delusional belief that his wife's cancer could be cured and her life saved only if the doctor would publicly acknowledge his error. Under these circumstances, we believe that the stalker might qualify for an insanity defense because a reasonable person, asked to assume that the stalker's irrational but sincerely held beliefs were factual, might well conclude that the stalker's behavior was his delusionally justified effort to save a life.

A second way that a mental disorder could impair recognition of wrongfulness is by generating symptoms that vitiate—from the stalker's psychiatrically disordered perspective—any intent to perform acts that would constitute a crime. For example, some stalkers whom Mullen and colleagues (1999) classify as "intimacy seeking" might deserve insanity acquittals because erotomanic delusions leave them convinced that their advances are desired. Some of the stalkers classified by Mullen and colleagues as belonging to the "incompetent" type might be criminally nonresponsible if they had mental illnesses that prevented them from recognizing that their awkward, persistent approaches were unwanted and disturbing. In other words, certain subgroups of stalkers may lack the requisite (subjective) mental state to commit an offense, given the way their mental condition alters their perceptions of the world.

The following pseudonymous case history, developed from public record documents available on the Internet (but with names and some case details changed), provides several instances of the sorts of ambiguous information that forensic examiners can encounter in assessing stalking defendants who raise an insanity defense. For purposes of this example, the reader should assume that the jurisdiction's insanity standard requires that a criminal defendant suffer from a severe mental disorder that renders him unable to know that his actions are wrong. The reader should then consider how events in the case history provide information for or against a valid insanity defense for the third of three instances in which the defendant was charged with stalking.

CASE EXAMPLE 7.4: MR. DRAKE

One morning, Ms. Verst, a reporter and columnist with the city's newspaper, received a voicemail message from Mr. Drake requesting a return call regarding a story that she had written about him. When

Ms. Verst returned the call, Mr. Drake tried to get her to remember a story that he said she had written about his candidacy for mayor. Ms. Verst told Mr. Drake that she had written no such story and ended the phone conversation. After this, Mr. Drake left many additional voicemail messages for Ms. Verst, and he sent many letters to her at the newspaper's office. Some letters referred to their (nonexistent) romantic relationship, with Mr. Drake stating that he loved Ms. Verst and wanted to be with her.

About 3 months after the first phone call, Ms. Verst received a letter from Mr. Drake in which he told her that human beings did not have much time left, that the end of the world was near, and that something would happen if they were not together. The letter alarmed Ms. Verst, and her editor sent her to a hotel until Mr. Drake could be located. Ms. Verst filed stalking charges and sought a civil protection order (CPO) against Mr. Drake. Five days after Ms. Verst obtained the CPO, Mr. Drake pled no contest to a misdemeanor charge of menacing by stalking, and was found guilty. A portion of his jail sentence was suspended on condition that he obey the CPO and not contact Ms. Verst further. In less than 4 weeks, however, Mr. Drake sent another letter to Ms. Verst, and he was quickly charged with aggravated menacing and menacing by stalking. This time, Mr. Drake was found not guilty by reason of insanity (NGRI) and sent for treatment to a state psychiatric hospital.

Mr. Drake remained hospitalized for several months, during which time he did not contact Ms. Verst. Upon learning that Mr. Drake would be released from the hospital, however, the newspaper sent Ms. Verst to a hotel and hired bodyguards to follow her around the clock until Mr. Drake was located. Three days after Mr. Drake's release, the newspaper printed a front-page article under Ms. Verst's byline. Later that day, Ms. Verst checked her office's voicemail and heard the following message left by Mr. Drake just after the article appeared: "Hi. You did a fine job with that article in this morning's paper. It looked great. Well, I'll call you and talk to ya' later, baby."

As a result of the above message, a police officer went to the home of Mr. Drake's mother and found Mr. Drake sitting on the porch. Mr. Drake told the officer that Ms. Verst had called him. The next day, Mr. Drake met with a police detective who advised Mr. Drake of his *Miranda* rights, which Mr. Drake waived. Mr. Drake told the detective that Ms. Verst had called him the previous morning, but that he had not answered the phone. He said he had known Ms. Verst had called because her name and number had come up on his caller ID. Mr. Drake provided other information about the previous day's events, and indicated his awareness of the CPO (which was still in effect) and his prior convictions.

Mr. Drake was arrested and charged with violating the CPO and with two felony counts of stalking. At his attorney's request, Judge Wedge of the trial court ordered an evaluation of Mr. Drake's competence to stand trial; shortly after this, a new attorney was appointed for Mr. Drake, and the order for the competence evaluation was withdrawn. Three months later, however, Judge Wedge, on his own motion, ordered Mr. Drake to undergo evaluation of his competence and ultimately ruled that Mr. Drake was not competent to stand trial. Mr. Drake then asked for a new attorney. Judge Wedge refused and ordered Mr. Drake back to the state psychiatric hospital for competence restoration.

After 3 months of inpatient treatment, Mr. Drake was found competent to stand trial. When Mr. Drake (through defense counsel) requested a bench trial, Judge Wedge had to disqualify himself, because while undergoing competence restoration at the hospital, Mr. Drake had sent Judge Wedge letters that contained self-incriminating statements.

Mr. Drake had a bench trial before a new judge at which no insanity defense was raised. The court found Mr. Drake guilty on both counts of menacing by stalking and violation of the CPO, and sentenced him to 18 months in prison. Mr. Drake appealed his conviction on several grounds, including a claim that his mental condition had prevented him from knowing the call would distress Ms. Verst.

The appeals court held, however, that in making the call Mr. Drake had indeed acted "knowingly." The court noted that the state's antistalking law did not require that a perpetrator threaten a victim explicitly (i.e., act with the purpose of threatening); the law required only that the stalker act knowingly and that the victim legitimately feel threatened. To act knowingly under the state's criminal code, an individual need be aware only that his conduct would probably lead to a particular result or that his conduct would probably be of a certain nature. Using reasoning similar to that contained in Iowa's *Neuzil* decision, the appeals court found that the prosecution had presented sufficient evidence to show that Mr. Drake had acted knowingly. Ms. Verst had repeatedly told him not to contact her again and that his contacts had distressed her. Mr. Drake had previously been accused of stalking Ms. Verst and had undergone post-NGRI hospitalization as a result. Ms. Verst had obtained a CPO against Mr. Drake, and Mr. Drake's statements to the police detective indicated that he knew he should not contact Ms. Verst. All this, in the appeals court's view, constituted sufficient evidence to allow the trial court to find that Mr. Drake had indeed acted knowingly.

The appeals court's reasoning is a good starting point for considering what a forensic examiner would have needed to address had Mr. Drake raised an insanity defense in his third stalking case. Assuming that Mr. Drake acted as the indictment charged, why did he call Ms. Verst—despite his previous conviction for calling her, and just 3 days after a long confinement in a psychiatric hospital for having called her? Did Mr. Drake know it was wrong and did he simply think he could get away with it? Was his leaving a message an act of hostility that he knew would bother Ms. Verst, but which Mr. Drake thought he could get away with because of the message's ostensibly benign content? Did Mr. Drake believe—despite the consequences he had suffered—that Ms. Verst loved him and wanted him to contact her? Did Mr. Drake have some other delusional idea that, had it been true, would make his action justifiable? After he left the hospital, did Mr. Drake use alcohol or other intoxicants that lowered his inhibitions about doing something he had often wanted to do, but that he knew was wrong and could refrain from doing when he was sober?

An evaluator might look into Mr. Drake's beliefs by examining materials generated around the time of the call and by interviewing individuals who had contact with him then. For example, documents or personnel from the hospital might help delineate the nature of Mr. Drake's psychiatric condition, might contain information about what he believed before he left the hospital, and might speak to how well his mental illness had responded to treatment shortly before he called Ms. Verst. Mr. Drake's mother might know what (if anything) her son had said about Ms. Verst after his hospital discharge, and whether he had continued to take medication (if any had been prescribed). A transcript or recording of the detective's interview of Mr. Drake might contain valuable information about Mr. Drake's understanding of the protection order, beyond his knowing that it existed. Additional information about this interview might also clarify why Mr. Drake said Ms. Verst had called him: was this Mr. Drake's rational attempt to avert guilt concerning an action that he knew was wrong, or did Mr. Drake honestly believe that Ms. Verst really had called him and that he was responding to her?

Other reported features of Mr. Drake's postarrest behavior suggest additional avenues for exploration and information-gathering. How did Mr. Drake respond to his first attorney's request for evaluations of his competence and sanity? Was the change in attorneys precipitated by the anger of a client who lacked insight into his psychiatric disorder and resented the suggestion that he was mentally ill? An examination of Mr. Drake's self-incriminating letters to the first trial judge might provide additional clues about his mental state. Did these letters suggest that Mr. Drake thought that his actions were innocent or justifiable, and that (despite his arrest and hospitalization) he could not grasp why his alleged action was grounds for criminal charges? Was he merely angry or disconsolate about the judge's ordering him back to the hospital?

Stalking and Volitional Control

Although the insanity tests of most U.S. jurisdictions require an analysis of a defendant's capacity to know or appreciate the wrongfulness of his alleged criminal conduct, a minority of states also include a "volitional" test in their insanity statutes. In general, volitional tests reflect the notion that certain defendants should not be held criminally responsible if, at the time of the alleged offense, they could not control their otherwise illegal conduct. Although several commentators regard the notion of impaired volition as philosophically problematic (American Psychiatric Association, 1983; Morse, 1994; Mossman, 1988), forensic evaluators who evaluate stalkers in jurisdictions that use volitional tests should be familiar with how psychiatric disorders might be conceptualized as impairing a stalker's ability to control conduct.

Two nineteenth-century cases serve as representative sources of volition-based insanity standards. In the 1840 trial of Edward Oxford, a man who attempted to assassinate Queen Victoria, the jury was instructed that "if some controlling disease was, in truth, the acting power within him which he could not resist, then he will not be responsible" (*Regina v. Oxford*, 1840, p. 850). In *Parsons v. State* (1887), the Alabama Supreme Court held that even when knowledge of right and wrong is present, a defendant may still lack criminal responsibility "if, by reason of the duress of mental disease, he has so far lost the power to choose between right and wrong as not to avoid doing the act in question, so that his free agency was at the time destroyed" (p. 597). A volitional "prong" appears in American Law Institute's (1962) insanity standard (*Model Penal Code* § 4.01), which defines a person as criminally nonresponsible for an otherwise criminal act "if at the time of such conduct as a result of mental disease or defect he lacks the substantial capacity to appreciate the criminality of his conduct or to conform his conduct to the requirements of the law."

Volitional insanity tests have generated significant controversy (English, 1988) and many U.S. jurisdictions removed them from their insanity defense standards following the highly controversial insanity acquittal of John Hinckley in 1982. When an insanity evaluation is requested in a jurisdiction that utilizes a volitional test, however, the evaluator must analyze clinical and forensic data to form an opinion about the defendant's behavioral self-control. Examples of the issues evaluators confront are described in the following pseudonymous vignette about a defendant charged with stalking in violation of a restraining order.

CASE EXAMPLE 7.5: MS. EPLET

Authorities charged Ms. Eplet with several counts of telephone harassment after she made hundreds of unwanted telephone calls to the home of Mr. Xenon, a former boyfriend. Ms. Eplet previously had been charged with assaulting Mr. Xenon, which had led to issuance of a restraining order. The telephone harassment charges included allegations that Ms. Eplet had threatened Mr. Xenon during some of the calls. While awaiting trial, Ms. Eplet called Mr. Xenon from jail until she was admonished by correctional officials.

When Ms. Eplet appeared in court, her defense attorney raised the question of her criminal responsibility, noting her history of receiving treatment for depression and hypomania, and her seemingly compulsive need to continue calling Mr. Xenon.

Ms. Eplet underwent the insanity evaluation at a hospital psychiatric unit, where staff members noted that she frequently engaged in provocative actions, such as making sexually flirtatious remarks to other patients. The forensic evaluator gathered information from Mr. Xenon's mother, who said that the defendant was "obsessed" with Mr. Xenon and that the restraining order obtained by Mr. Xenon had not affected the frequency of Ms. Eplet's calls. The evaluator also learned about similar behavior in a prior relationship that resulted in a restraining order, which Ms. Eplet had obeyed.

Before the evaluation, Ms. Eplet had not undergone psychiatric hospitalization, but doctors had prescribed medications for her for many years. During the evaluation, she did not appear psychotic. However, she reported feeling depressed, and clinicians observed objective signs of severe mood problems, including irritability, intrusiveness, and diminished need for sleep. Ms. Eplet continued to call Mr. Xenon from a telephone at the hospital until staff members intervened.

A threshold question in any evaluation of criminal responsibility is whether the defendant has a mental disorder that meets the jurisdiction's insanity standard. The evaluator concluded that Ms. Eplet suffered from bipolar II disorder and was hypomanic when the alleged offense occurred, a condition that satisfied the jurisdiction's insanity requirement that the defendant have a "substantial mental disease" at the time of the alleged offense. Yet Ms. Eplet had demonstrated in the past that, despite suffering from this serious impairment, she could refrain from telephoning a previous boyfriend after that boyfriend had obtained a restraining order against her. Moreover, following sanctions in jail and in the hospital, Ms. Eplet stopped calling Mr. Xenon, demonstrating a capacity to "conform her conduct" or at least delay calling under certain circumstances. Finally, Ms. Eplet's actions did not appear motivated by any psychotic beliefs or by beliefs that if she did not call Mr. Xenon, something adverse would occur.

These areas of analysis, highlighted by Rogers (1987), exemplify the types of issues evaluators should consider in evaluating the volitional controls of a defendant charged with stalking. Melton, Petrila, Poythress, and Slobogin (1997) note that courts have often viewed passion-driven, nonpsychotic actions as not qualifying for an insanity defense. Some courts have scrutinized carefully the degree of impulsiveness displayed by the defendant and have tended to regard evidence of planning before the criminal act as negating the possibility that the act was beyond the defendant's volitional control (*Rollins v. Commonwealth*, 1966; *Thompson v. Commonwealth*, 1952). Almost all instances of criminal stalking are, by definition, repeated behaviors (and thus do not seem impulsive), and most acts of stalking involve deliberation or at least preplanned action. These features of stalking, when present, would therefore militate against a conclusion that a stalker lacked volitional control.

On the other hand, many stalkers act from motives that clearly deviate from reality and that reflect severe mental illnesses. One can conceive of defendants who, despite retaining their general sense of right and wrong, might qualify for a volition-based excuse from criminal responsibility because of a clearly psychotic motivation for their acts, or because their behavior reflected a significant mental disease or defect (e.g., mania, brain trauma causing frontal lobe injury, or severe mental retardation accompanied by compulsive or stereotypic behavior). As a practical matter, most defendants who can recognize the wrongfulness of their actions will not qualify for an insanity defense based on their lack of ability to conform their conduct to the law's requirements. Yet the driven, relentless, explanation-defying persistence of some stalkers—exemplified by stalkers who continue to contact their victims despite restraining orders and unambiguous threats of legal consequences—suggests that their mental conditions may, in a few cases, specifically impair behavioral control while leaving other cognitive capacities intact.

CONCLUSION

Individuals who stalk do so for reasons that range from rational (if unsavory) to clearly psychotic. For more than a quarter century, clinicians have recognized that "forensic romances" generated by erotomanic delusions are a potential source of illegal behavior (Goldstein 1978, 1987) and of questions about the competence or sanity of accused perpetrators (Leong, 1994). Available studies suggest that a substantial fraction of stalkers act as they do because they suffer from psychiatric conditions that severely impair their judgment. The same conditions may so disorder some stalkers' thinking and perceptions as to render them incompetent to stand trial and/or criminally nonresponsible.

Now that stalking is statutorily recognized as a distinct criminal offense, forensic clinicians may expect increasing numbers of referrals for evaluation and treatment of defendants who face stalking charges. As they conduct forensic evaluations, clinicians should expect to face an assortment of intriguing intellectual challenges.

REFERENCES

American Law Institute. (1962). *Model penal code: Proposed official draft.* Philadelphia: The Institute.

American Psychiatric Association. (1983). American Psychiatric Association statement on the insanity defense. *American Journal of Psychiatry, 140*, 681–688.

American Psychiatric Association. (2000). *Diagnostic and statistical manual of mental disorders* (4th ed., Text Rev.). Washington, DC: Author.

Blackstone, W. (1765–1769). *Commentaries on the laws of England*. Oxford: Clarendon Press.

Brüne, M. (2003). Erotomanic stalking in evolutionary perspective. *Behavioral Sciences and the Law, 21*, 83–88.

Chadwick, P. D., & Lowe, C. F. (1990). Measurement and modification of delusional beliefs. *Journal of Consulting and Clinical Psychology, 58*, 225–232.

Chadwick, P. D., & Lowe, C. F. (1994). A cognitive approach to measuring and modifying delusions. *Behaviour Research and Therapy, 32*, 355–367.

Commonwealth v. Duncan, 239 Pa. Super. 539 (1976).

Drope v. Missouri, 420 U.S. 162 (1975).

Dusky v. United States, 362 U.S. 402 (1960).

English, J. (1988). The light between twilight and dusk: Federal criminal law and the volitional insanity defense. *Hastings Law Journal, 40*, 1–52.

Esquirol, J. E. D. (1976). *Des maladies mentales considérées sous les rapports médical, hygiénique et médico-légal*. New York: Arno Press. (Original work published 1845)

Gillett, T., Eminson, S. R., & Hassanyeh, F. (1990). Primary and secondary erotomania: Clinical characteristics and follow-up. *Acta Psychiatrica Scandanavica, 82*, 65–69.

Goldstein, R. L. (1978). De Clérambault in court: A forensic romance? *Bulletin of the American Academy of Psychiatry and the Law, 6*, 36–40.

Goldstein, R. L. (1987). More forensic romances: De Clérambault's syndrome in men. *Bulletin of the American Academy of Psychiatry and the Law, 23*, 219–230.

Hale, M. (1736). *Historia placitorum coronae: The history of the pleas of the crown*. London: Gyles, Woodward, and Davis.

Harmon, R. B., Rosner, R., & Owens, H. (1995). Obsessional harassment and erotomania in a criminal court population. *Journal of Forensic Sciences, 40*, 236–249.

Iowa State Bar Association, Special Committee on Uniform Court Instructions. (1988–2004). *Iowa criminal jury instructions*. Des Moines, IA: The Association.

Jason, L. A., Reicher, A., Easton, J., Neal, A., & Wilson, M. (1984). Female harassment after ending a relationship: a preliminary study. *Alternative Lifestyles, 6*, 259–269.

Kesavarajah v. R., 181 C.L.R. 230, 123 A.L.R. 463 (1994).

King v. Pritchard, 7 Car. & P. 303, 173 Eng. Rep. 135 (1836).

Leong, G. B. (1994). De Clérambault syndrome (erotomania) in the criminal justice system: Another look at the recurring problem. *Journal of Forensic Sciences, 39*, 378–385.

Leong, G. B., & Silva, J. A. (1988). The right to refuse treatment: an uncertain future. *Psychiatric Quarterly, 59,* 284–292.

Melton, G. B., Petrila, J., Poythress, N. G., & Slobogin, C. (1997). *Psychological evaluations for the courts: A handbook for mental health professionals and lawyers* (2nd ed.). New York: Guilford Press.

M'Naghten's Case, 10 Cl. & F. 200, 8 Eng. Rep. 718 (H.L. 1843).

Morse, S. J. (1994). Causation, compulsion, and involuntariness. *Bulletin of the American Academy of Psychiatry and the Law, 22,* 159–180.

Mossman, D. (1988). *United States v. Lyons:* Toward a new conception of legal insanity. *Bulletin of the American Academy of Psychiatry and the Law, 16,* 49–59.

Mullen, P. E., & Pathé, M. (1994). The pathological extensions of love. *British Journal of Psychiatry, 165,* 614–623.

Mullen, P. E., Pathé, M., & Purcell, R. (2001a). Stalking: New constructions of human behaviour. *Australian and New Zealand Journal of Psychiatry, 35,* 9–16.

Mullen, P. E., Pathé, M., & Purcell, R. (2001b). The management of stalkers. *Advances in Psychiatric Treatment, 7,* 335–342.

Mullen, P. E., Pathé, M., Purcell, R., & Stuart, G.W. (1999). Study of stalkers. *American Journal of Psychiatry, 156,* 1244–1249.

Munro, A., & Mok, H. (1995). An overview of treatment in paranoia/delusional disorder. *Canadian Journal of Psychiatry, 40,* 616–622.

Nadkarni, R., & Grubin, D. (2000). Stalking: Why do people do it? *British Journal of Psychiatry, 320,* 1486–1487.

National Criminal Justice Association. (1993). *Model antistalking code.* Retrieved March 31, 2005, from http://www.ojp.usdoj.gov/ocpa/94Guides/DomViol/appendb.htm

Odom-White, A., de Leon, J., Stanilla, J., Cloud, B. S., & Simpson, G. M. (1995). Misidentification syndromes in schizophrenia: Case reviews with implications for classification and prevalence. *Australian and New Zealand Journal of Psychiatry, 29,* 63–68.

Parsons v. State, 81 Ala. 577 597 (1887).

People v. Stuart, 100 N.Y.2d 412, 797 N.E.2d 28, 765 N.Y.S.2d 1 (2003).

Pinals, D. A. (2005). Where two roads meet: Restoration of competence to stand trial from a clinical perspective. *New England Journal on Criminal and Civil Confinement, 31,* 81–108.

Regina v. Oxford, 173 Eng. Rep. 941 (N. P. 1840).

Rogers, R. (1987). APA's position on the insanity defense: Empiricism versus emotionalism. *American Psychologist, 42,* 840–848.

Rollins v. Commonwealth, 151 S.E.2d 625 (Va., 1966).

Rosenfeld, B. (2000). Assessment and treatment of obsessional harassment. *Aggression and Violent Behavior, 5,* 529–549.

Rosenfeld, B. (2003). Recidivism in stalking and obsessional harassment. *Law and Human Behavior, 27,* 251–265.

Segal, J. H. (1989). Erotomania revisited: From Kraepelin to *DSM-III-R. American Journal of Psychiatry, 146,* 1261–1266.

Sell v. United States, 539 U.S. 166 (2003).

Singer, I. (1987). *The nature of love: Vol. 2. Courtly and romantic.* Chicago, IL: University of Chicago Press.

Slobogin, C. (2000). An end to insanity: Recasting the role of mental disability in criminal cases. *Virginia Law Review, 86,* 1199–1247.

State v. Neuzil, 589 N.W.2d 708 (Iowa 1999).

Thompson v. Commonwealth, 70 S.E.2d 284 (Va. 1952)

U.S. Department of Justice, Office of Justice Programs. (2002, January). *Strengthening antistalking statutes.* Retrieved January 30, 2007, from http://www.ojp. usdoj.gov/ovc/publications/bulletins/legalseries/bulletin1/welcome.html

Warren, L. J., MacKenzie, R., Mullen, P. E., & Ogloff, J. R. (2005). The problem behavior model: The development of a stalkers clinic and a threateners clinic. *Behavioral Sciences and the Law, 23,* 387–389.

Zona, M., Sharma, K., & Lane, J. (1993). A comparative study of erotomanic and obsessional subjects in a forensic sample. *Journal of Forensic Sciences, 38,* 894–903.

PART IV

Special Issues

8 Juvenile Aspects of Stalking

Charles L. Scott
Peter Ash
Todd Elwyn

Stalking that elicits fear in the target is relatively rare below age 16. Case reports reveal that some children and adolescents exhibit stalking behavior, and research on college populations suggests that stalking behavior in late adolescence is not uncommon. Stalking is a theme seen in movies and children's literature. The definition of stalking is used to distinguish stalking from developmentally normal following behavior commonly seen as a component of adolescent courtship, admiration, or crushes. This chapter reviews the literature on juvenile stalkers, including the frequency and patterns of juvenile stalking and the characteristics of juvenile stalkers. The chapter also provides suggestions for assessment, interventions, and legal responses in the management of the juvenile stalker.

INTRODUCTION

Some stalking-like behaviors are common in immature courtship behaviors of children and adolescents, but stalking characterized by repeated unwanted intrusion and communications that elicit fear in the target is relatively rare. In recent years, a number of published case reports suggest that some children and young adolescents exhibit stalking behavior, and research on college populations suggests that stalking behavior in late adolescence is not so uncommon. To help illustrate how pathological stalking overlaps with themes in normal development, this chapter begins with a survey of stalking in movies and children's literature. The chapter then uses the definition of stalking to distinguish stalking from developmentally normal following behavior commonly seen as a component of adolescent courtship, admiration, or crushes. Literature on juvenile stalkers is then reviewed to provide a picture of how commonly stalking occurs, as well as the characteristics of juvenile stalkers. The chapter then considers certain other behaviors that resemble stalking and examines theories about how stalking behavior develops. Finally, the chapter discusses the important topic of managing the juvenile stalker, including assessment, interventions, and legal responses.

JUVENILE STALKING IN MOVIES AND CHILDREN'S LITERATURE

Children and adolescents may be exposed to stalking behaviors and themes through television, books, and movies. The influence of media representations of crime and violence is an important avenue of exploration in general clinical work with children and adolescents. In our discussions we have noted that representations of juvenile and adolescent stalking in the media are not uncommon, and although there are no data linking them directly to stalking behavior, we have felt that awareness of these portrayals can be important for assessment of stalking risk and effects for stalking victims. For decades young children have witnessed the persistent, intimacy-seeking, amorous behaviors of the cartoon skunk Pepé Le Pew (Jones, 1945), who was enamored of the cat Penelope. Predatory stalking behaviors are a staple of movies and television stories directed at older children and adolescents. Teen horror films from *Halloween* (Carpenter, 1978) to *Scream* (Craven, 1996) regularly build suspense and heighten the tension by having the unidentified killer secretly follow and stalk adolescent victims as a prelude to killing them. In the teen thriller *Swimfan* (Polsono, 2002), a rejected high school girl stalks a male peer with whom she had a brief sexual encounter, reminiscent of the adult-oriented film *Fatal Attraction* (Lyne, 1987).

Works of fiction for juveniles, particularly older children and teenagers, contain a variety of stalking themes. In the book *I'm Not Who You Think I Am* (Kehret, 1999), targeted toward 9- to 12-year-olds, a delusional woman believes a 13-year-old girl is her daughter and attempts to kidnap her. Another story directed at preteens, *Disappearing Act* (Fleischman, 2003), illustrates how the term "stalking" is popularly used to describe following or harassing behaviors by an unknown person, regardless of motive. In this book, the mysterious "stalker" follows and threatens a 12-year-old boy and his sister, and is interested only in a map he assumes they possess. In *Pursued* (Rushford, 1994), a popular high school girl is stalked and then kidnapped for ransom by her ex-boyfriend and his new girlfriend, who are stalking their victim so that the police will suspect another boy who is romantically pursuing the girl. In *Stalker* (Cray, 1998), a 17-year-old girl who has won a celebrity look-alike contest is kidnapped by a mentally disturbed woman who has been stalking the celebrity. *Are You in the House Alone?* (Peck, 1976) tells the story of a high school girl who receives threatening notes and repeated phone calls before being raped by a male classmate. These and other similar books generally are classified under the heading "mystery" or "suspense."

Some video games engage children in simulated predatory stalking. For example, in *Predator: Concrete Jungle* (Vivendi Universal Games, 2004), players assume the perspective of the alien Predator, who roams the city landscape stalking human prey. In this game, as in many such games, players may also experience what it is like to be stalked. In the very violent game *Manhunt* (Rockstar Games, 2003), players advance by stalking and murdering men who have been hired to hunt down and kill them. The murders are shown in graphic detail. In *Silent Hill 4: The Room* (Konami Digital Entertainment, 2004), a man awakens to find himself trapped in his apartment and stalked by dangerous ghostly apparitions. Some have argued that violent video games, movies, and television shows contribute to the development of violent behavior in youth (Browne & Hamilton-Giachritsis, 2005). Video games and media depictions of following and stalking behaviors might serve to normalize them. However, whether they serve to encourage the development of stalking behaviors by juveniles has not been studied and is not known.

WHAT IS JUVENILE STALKING AND WHAT IS NOT?

Definitions of stalking vary, and there is no consensus definition at this time. As noted in chapter 1, Mullen, Pathé, and Purcell (2000) describe stalking as "those repeated acts, experienced as unpleasantly intrusive, which create apprehension and can be understood by a reasonable fellow citizen . . . to be grounds for becoming fearful." Westrup (1998) proposed using a *DSM*-type definition in which stalking was defined as "a constellation of behaviors that (a) are directed repeatedly towards a specific individual (the target), (b) are experienced by the target as unwelcome and intrusive, and (c) are reported to trigger fear or concern in the target." These definitions have been described based on work with adult populations.

The stalking behaviors of youth described in reports of high school aged and younger juveniles (Emer, 2001; McCann, 1998; Snow, 1998; Urbach, Khalily, & Mitchell, 1992; Vaidya, Chalhoub, & Newing, 2005) appear to follow patterns similar to those of adults (see chapter 1). Stalkers are typically male, and their targets typically female. Behaviors included telephone calls, repetitive letter writing, and physical approach. Threats were found in over half the cases. In the college age group, intrusive or unwanted pursuit most commonly followed the breakup of a romantic relationship. In a significant minority of cases, however, the victim was a professor or someone other than a romantic partner.

Developmentally Normal Following Behavior

Many developmentally appropriate behaviors exhibited by children and adolescents superficially resemble adult stalking behavior. For example, both school aged children and adolescents commonly develop crushes on their teachers and write notes or present small gifts to them in an attempt to garner their attention. Many youth idolize celebrity figures such as movie or rock stars and make repeated attempts to be closer to them through letter writing or attending concerts.

Children and adolescents also develop intense romantic feelings toward other peers in their environment, often at school. Following the object of their affections around school is common early adolescent courtship behavior. Behaviors such as calling repetitively on the phone, writing multiple notes, waiting in locations where the loved person is likely to come, and following the love object are generally viewed as a normal part of development. Such behavior is rarely experienced as threatening by the target. We are not aware of any systematic study of these behaviors in precollege youth, nor are we aware of the degree to which adult pathological stalkers engaged in developmentally normal following as children or adolescents. The following case example illustrates how an adolescent romantic crush can involve elements of intrusive or unwanted attention that may not qualify as actual stalking.

CASE EXAMPLE 8.1: MARK AND LAURA
Laura is a 13-year-old girl who tells all of her friends that she is "totally in love" with Mark, a 16-year-old boy who is a sophomore in high school. She leaves Mark "secret love notes" in his locker. She finds out his cell phone number and frequently calls him "just to hear his voice" that is on his phone message. One day, Mark notices a number on his caller ID that is associated with frequent hang-ups. He calls the number and Laura answers. He tells her to stop calling him and hangs up. Laura is embarrassed and mortified not realizing that her number had shown up on his phone.

Laura's behavior is characteristic of a teenage girl who develops a romantic "crush" on an older popular male peer. Although she has repeated behaviors to establish some type of contact with Mark, when confronted she is extremely embarrassed and vows to stop all attempts to contact him. Mark experiences annoyance, rather than fear. Laura does not represent a high risk of continued following behavior although she may need some emotional reassurance to overcome her personal shame.

College dating behavior has received more attention than earlier age courtship. One study found frequent forms of intrusion reported by over 60% of an undergraduate sample, including making hang-up telephone calls, calling on the telephone and arguing, watching from a distance, and failing to take hints that one is unwelcome (Cupach & Spitzberg, 1998). Less common behaviors in this sample included sending offensive pictures, sending excessive e-mails, making threatening communications, breaking into someone's home, tape-recording conversations without permission, and taking photographs without consent. A second study found that 20% of undergraduates surveyed had been the target of intrusive contact, and 20% of those had feared for their safety as a result (Haugaard & Seri, 2003). It does appear that such intrusive contact can lead to PTSD symptoms in the target (Westrup, Fremouw, Thompson, & Lewis, 1999).

EPIDEMIOLOGY AND PATTERNS OF JUVENILE STALKING

Juvenile Stalking: How Common Is It?

Actual pathological stalking by youth under age 18 occurs, but appears to be uncommon. Isolated case reports of child stalkers as young as 9 and 10 have been published (Brewster, 2003; McCann, 2000; Snow, 1998). A study of restraining orders issued by a Massachusetts family court over a 10-month period indicates that 757 restraining orders were issued to juveniles who exhibited threatening, abusive, or stalking behavior (National Victim Center, 1995). Although this study did not separate those restraining orders issued for stalking behavior from other threatening behaviors, this report nevertheless suggests that a significant number of adolescents demonstrate stalking-like behavior (McCann, 2001) that may not rise to the level of criminal or delinquent stalking charges. In the largest sample of juvenile stalkers published to date, McCann (2000) reviewed 13 cases of stalking by children and adolescents that he obtained from his case files, published literature, and media reports. This particular sample had a mean age of 14.1 years, with ages of offenders ranging from 9 to 18. McCann described these youth as "obsessional followers" and noted that the majority of perpetrators were male and the majority of the victims were female. In this same sample, nearly half of the victims were adults and the other half were same age peers. The most common method of stalking noted was physical approach toward the victim. Other forms of stalking include making unwanted sexual advances, telephone calls, letter writing, and vandalism.

McCann's study (2000) found that the most common type of perpetrator-victim pattern involved casual acquaintances (64%), followed by strangers (21%) and prior intimate partners (14%). He contrasts this perpetrator-victim pattern to that of adult stalkers described by Meloy (1998). Meloy found that the majority of adult stalkers' victims were from prior intimate relationships, in contrast to McCann's findings that juvenile perpetrators were more likely to stalk casual acquaintances. McCann (2000) theorizes that this difference stems from particular developmental issues faced by adolescents. In particular, he proposes that because adolescents are exploring their self-identity and emerging sexual feelings, their obsessive fixations are more commonly directed toward casual acquaintances rather than prior intimate partners (McCann, 2001). This theory would appear to apply better to those in early to mid-adolescence than to those in late adolescence.

Little is known about how often juveniles are arrested or prosecuted for stalking. One study in Hawaii examined the legal records of youth committed to the state's youth correctional facility during a 1-year period. The study found that none of the incarcerated youth were charged with, nor had a history of being charged with, harassment by stalking or aggravated harassment by stalking. However, a small percentage of youth (5.5%) had been adjudicated for harassment, which under Hawaii law may include some stalking behaviors such as making repeated communications after being told to stop (Elwyn, Wang, Geobert, Johal, & Kim, 2004).

Patterns of Juvenile Stalkers

McCann (1998) noted three subtypes of stalking in juveniles that matched the typology developed by Zona, Sharma, and Lane (1993): erotomanic, love obsessional, and simple obsessional (for a further clarification of this and other typologies, see chapter 2). A person with erotomanic subtype delusionally believes that another person, usually of higher social status, loves him or her. Love obsessional stalkers maintain an intense love for someone, and although they may recognize that the person does not return their love, they often believe that the love object will eventually return their love if the stalker's feelings are made known. For the simple obsessional stalker, a prior relationship actually existed and the individual seeks to reunite with the victim or seek revenge for being rejected.

As described in chapter 2, the typology developed by Mullen et al. (2000) classifies stalkers into categories based on the motivation of the stalker. Although our GAP Committee on Psychiatry and the Law felt that their five categories (rejected, intimacy seeking, incompetent, resentful, or predatory) could theoretically apply to juveniles, no research has yet examined their applicability.

Other Behaviors That Resemble Stalking Among Juveniles

Other behaviors that may overlap juvenile stalking include bullying and sexual harassment. In the United States, the percentage of students that report being bullied ranges from 25% (Duncan, 1999) to 75% (Hoover, Oliver, & Hazler, 1992). Bullying has been defined as occurring when a person "is exposed, repeatedly and over time, to negative actions on the part of one or more other students" (Olweus, 1993). McCann (2001) notes that similarities between stalking and bullying include: (1) more than one incident of threat, harassment, or intimidation; (2) a perpetrator who threatens or evokes fear in the victim; and (3) an awareness by the victim that he or she is being threatened. Differences between bullying and stalking noted by McCann include the following: (1) bullying can be perpetrated by a group rather than an individual; (2) the motivation of bullying centers on dominating the victim, whereas stalking indicates a disturbance of attachment; and (3) a bully's attempts to exclude the victim from a peer group is not a common feature of stalkers. Although there are differences between bullying and stalking, a victim of bullying may nonetheless be allowed to pursue civil protection orders and possible criminal charges of stalking against the perpetrator when the bullying behavior meets a state's legal definition for stalking.

In some cases, stalking may be a component of dating violence. Studies report that between 20% to 40% of college aged girls have experienced some dating violence (Neufeld, McNamara, & Ertl, 1999; Straus, 2004). Although sexual harassment and stalking are not equivalent, certain types of sexual harassment by youth may closely resemble stalking behavior. In their study of 561 students age 11 to 16, Roscoe, Strouse, and Goodwin (1994) noted that 50% of girls and 37% of boys described having experienced some form of sexual harassment. Of this sample, approximately 20% of students received harassing telephone calls, letters, or notes perceived as sexually harassing. Because these types of behaviors have also been described in child and adolescent obsessional followers, McCann (1998) suggests that a subset of sexual harassers may also meet the definition of stalking (McCann, 2001). When considering intervention, the presence of sexual harassment is important to recognize because additional school and legal interventions are available to juvenile victims of sexual harassment.

How Does Juvenile Stalking Develop?

A number of dynamic theories regarding the development of adult stalkers have been proposed (see chapters 1 and 2 for discussions related to dynamic theories and understanding motivation behind various stalking types). Although it is likely that many of these factors also play a role in juvenile stalking, no empirical research tells us whether similar factors give rise to juvenile stalking. One theory of stalking suggests that it is a variant of intimate violence. Logan, Leukefeld, and Walker (2000) found a high level of association in victims of stalking with prior physical or emotional abuse victimization.

The development of pathologic childhood attachments has been proposed as a possible etiology of stalking behavior (Meloy, 1992, 1996), and these theories may also be understood in the context of juvenile stalking. First, Bowlby's theory of childhood attachment centers on the importance to the child of maintaining the affectional bond to the caregiver. As a result, the child demonstrates a range of behaviors in an effort to preserve this bond and keep the attachment figure readily available. Crying, clinging, temper tantrums, and angry demands serve to attract the caregiver's attention with the desired reunion following (Bowlby, 1980). These infantile behaviors have been compared to those behaviors of adult stalkers who attempt to woo their love objects through the use of letters, phone calls, following, and increasingly angry protests.

Another theory posits that deficits in different subphases of Mahler, Pine, and Bergman's (1975) separation-individuation paradigm contribute to adult stalking behavior (Kienlen, 1998). For example, Meloy (1996) theorizes that disturbances in the differentiation and practicing subphases are important in the development of obsessional following, whereas Dutton and Golant (1995) proposes that deficits in the rapprochement phase played a significant role.

Kienlen (1998) proposes that disturbed childhood relationships with a parent or caregiver can result in a preoccupied attachment pattern in adulthood. In some individuals, this preoccupied attachment ultimately erupts into stalking behavior. In their study of childhood relationships among individuals who exhibit adult criminal stalking behavior, Kienlen found that more than 60% of adult stalkers experienced a loss or change in a primary caregiver during their childhood. Among juvenile and adolescent stalkers, these dynamic contributing factors may play a role.

MANAGING THE JUVENILE STALKER

Evaluation of the Alleged Juvenile Stalker

There has been little research conducted regarding the psychiatric assessment of juveniles referred for stalking. Evaluation of a potential juvenile stalker utilizes general violence risk assessment approaches (see chapter 3), research from adult stalkers, and data published from McCann's small samples of adolescent obsessional followers. Based on our own clinical and forensic work, we recommend the use of a comprehensive approach when evaluating a juvenile referred for stalking. Important components of the psychiatric assessment are listed in Table 8.1.

The evaluator should take a detailed history from the youth regarding all alleged verbal or written threats. Other sources of information to consider in evaluating juvenile threats include the victim's account, notes, letters, diaries, pictures of graffiti, recorded audio/videotapes, school records, juvenile arrest records, juvenile probation reports, counseling records, computer website visits, and

Table 8.1. Components to Be Assessed in Possible Juvenile Stalkers

- Detailed history of present behavior
- Peer influences
- Intent of behavior
- Environmental access to target
- Fit between behavior and applicable legal definition of stalking
- History of prior attachments and prior stalking
- Presence of psychiatric disorder
- Violence risk assessment

e-mail correspondence. Collateral interviews with the potential victim, juvenile's parents/caretakers, peers, counselors, and schoolteachers may yield useful information. In examining these data, the evaluator should consider the following:

- the potential target(s) of the threat
- the relationship of the potential target to the juvenile
- the type and nature of the threat
- the situation(s) that have triggered threat
- escalation of the threat over time
- attempts to act on the threat
- previous interventions to manage the threat
- involvement of others in making the threat
- any suggested use of weapons
- the attitude by the juvenile when confronted

Because most juveniles reside with their parents or legal guardians, the clinician should ask about parental and guardian attempts to control or manage the juvenile's behavior. Because some adult stalkers ultimately harm those individuals who prevent them from contacting their victim, parents may be at increased risk from juveniles who stalk.

The examiner needs to determine peer influences on the youth's behavior. Peer relationships are extremely influential in adolescence, and the evaluator must determine whether peers play a role, either directly or indirectly, in the stalking behavior. In particular, the evaluator should ask whether other peers participate with the juvenile in stalking and, if not, whether peers are providing encouragement to the juvenile to continue the stalking behavior.

The examiner should consider the youth's emotional, cognitive, and psychological maturity when determining the juvenile's capacity to form the specific intent for stalking outlined in their jurisdiction (McCann, 2001). Some antistalking statutes require that the perpetrator intend to cause fear of harm or injury to the victim (for a further discussion of these matters, see Part III: Stalking and the Law, chapters 6 and 7). Intent is also relevant for treatment considerations. Therefore, the examiner must address the youth's understanding of and beliefs about the purpose of their behavior.

The evaluator should determine whether the behavior triggering the referral is consistent with the legal definition of stalking. Other behaviors sometimes confused with stalking include bullying, sexual harassment, and general threats to harm others such as bombing or shooting up a school. Although threats may not technically meet the statutory criteria for stalking, a violence risk assessment may nevertheless be warranted.

The examiner should carefully review any prior history of stalking behavior or obsessional attachments by the juvenile, including behaviors toward other peers, celebrities, or teachers. The clinician should attempt to determine whether the youth's thoughts are consistent with developmentally appropriate fantasies that often include unrealistic expectations that a teacher, peer, or other person will return their love. Indications that the behavior is in excess of expected fantasy includes a youth's persistent fixation despite feedback or intervention, a youth's continued attempts to access the victim in violation of agreements not to do so, and escalating intrusions (such as making threatening communications or repeatedly following).

The clinician should carefully screen for the presence of any psychiatric disorder, with particular consideration to the possibility of a first episode of a developing psychotic disorder. In addition, the examiner should review the impact on the youth's reported stalking of any other mental disorder, cognitive impairment, or behavioral difficulty.

The examiner should explore the various environments familiar to the juvenile to determine the proximity risk to the alleged stalking victim. This inquiry may be particularly important for those youth who target other youth. Common locations where juveniles can easily stalk other peers include school, the local neighborhood, parks, malls, clubs, concerts, and sporting events.

The evaluator should conduct a thorough general violence risk assessment of the youth. McCann (2001) notes that many risk factors for future violence by stalkers appear similar to those associated with violence in general. In his sample of child and adolescent obsessional followers, McCann (2000) found that 31% eventually acted violently after having expressed a threat. In general, risk factors for future violence in juveniles include a past history of violence, early onset of offending, chronicity of offending, diversity of law-violating behaviors, access to weapons, involvement with gangs, cognitive impairment, use of alcohol and drugs, presence of a conduct disorder, and disturbed family relationships (Scott, 1999). A possible risk factor for future violence in adolescents with erotomania is a youth's fixations on multiple people. For example, Urbach et al. (1992) describe an adolescent male with multiple object fixations who ultimately demonstrated at least one act of violence. McCann (2001) has proposed that a youth's fragile developing sense of self-identity may increase the likelihood of his developing multiple and changeable object fixations. However, the exact relationship, if any, of multiple object fixations to future violence remains unclear.

In the wake of Columbine, schools have become highly sensitized to threats of potential violence, and may suspend youth whom they suspect of being at risk "pending a psychiatric evaluation." These youth may be brought by school personnel or parents to emergency rooms for "clearance" that they are safe to return to school. Adolescents who stalk are sometimes referred in this way. One critical limitation in an evaluation conducted in an emergency room is that collateral information, especially from peers, is seldom available. The patient himself may minimize or conceal his behavior and thoughts. The evaluating clinician should therefore be very cautious in making determinations of risk with such limited information.

Interventions With a Juvenile Stalker

There is no "one size fits all" approach to juveniles who stalk; stalkers must be evaluated on a case-by-case basis. Treatment of any underlying psychiatric disturbance represents one general principle that should be implemented. Although some youth will have mental illnesses responsive to psychotropic medication, the vast majority of youthful offenders will also require other types of therapy and intervention. Self-management approaches described by Wexler (1991) represent one potential therapy that may be useful with adolescents whose obsessional following begins after a breakup from an intimate relationship (McCann, 2001). The self-management approach includes a combination of cognitive behavioral and psychoanalytic self-psychology techniques. This approach may be effective in those adolescents who react with anger and jealousy after a breakup. McCann (2001) proposes that juveniles who stalk acquaintances or strangers do so in response to their feelings of depression, anxiety, and envy. He recommends therapies designed to increase the youth's social skills and feelings of competence.

Minimizing contact between the alleged stalker and victim may be useful. When the perpetrator attends the same school as the victim, a change in schools may be necessary to avoid ongoing contact. Sometimes, this will mean that the victim must change schools. Although this may seem like "punishing the victim," in some cases it may be the safest and simplest option.

A variety of school interventions can help prevent the stalker from reaching the intended victim should the stalker come to the victim's school. First, the security staff at the school can be educated regarding the identity of the alleged stalker, the importance of early identification and apprehension should the stalker enter campus, and the significance of preventing contact between the stalker and victim. Second, the front desk, reception, and administrative staff can be similarly educated with an emergency action plan in place should the stalker be noted to enter the school. Third, the intended victim's teachers can be made aware of a potential stalking situation involving one of their students and the importance of minimizing contact with the perpetrator. All the above parties should have a photograph of the alleged stalker to assist in immediate identification. Fourth, emergency contact numbers should be readily available to everyone involved.

A juvenile's parents can also impose restrictions to help decrease activity by a child or adolescent who is stalking. Such restrictions can include limitations on telephone and computer use, denial of car privileges, and close monitoring of after-school and weekend activities. In small communities where youth are often involved in the same activities outside of school, cessation of contact can be very difficult. In designing an intervention plan, it is important to consider the likely situations in which the stalker can readily find his victim. In those circumstances in which the victim is not aware of being stalked and the perpetrator communicates a desire to harm the victim, clinicians should try to protect the victim in a manner that comports with the local jurisdiction's laws regarding confidentiality and duties to third parties.

Legal remedies to stalking are discussed in detail in chapter 6. Some states have enacted legislation that permits issuing restraining orders against juvenile stalking offenders. For example, in Colorado, any municipal or district court can issue a temporary or permanent civil restraining order against a juvenile who is 10 years of age or older to prevent stalking (Col. Rev. Stat. Ann., 2004). As with interventions targeted toward adult stalkers, careful consideration must also be given to the possibility that a restraining order may escalate the behavior of some juvenile stalkers. To date, there is no research that examines the efficacy of restraining orders when applied against children or adolescents.

Legal Responses to Juvenile Stalkers

Juveniles who have been charged with stalking may be addressed by the juvenile justice system or by adult criminal courts, depending on applicable state laws. In some states, such as Florida, prosecutors have the authority to prosecute as adults adolescents charged with aggravated stalking who are 14 or older at the time of the offense (Fla. Stat. § 985.227(1)(a), 2004).

Juveniles who have been adjudicated delinquent for stalking in juvenile court face a variety of consequences depending on their state's statutes. These consequences can range from outpatient monitoring (probation) to a requirement that the juvenile be placed in a secure residential treatment facility. Outpatient supervision can include special curfews, driving restrictions, no victim contact, ongoing counseling, and periodic risk assessments of violence. A juvenile court judge may also place a youth in intensive residential treatment. For example, in Florida, children who are less than 13 years of age and are adjudicated delinquent on aggravated stalking are eligible for intense residential treatment program (Fla. Stat. § 985.03, 2004).

Other restrictions may also be placed on the juvenile. In Washington State, any juvenile who has committed a felony while stalking a family or household member may not lawfully possess a firearm (Rev. Code Wash. Ann. § 9.41.040(2)(a)(i), 2004). In Arkansas, stalking is included among a list of crimes defined as sex offenses (Ark. Code Ann. § 12–12–903, 2004).

When a youth is adjudicated delinquent for a stalking offense, his juvenile court records may lose their traditional confidential status. In Minnesota, if a juvenile has been adjudicated delinquent of stalking, the juvenile's probation officer must transmit a copy of the court's disposition order to the superintendent of the juvenile's school district or the chief administrative officer of the juvenile's school (Minn. Stat. § 260B.171, 2004). In Washington State, when a juvenile adjudicated delinquent for stalking is released from a juvenile facility, written notice is sent to law enforcement agencies and schools where the juvenile intends to reside or the last school attended by the juvenile (Rev. Code Wash. Ann. § 13.40.215, 2004). In addition, if the juvenile resides in a residential facility, the statute authorizes notification of any employer that employs the offender while residing at the residential facility. If requested in writing, any witness who testified against the juvenile as well as any person specified in writing by the prosecuting attorney may also receive notice regarding the release of the juvenile.

A charge of stalking against an adult may also affect the confidentiality of that person's juvenile court records. In Minnesota, mental health professionals evaluating adults convicted of stalking are granted access to the person's juvenile court records if relevant and necessary for the assessment (Minn. Stat. § 609.749, 2004). In Virginia, the probation officer has the authority to include information from available juvenile court records when a person is tried in a circuit court for stalking (Va. Code Ann. § 19.2-299, 2000).

CASE EXAMPLE 8.2: JOHN AND LISA

John is a 16-year-old boy who had been involved for 2 years with Lisa, a same aged peer who attends his same school. Lisa told John that she was no longer interested in dating him after John found Lisa "making out" with his best friend behind the bleachers at a school football game. Although Lisa has told John that "it is over," he continues to call her on her cell phone, send her e-mails, and attempt to text message her.

When Lisa does not return John's phone calls or e-mail messages, he begins waiting after class to talk to her to convince her that they should "get back together." He tells her that he "forgives her" and emphasizes that "you are the only one for me." Lisa informs John that their break up is final and to "get over it."

Over the next month John becomes increasingly depressed and has thoughts of committing suicide combined with fantasies of killing Lisa and her new boyfriend. One evening while watching television with her new boyfriend at his house, Lisa looks out the window and sees John sitting outside in his car watching them. When John sees Lisa looking out the window, he drives away while she calls the police. The police pull John over and find a loaded registered .45 revolver in the glove compartment of the car. John denies any intent to harm Lisa and states that he was just driving by to "see if she was home so that he could talk to her."

John's initial behaviors following the breakup with Lisa are not atypical for a teenager who feels emotionally bruised regarding the ending of a relationship. However, John's increasing depression and inability to stop thinking about Lisa indicate that he has become inappropriately preoccupied with his former girlfriend. John develops suicidal and homicidal fantasies and as a result, his risk of aggression and violence increase substantially. His driving to Lisa's home to watch her and her new boyfriend indicates that he is taking active steps to monitor her new relationship.

Lisa, her new boyfriend, and both families should consider several interventions to minimize any future risk. First, all parents need to be notified regarding the concern about John's behavior to help enact additional recommendations. Second, Lisa and her new boyfriend must cease all contact with John to prevent any encouragement or escalation of behaviors. Third, John should be taken immediately to a mental health professional to evaluate and treat his depression and suicidality. A decision regarding immediate inpatient hospitalization should be considered. Fourth, all firearms and weapons should be removed from John's environment to minimize the risk impulsive aggression. Fifth, a determination needs to be made about whether to prosecute John, a 16-year-old, for being in possession of a handgun. Sixth, careful consideration should be given for a restraining order against John. The risks and benefits of such an order would need to be reviewed to determine if the implementation of such order could potentially further increase violence. Considerations might include any history of prior responses to limit setting or prior restraining orders, antisocial tendencies and relationship with local police or authority who would be delivering the restraining order and monitoring it. Seventh, Lisa's family may wish to consider notifying the local police so that they are aware of the situation should emergency intervention be required. Eighth, the school should consider a transfer of John to another school to minimize his contact with Lisa and assist in lessening his obsessive attachment. Less desirable, but occasionally indicated, would be to transfer Lisa to another school. Ninth, appropriate school officials, security, and teachers at Lisa's school should be educated about John's behavior toward Lisa and an emergency preparedness plan devised should John come to the school campus in the future.

CONCLUSION

Although important research regarding adult stalkers has been conducted in the past 20 years, juvenile stalkers have received little attention. Recent research on child and adolescent obsessional followers represents an important first step in understanding the characteristics of both juvenile perpetrators and the interpersonal context in which stalking occurs. Future research will help guide not only assessments of such youth but also appropriate interventions for them.

REFERENCES

Ark. Code Ann. § 12–12–903 (2004).
Bowlby, J. (1980). *Attachment and loss: Vol. III. Loss, sadness, and depression.* New York: Basic Books.

Brewster, M. P. (2003). Children and stalking. In M. P. Brewster (Ed.), *Stalking: Psychology, risk factors, interventions, and law* (pp. 9.1–9.22). Kingston, NJ: Civic Research Institute.

Browne, K. D., & Hamilton-Giachritsis, C. (2005). The influence of violent media on children and adolescents: A public-health approach. *Lancet, 365,* 702–710.

Carpenter, J. (Director), & Hill, D. (Producer). (1978). *Halloween* [Motion Picture]. United States: Compass International Pictures.

Col. Rev. Stat. Ann. 13–14–102 (2004).

Craven, W. (Director), Konrad, C., & Woods, C. (Producers). (1996). *Scream* [Motion Picture]. United States: Dimension Films.

Cray, J. (1998). *Stalker.* New York: Aladdin.

Cupach, W. R., & Spitzberg, B. H. (1998). Obsessive relational intrusion and stalking. In W. R. Cupach & B. H. Spitzberg (Eds.), *The dark side of close relationships* (pp. 233–263). Mahwah, NJ: Erlbaum.

Duncan, R. D. (1999). Peer and sibling aggression: An investigation of intra- and extra-familial bullying. *Journal of Interpersonal Violence, 14,* 871–886.

Dutton, D. G., & Golant, S. K. (1995). *The batterer: A psychological profile.* New York: Basic Books.

Elwyn, T. S., Wang, E., Geobert, D., Johal, S., & Kim, S. P. (2004, October). *Youth incarcerated in Hawaii for stalking offenses.* Paper presented at the poster session of the annual meeting of the American Academy of Psychiatry and the Law, Scottsdale, AZ.

Emer, D. M. (2001). Obsessive behavior and relational violence in juvenile populations: Stalking case analysis and legal implications. In J. A. Davis (Ed.), *Stalking crimes and victim protection: Prevention, intervention, threat assessment, and case management* (pp. 33–68). Boca Raton, FL: CRC Press.

Fla. Stat. § 985.03 (2004).

Fla. Stat. § 985.227(1)(a) (2004).

Fleischman, S. (2003). *Disappearing act.* New York: Greenwillow Books.

Haugaard, J. J., & Seri, L. G. (2003). Stalking and other forms of intrusive contact after the dissolution of adolescent dating or romantic relationships. *Violence & Victims, 18,* 279–297.

Hoover, J. H., Oliver, R., & Hazler, R. J. (1992). Bullying: Perceptions of adolescent victims in the Midwestern USA. *School Psychology International, 13,* 5–16.

Jones, C. (Director). (1945). *The odor-able kitty* [Theatrical Animation]. United States: Warner Bros.

Kehret, P. (1999). *I'm not who you think I am.* New York: Dutton Children's Books.

Kienlen, K. K. (1998). Developmental and social antecedents of stalking. In J. R. Meloy (Ed.), *The psychology of stalking: Clinical and forensic perspectives* (pp. 51–67). San Diego: Academic Press.

Konami Digital Entertainment. (2004). *Silent hill 4: The room* [Video Game]. Redwood City, CA: Konami Digital Entertainment.

Logan, T. K., Leukefeld, C., & Walker, B. (2000). Stalking as a variant of intimate violence: implications from a young adult sample. *Violence and Victims, 15*, 91–111.

Lyne, A. (Director), Lansing, S., & Jaffe, S. R. (Producers). (1987). *Fatal attraction* [Motion Picture]. United States: Paramount Pictures.

Mahler, M. S., Pine, F., & Bergman, A. (1975). *The psychological birth of the human infant: Symbiosis and individuation.* New York: Basic Books.

McCann, J. T. (1998). Subtypes of stalking (obsessional following) in adolescents. *Journal of Adolescence, 21*, 667–675.

McCann, J. T. (2000). A descriptive study of child and adolescent obsessional followers. *Journal of Forensic Sciences, 45*, 195–199.

McCann, J. T. (2001). *Stalking in children and adolescents: The primitive bond.* Washington, DC: American Psychological Association.

Meloy, J. R. (1992). *Violent attachments.* Northvale, NJ: Jason Aronson.

Meloy, J. R. (1996). Stalking (obsessional following): A review of some preliminary studies. *Aggression and Violent Behavior, 1*, 147–162.

Meloy, J. R. (Ed.). (1998). *The psychology of stalking: Clinical and forensic perspectives.* San Diego: Academic Press.

Minn. Stat. § 260B.171 (2004).

Minn. Stat. § 609.749 (2004).

Mullen, P. E., Pathé, M., & Purcell, R. (2000). *Stalkers and their victims.* Cambridge, UK; New York: Cambridge University Press.

National Victim Center. (1995). *School crime: K–12.* Arlington, VA: Author.

Neufeld, J., McNamara, J. R., & Ertl, M. (1999). Incidence and prevalence of dating partner abuse and its relationship to dating practices. *Journal of Interpersonal Violence, 14*, 125–137.

Olweus, D. (1993). *Bullying at school: What we know and what we can do.* Cambridge, MA: Blackwell.

Peck, R. (1976). *Are you in the house alone?* New York: Viking Press.

Polsono, J. (Director), Caracciolo, J., Segan, A. L., & Penotti, J. (Producers). (2002). *Swimfan* [Motion Picture]. United States: 20th Century Fox.

Rev. Code Wash. Ann. § 9.41.040 (2)(a)(i) (2004).

Rev. Code Wash. Ann. §13.40.215 (2004).

Rockstar Games. (2003). *Manhunt* [Video Game]. New York: Rockstar Games.

Roscoe, B., Strouse, J. S., & Goodwin, M. P. (1994). Sexual harassment: Early adolescents' self-reports of experiences and acceptance. *Adolescence, 29*, 515–523.

Rushford, P. H. (1994). *Pursued.* Minneapolis, MN: Bethany House.

Scott, C. L. (1999). Juvenile violence. *Psychiatric Clinics of North America, 22*, 71–83.

Snow, R. L. (1998). *Stopping a stalker: A cop's guide to making the system work for you.* New York: Plenum Trade.

Straus, M. A. (2004). Prevalence of violence against dating partners by male and female university students worldwide. *Violence Against Women, 10*, 790–811.

Urbach, J. R., Khalily, C., & Mitchell, P. P. (1992). Erotomania in an adolescent: Clinical and theoretical considerations. *Journal of Adolescence, 15*, 231–240.

Va. Code Ann. § 19.2–299 (2000).

Vaidya, G., Chalhoub, N., & Newing, J. (2005). Stalking in adolescence: A case report. *Child and Adolescent Mental Health, 10,* 23–25.

Vivendi Universal Games. (2004). *Predator: Concrete jungle* [Video Game]. Paris: Vivendi Universal Games.

Westrup, D. (1998). Applying functional analysis to stalking behavior. In J. R. Meloy (Ed.), *The psychology of stalking: Clinical and forensic perspectives* (pp. 275–294). San Diego, CA: Academic Press.

Westrup, D., Fremouw, W. J., Thompson, R. N., & Lewis, S. F. (1999). The psychological impact of stalking on female undergraduates. *Journal of Forensic Sciences, 44,* 554–557.

Wexler, D. B. (1991). *The adolescent self: Strategies for self-management, self-soothing, and self-esteem in adolescents.* New York: Norton.

Zona, M. A., Sharma, K. K., & Lane, J. (1993). A comparative study of erotomanic and obsessional subjects in a forensic sample. *Journal of Forensic Sciences, 38,* 894–903.

9   Cyberstalking

Graham D. Glancy
Alan W. Newman
Mordecai N. Potash
John Tennison

Cyberstalking involves the use of the Internet or other electronic communication to stalk another person. Already common, it is likely to become more common as the use of the Internet continues to grow. The characteristics of online stalkers and their victims have some differences from those of the offline stalker. Mullen, Pathé, Purcell, and Stuart's (1999) classification may apply to cyberstalkers except for the apparently common phenomenon of child luring that may be a new category. The methods of cyberstalking, as described in this chapter, are particularly ingenious. We know little about the effect on victims, but postulate that it is similar to offline stalking. We make some suggestions that may prevent cyberstalking, as well as offer some steps to bear in mind once cyberstalking occurs.

INTRODUCTION

The proliferation of personal computers with Internet access in the last decade has raised concerns about a new phenomenon known as cyberstalking. The Internet can be used to annoy and harass large numbers of victims in a generic manner by disseminating computer viruses, Internet scams, and "spamming" people with unsolicited e-mail. In 1999 Janet Reno, the attorney general of the United States, defined cyberstalking as the use of the Internet, e-mail, or other electronic communications devices to stalk another person (Reno, 1999).

Barak (2005) looked at the issue of sexual harassment on the Internet. He characterizes cyberstalking as one type of sexual coercion. He notes that online behavior is characterized by disinhibition, openness, venture, and bravado—an atmosphere characterized by typical masculine attitudes. He argues that the lack of legal boundaries or enforcement vehicles encourage people to do what they would not have done in offline situations. He notes the near impossibility of implementation of legal procedures on a large scale.

In this chapter we will discuss what is known about the prevalence of this phenomenon, the types of cyberstalking, and what is known about the perpetrators. In addition, we will generate some hypotheses about the comparison between online and offline stalkers. We will also discuss the effects on victims and current thoughts and resources for dealing with cyberstalking. Finally, we will make some suggestions about future directions for research in this field.

PREVALENCE

Reno (1999), extrapolating from general surveys of stalking victims, estimated that there may be as many as 475,000 online stalking victims in the United States each year; however, she cautioned that this figure is mere speculation. She also quoted estimates by various police departments that 20% of stalking cases involve cyberstalking. The forensic psychiatrist attached to the Ontario Threat Assessment Unit (P. I. Collins, personal communication, June 15, 2005) estimated a much smaller figure, perhaps 1 in 20 (5%), despite the fact that the use of technology is assumed to be equivalent in Ontario and the United States.

Alexy, Burgess, Baker, and Smoyak (2005) studied 756 students from two universities. They found that male students were more likely to have been cyberstalked. The perpetrators were most likely to have been a former intimate partner. The stalking was likely to include threats of suicide. It was noted that these victims were less likely to do anything about the situation because they believed that it would resolve itself.

In a review of the literature on stalking, we could find only a few references to cyberstalking. Mullen et al. (1999) made passing reference to the fact that e-mails were used in 2 of their 145 cases. This is similar to a Dutch study of 235 stalking victims that found 2% reported stalking by means of the Internet (Kamphuis & Emmelkamp, 2001). A survey of 4,446 women found that 581 reported some form of stalking and in 25% of these incidents e-mail "was used" (Fisher, Cullen, & Turner, 2002).

Fremouw, Westrup, and Pennypacker (1997) noted that 24.2% of students in psychology courses reported being victims of stalking in general. In an attempt to compare these results in a university that was highly ranked among America's most wired colleges, Leblanc, Levesque, Richardson, and Berka (2001) found that 12% of female and 2% of male students reported being stalked. E-mails ranked fifth among the methods listed, in that 58% reported repeated e-mails as a method used. Leblanc et al. noted that their results showed a lower rate of stalking despite having a highly wired campus. A survey conducted by the National Center for Missing & Exploited Children found that 6 percent of youths reported being harassed online and 19% reported unwanted sexual solicitation. Forty-eight percent of the perpetrators were under age 18, and at least 25% were female (Finkelhor, Mitchell, & Wolak, 2000). Thus, it can be concluded that data on the prevalence of cyberstalking in the academic literature is particularly sparse. Some authors have suggested there are no credible statistics on prevalence at this time (Bocij & McFarlane, 2003). In our discussions among members of the GAP Committee on Psychiatry and the Law, we postulated that this is a dynamic situation and that, at any point, prevalence may be inaccurate 1 year later due to the increasing use of computers for communication.

CHARACTERISTICS OF CYBERSTALKERS

CASE EXAMPLE 9.1: MAN CHARGED AFTER 5 MONTHS OF CYBERSTALKING

A Cambridge graduate, who became the first person in Britain to be convicted of using the Internet to stalk a former girlfriend, was jailed for 3 months after he continued to harass his victim. Despite a court order that prevented him from going within a mile of his former girlfriend's home, the subject, a 24-year-old university graduate, turned up on her doorstep clutching a bottle of champagne only weeks after his conviction. When he rang the buzzer for the specially installed video entry system at her flat, she immediately called the police. He tried to escape but was rugby tackled by officers when he ran off. When charged, he told the police that he was an entirely friendly person. He was sentenced to 3 months in prison for breaching a restraining order and was told by the judge that this would be a lesson to him.

He had previously been convicted, under new antistalking legislation, of harassing the victim, whom he met while they were students at university. Evidence in court revealed that he had used the Internet to wage a malicious and unrelenting campaign against her over 5 months. He would send offensive e-mails to the children's charity where she worked, featuring sinister and frightening messages including references to *The Shining*, the film starring Jack Nicholson wherein the lead character attempts to kill his wife and child in a deserted hotel. He was sentenced to a 2-year conditional discharge with a restraining order. Five weeks later he turned up at her home. The victim testified that she loathed and hated him and was deeply frightened by his references to *The Shining*. She also reported how stressful and distressing the past year had been. (Senan, 1999)

Most examples of cyberstalking appear in the media or anecdotal reports. Only one systematic study exists (Lucks, 2004). It is widely assumed that the majority of cyberstalkers are male, whereas the group Working to Halt Online Abuse (WHOA) reports that 61.5% of victims are female (WHOA, 2003). This is similar to the figures for victims of offline stalking—72% found by Meloy and Gothard (1995) and 95% found by Schwartz-Watts, Morgan, and Barns (1997). WHOA notes that 49.2% of victims had no prior relationship with their stalker, whereas 46.3% had some prior contact. This could be consistent with the finding from a sample of offline stalking cases that 30% of victims were stalked by ex-partners and 23% had a professional relationship with the stalker (Mullen et al., 1999). Reno (1999) states that cyberstalkers were formerly involved in an intimate relationship with their victim and that their motivation is a desire to control the victim. However, no studies are quoted to support this and she is apparently describing a stereotypical stalker. Her description is challenged by Finkelhor's et al.'s (2000) findings above.

It has been argued that cyberstalking is an entirely new form a deviant behavior (Bocij & McFarlane, 2003). This gained some support from a study by Lucks (2004), who randomly selected 20 stalking cases filed with the district attorney's office in San Diego. She divided them into stalkers or cyberstalkers and compared the two groups. She found that cyberstalkers had younger victims, were technologically sophisticated, used pornography, were above average intelligence and better educated, had multiple victims who were unknown to them, remained anonymous, had brief stalking careers, were addicted to the Internet, and engaged in interstate stalking. They had no history of criminality, substance abuse, or restraining orders and were either employed or were college students.

Various classifications of stalkers have been proposed (see chapter 2), including the obsessional followers classification, which defines stalkers by the nature of the attachment and the type of previous relationship. Harmon, Rosner, and Owens (1998) examined related stalker subtypes, and thence Mullen et al. (1999) developed these classifications into five groups based on context and motivation: the rejected, the intimacy seeking, the incompetent, the resentful, and the predatory. (As noted, for a detailed review of stalking typologies, see chapter 2.) Bowker and Gray (2005) propose that there are three types of cybersex offenders: dabblers, preferential offenders, and a miscellaneous group comprising pranksters or misguided individuals.

For the purposes of this chapter, we perused the popular press for cyberstalking cases and selected 14 at random. We then attempted to fit them into the classification proposed by Mullen and colleagues (1999) and found that they all could fit quite easily. Due to the unscientific nature of this brief survey, we could not make any direct comparison to Mullen et al.'s cohort. Neither could we confirm any of the particular hypotheses regarding distinct cyberstalking subtypes noted above. We did, however, form certain impressions based on the 14 cases. First, that the motivations and contexts were not dissimilar to Mullen et al.'s group. Second, 11 out of our 14 cases involved men stalking women. In the other three, the perpetrators were men but the victims were, in turn, a married couple representing an Internet company, an ethnic group, and a male supervisor. This suggests a greater male-to-female ratio than is found in most studies of stalkers in general. A striking finding was the ingenuity used in some of the cases. Case Example 9.2 illustrates this observation.

A third impression from the 14 cases was that luring prospective victims, especially child victims (Finkelhor et al., 2000), is particularly common on the

Internet. It appears that pedophilic or predatory stalkers are a higher proportion of cyberstalkers compared with groups of general stalkers. Predatory behavior is well known among rapists and sexual sadists but not as commonly seen among pedophiles, although it certainly exists. However, there seems to have been an explosion of this particular behavior on the Internet. It is unclear whether a separate category should be used for this type of behavior or whether we should consider these perpetrators predatory cyberstalkers. Many of them are simply taking advantage of a convenient medium to contact prospective victims. By using the Internet, the grooming behavior of the pedophile, analogous to the normal courtship behavior of the heterophile, is achieved by electronic means, dispensing with face-to-face interaction. However, this behavior appears somewhat paradoxical because in the majority of pedophilic acts, the perpetrator knows the victim and a relationship is established, whereas in cyberstalking the stalker contacts an individual whom he has never met. This is different from the pedophile becoming attracted to a victim over whom he has power and control in that the relationship is purely in fantasy. The Internet is popular for cyberstalkers because it provides an easy cover for deceit and anonymity.

CASE EXAMPLE 9.2: CYBERSTALKER SOLICITS SEXUAL ASSAULT OF VICTIM

A 50-year-old former security guard pleaded guilty to one count of stalking and three counts of solicitation for sexual assault. The case involved the stalker terrorizing a 28-year-old woman who had spurned him. He did this by posting personal advertisements in her name on various Internet services in which he made it appear that she had fantasies of being raped. On at least six occasions men responding came knocking on her door, often in the middle of the night, saying they were there to rape her. Using log-ons such as "KinkyGa130" he placed online advertisements that included the victim's address, telephone number, and details about her apartment's layout. The victim, who did not own a computer, had no clue why she was being targeted by these men. When she learned of the scheme, she placed a note on her apartment door saying that the messages were fake. The perpetrator then sent e-mails to respondents saying the note was part of the fantasy and even offered instructions on how to get past her security lock. (Miller & Maharaj, 1999)

It could be argued that the behavior becomes cyberstalking only when the electronic transmission is intended to coerce, intimidate, or harass the person causing substantial emotional distress, as seen in Case Example 9.3. This differentiates the cyberstalker from the online luring perpetrator who does not necessarily instill fear directly in the victim. However, this type of online luring perpetrator appears to have the intention of, superficially at least, sexually assaulting the child victim who is below the age of consent. It is, therefore, a point for argument whether the luring perpetrator belongs in the cyberstalking group.

It could also be argued that the cyberstalker instills fear by proxy, perhaps to the child's guardian or parent rather than the child directly, or would instill such fear if they were aware of the behavior. This behavior should be recognized at the least as a serious phenomenon that occurs in online behavior but is not within the usual definition of stalking.

It is also unknown what proportion of luring perpetrators actually approach a real victim and how many simply indulge in fantasy. A few well publicized cases in which the perpetrator and victim actually meet, as well as many instances in which police encourage a meeting to apprehend the perpetrator, do not present a pool of sufficient data to come to any conclusions.

Mitchell, Finkelhor, and Wolak (2005) looked at the Internet lurer as part of the National Juvenile Online Victimization Survey. They compared characteristics of proactive investigations (fake child victims) to a number of cases involving online meetings between offenders and actual juvenile victims. They found offenders caught with fake victims were of higher social class, were less sexually deviant, and had less criminal history than those arrested for Internet crimes against actual juvenile victims. They noted that proactive investigations generally resulted in convictions and subsequent stiff sentences against the perpetrators. They concluded that these targeted investigations were a creative, successful, and sophisticated response to Internet crimes. However, the research did not negate the argument that it is possible that these offenders would never have acted out their fantasies except for the encouragement of police officers posing as juveniles.

METHODS OF CYBERSTALKING

It is likely that there are as many methods of cyberstalking as the technology will allow. It is a paradox that stalkers will often show amazing application, ingenuity, and dedication in their stalking behavior that is in stark contrast to their failure in all other facets of their lives (Mullen et al., 1999; Pathé & Mullen, 1997).

Electronic communication technology can also provide a vehicle whereby a cyberstalker can encourage third parties to harass or threaten a victim. To effect this, the stalker impersonates the victim and posts inflammatory messages on bulletin boards and in chat rooms, causing viewers to send threatening messages back to the victim who they believe to be the author. It is likely that the intended objectives of instilling fear are achieved, although no academic literature specifically supports this.

CASE EXAMPLE 9.3: CYBERSTALKER USES
eBAY TO HARASS VICTIM

A former employee of eBay was sued over allegations that he used his position at eBay to obtain personal information about the plaintiff and then used this information to stalk her online for over 2 years.

The couple met each other online via an e-mail dating service. She claims the cyberstalking began after she ended their relationship. It is alleged that he used her eBay password to post items for sale on the auction site associating her with an Internet pornography site. He also contacted her eBay customers to disparage her. Additionally, she claims that he hacked into her financial records. (Knott, 1999)

More common methods of cyberstalking include leaving harassing and threatening e-mails or messages in the guestbook of a website. Stalkers may also send inappropriate electronic greeting cards or post personal advertisements in the victim's name. There are other instances in which websites have been created that may include digitally altered pornographic photographs that lead to threatening or harassing behavior directed at the victim. Specific Internet viruses are sometimes sent to victims to annoy and interrupt personal and business activities. Likely this behavior has a significant psychological impact because of its very specificity. It was reported that Bill Gates, founder of Microsoft, receives eight million harassing e-mails each day (Fox Headline News, 2004).

More sophisticated cyberstalking occurs when the perpetrator uses spyware to track websites that the victim visits or even to record each keystroke the victim makes. Other instances have involved the stalker hacking into the victim's computer via the Internet or using the victim's name and handle to order services or buy products that embarrass, overwhelm, or frighten the victim (Hitchcock, 2003).

EFFECT OF CYBERSTALKING ON VICTIMS

The effect of stalking on victims in general is reviewed in chapter 5. Pathé and Mullen (1997), in a nonstandardized, self-report study of 100 victims of stalking in general, noted that 83% suffered from anxiety, panic, and hypervigilance, 74% from sleep disorders, 55% from intrusive recollections and flashbacks, and that 37% satisfied the criteria for posttraumatic stress disorder. All but six had to make major changes in their work and social lives. In a study of 201 self-identified stalking victims, 2% of whom were stalked on the Internet, Kamphuis and Emmelkamp (2001) noted that the trauma symptoms were comparable to victims of general trauma or major airplane crashes. There is little room for doubt that offline stalking in general causes emotional distress.

Generally speaking, the intent of stalking is to harass, threaten, or instill fear. On the subject of cyberstalking, Vice President Al Gore said, "Make no mistake: this kind of harassment can be as frightening and as real as being followed and watched in your neighborhood or in your home" (Reno, 1999, p. 1).

No studies to date have looked at victims of Internet stalking as a group. Three possible hypotheses have been generated in our committee's review of the literature.

1. Victims of stalking on the Internet experience identical psychological consequences to stalking victims in general.
2. Victims of cyberstalking experience increased psychological distress compared to stalking victims in general.
3. Victims of Internet stalking experience less psychological distress than stalking victims in general.

No data exist to support or refute any of these hypotheses. It could be argued that cyberstalkers cause less impact because the stalking is more removed and anonymous, perhaps lessening the risk of face-to-face contact. However, a contrary argument could also be used—that cyberstalking involves a pervasive, sometimes anonymous, form of stalking, creating a fear of the unknown that is not controllable by the victim. This could be the case particularly if significant amounts of personal information are disclosed or if sophisticated spyware is used. Cyberstalking also makes it easier to harass the victim at work and at home without inconvenience to the stalker. This is yet another area that awaits research initiatives in order to resolve. Currently, our prevailing hypothesis is that victims of cyberstalking experience similar psychological consequences to victims of stalking in general.

DIFFERENCES BETWEEN CYBERSTALKING AND STALKING IN GENERAL

It has been suggested that online stalkers are likely to be of higher social class and to be more sophisticated than stalkers in general (Deirmenjian, 1999). These hypotheses await empirical validation. Although the individual would need access to a computer, there are numerous ways that people can have access to a computer at fairly minimal expense nowadays. In fact, Cooper (1997) notes affordability as a factor constituting growth. Nonetheless, Mitchell et al. (2005), in a study of family and acquaintance sexual abuse entailing Internet use, found that 65% of their group had annual incomes of less than $50,000.

As the use of the Internet and electronic communications continue to grow, it is likely that cyberstalking will grow at the same if not higher rate. A study of college women suggested a much higher rate of Internet stalking than the rate found in other studies (Fisher, Cullen, Belknap, & Turner, 1999). This may suggest a trend (at least among college students) toward more frequent cyberstalking in the future. On the surface, there are certain differences between cyberstalking and stalking in general. One of the primary differences is that, by definition, cyberstalking does not involve face-to-face contact. It is hypothesized that there is, therefore, less disincentive than might be found ordinarily in stalking. As well as avoiding the embarrassment and possible danger of facing the victim, it may appear to the stalker that there is less chance of being caught. The stalker does not necessarily even need to be in the same jurisdiction, or even the same country as the victim. It would also seem easier to use a false identity and even a fictional personality.

The fact that cyberstalking is so simple suggests that it is likely to become more common than other forms of stalking. As noted above, the impersonal and nonconfrontational nature of stalking does not require a great deal of effort or expense on the part of the stalker and may involve less chance of being apprehended. Although some cyberstalkers are ingenious and may have sophisticated computer skills, cyberstalking can be accomplished with fairly minimal computer savvy. Moreover, stalkers can devote a lot of time to considering ways to effect their goals (Mullen et al., 1999), seemingly implying that a limited knowledge of technology would be only a small hurdle to surmount.

A significant question is whether cyberstalking may lead to offline stalking and thence to violence. It could be hypothesized that cyberstalking is more removed from the victim and that the stalker has deliberately chosen a nonconfrontational approach. However, the situation is rarely so simple. For example, Dietz et al. (1991) found that inappropriate letter writers who did not threaten were more likely to pursue a personal encounter. It is difficult to know whether this applies to cyberstalkers. As noted, cyberstalkers could be located in a different state or even a different continent, creating major barriers to personal contact, although this does not provide total protection.

Taking this argument one step further, one can ask, do cyberstalkers who threaten a victim follow through on their threats to harm the victim? Regretfully, the literature thus far does not help us answer this question, either. Though we believe that cyberstalkers have deliberately chosen a nonconfrontational route, it would be nevertheless improper to suggest that threats should not be taken seriously. In these cases a thorough risk assessment and risk management investigation, as well as a possible security consultation, should be undertaken (see chapter 4 for further discussion related to risk management).

STRATEGIES FOR DEALING WITH CYBERSTALKING

A plethora of online organizations have emerged to address the problems associated with cyberstalking. One organization, WHOA (Working to Halt Online Abuse), was founded in 1997 to fight online harassment by educating the general public and law enforcement personnel. We refer the reader to chapter 4, Risk Management of Stalking, in this book for suggestions regarding risk management of stalking in general. Although the strategies delineated for general stalking may be relevant, in cases of cyberstalking, specific strategies should be taken into consideration. To reduce the likelihood that one will become a victim of cyberstalking, the steps listed in Table 9.1 should be considered.

Hitchcock (2003) notes that the first thing a possible victim of cyberstalking should do is determine whether an electronic message is a spam message

Table 9.1. Preventing Cyberstalking

1. Keep your primary e-mail address private.
2. Do not fill out online profiles.
3. Watch what you say online.
4. Avoid chat rooms.
5. Use firewall/antivirus protection.

or whether the victim is being specifically targeted. A victim of cyberstalking should, as a first step, notify the Internet service provider (ISP) from which the e-mail originates. According to Reno (1999) most major ISPs have established an address to which complaints can be sent (generally "abuse@[ISPdomain]"). Most ISPs do have clear online agreements specifically prohibiting abusive or harassing conduct and have the right to terminate an account should this policy not be followed. However, for some ISPs the procedures for lodging complaints are difficult to locate and some do not have clear policies. It can take considerable time, effort, and cost to provide protection, and the online industry associations have not always been willing to make these efforts.

Certain ISPs provide options to block e-mails containing certain language or that originate from specific designated addresses. One of the problems with this is that the victim may not know that they are being threatened and therefore may not take appropriate precautions to manage the risk. Similarly, chat rooms often have facilities to block or stifle those who attempt to bother or harass other users. Increasingly, chat rooms have become "gated communities" thereby refusing admission to unknown persons.

General precautions that many people use include using great discretion in giving out a private e-mail address and using different e-mail addresses for business and private purposes. However, in practice this can lead to a great deal of confusion and if business activity is interrupted by a stalker it could add to the hardships that a victim endures.

It is important to monitor and save the stalker's communications in order to provide this information to an expert in risk assessment. By saving these communications, much information can usually be gleaned about the mental state and intentions of the stalker. Every communication from a cyberstalker should also be saved for legal purposes.

It is vital, at the earliest opportunity, to inform the harasser that his or her behavior is unacceptable and that you do not want to receive any further communication. Most stalking victims feel angry. As such, this warning should be given clearly, but in neutral language. Meloy (2004) suggests that mental health professionals should not reply to any communications from ex-patients and should have a standard administrative response saying further contact is not allowed by the administration. This is an intriguing but drastic proposition that

Table 9.2. Steps to Take if Cyberstalking Begins

1. Tell the subject in neutral language to cease communication.
2. Do not have any further contact.
3. Save everything.
4. Contact stalker's ISP.
5. Contact police.

has a preventative role, in addition to being a good strategy for attempting to stop harassment. It is important to keep a copy of this notice for possible future legal proceedings. However, our committee has viewed this approach as being somewhat too rigid for general use, although some may see the wisdom of it.

Following this single communication to the cyberstalker to stop, the victim should have no further communication with the cyberstalker because this would serve only to encourage him or her. At the point when the harassment becomes cyberstalking, the police should usually be called. Police organizations are becoming increasingly sophisticated (Hitchcock, 2003) at dealing with these situations.

In their management of cyberstalking, many police forces now have specific officers who are experts in assessing threats, and in particular, computer harassment. Even if the ISP has been unhelpful to an individual, they are often more helpful when the police become involved. It should be noted, however, that sophisticated users of the Internet can maintain anonymity by using a variety of means including anonymous e-mail services, ISPs, Internet cafés, and libraries. This can pose a problem for victims and investigators. Reno (1999) suggests that ISPs should become increasingly responsible for cyberstalking and increase the steps that they take. Table 9.2 summarizes the steps that should be taken if cyberstalking occurs.

Legal Recourse

Many countries have cyberstalking or related laws, as do the United Kingdom, Australia, and India (Hitchcock, 2003). Some jurisdictions have antistalking laws that are flexible enough to take into account cyberstalking (Merschman, 2001; Reno, 1999), and other jurisdictions have explicitly worded statutes that cover electronic communication. However, Merschman makes the point that the U.S. federal statute (see chapter 6, this volume) had not been sufficiently flexible, including loopholes that may not have protected victims. However, as discussed in chapter 6, newer federal legislation was crafted to provide better protections. Internationally, the European Union and UNESCO have set up broader based international initiatives to deal with illegal use of the Internet (Le Toquin, 2001).

Cyberstalking is, therefore, defined by law differently across individual jurisdictions. Although definitions may vary, these laws contain certain common

Table 9.3. Major Elements in Cyberstalking Laws

1. Electronic transmission
2. Sent to and received by specific person
3. Intent to coerce, intimidate, or harass
4. Content is obscene, suggestive, and so on, or threatening

elements (see Table 9.3). First, electronic transmission of information is used in every case to delineate the means of communication. Second, the illegal transmission would generally be one sent to a specific person and received by that person, although in one well-publicized case, a cyberstalking hate crime was perpetrated by targeting a specific ethnic group (Miller & Maharaj, 1999). Third, the laws usually require evidence of intent to coerce, intimidate, or harass the person. Finally, there is typically a requirement that the transmission of content is obscene, vulgar, profane, lewd, lascivious or suggestive, or threatening of any illegal or immoral act (Hitchcock, 2003).

Another unique aspect of cyberstalking laws is based on the fact that cyberstalking can cross jurisdictional boundaries. Mahoney (2001) notes that child predators are forming an online community network and virtual bond that is unparalleled in history. Although the law in the original jurisdiction can be used, boundary issues engender problems in terms of investigation, search warrants, and the use of evidence (D'Ovidio & Doyle, 2003; Hitchcock, 2003; Laycock, 2004; Lee & Lynch, 2005; Merschman, 2001; Ryan, Wallace, Lusthaus, & Kim, 2005).

CONCLUSIONS

It is widely believed that cyberstalking is exponentially increasing as a phenomenon proportional to the rise in the use of the Internet and electronic media. However, only recently have some data emerged about the prevalence of cyberstalking. Thus, specific conclusions about the growth of the phenomenon and its frequency remain limited. We suggest that existing typologies may be suitable for cyberstalkers but note that there are certain differences between cyberstalkers and stalkers in general. Primarily these include the ingenuity and choice of methods used by cyberstalkers. An issue that awaits research is whether cyberstalkers prefer to remain removed and anonymous from their victims or whether they are equally likely to approach and finally physically assault victims. Cyberstalking, in our view, appears to invoke at least the same responses in victims as other types of stalking, although this too awaits empirical research.

Luring potential victims, and most particularly children, seems to be a relatively common and significant phenomenon among stalkers that is being increasingly recognized, and disproportionately seems to involve the Internet. This phenomenon is as yet incompletely understood.

We have concluded this chapter with some suggested strategies for dealing with cyberstalking. It is anticipated that future research will clarify some of the issues regarding this and delineate additional strategies based on a better understanding of cyberstalkers, risk assessment related to cyberstalking, and the aspects of cyberstalking that are unique among stalkers.

APPENDIX

Key References

- Fisher, B. S., Cullen, F. T., Belknap, J., & Turner, M. G. (1999). *Being pursued: Stalking victimization in a national study of college women.* Washington, DC: U.S. Department of Justice.
- Reno J. (1999). *Report on cyberstalking: A new challenge for law enforcement and industry—A report from the U.S. attorney general to the vice-president.* Washington, DC: U.S. Department of Justice. (http://www.usdoj.gov/criminal/cybercrime/cyberstalking.htm)

Online Resources

- CyberAngels (http://www.cyberangels.org)
- WiredSafety (http://wiredsafety.org/cyberstalking_harassment). A compilation of useful guidelines about cyberstalking and harassment.
- Working to Halt Online Abuse (WHOA) (http://www.haltabuse.org)

REFERENCES

Alexy, E. M., Burgess, A. N., Baker, T., & Smoyak, S. A. (2005). Perceptions of cyberstalking among college students. *Brief Treatment and Crisis Intervention, 5*(3), 279–289.

Barak, A. (2005). Sexual harassment on the Internet. *Social Science Computer Review, 23*(1), 77–92.

Bocij, P., & McFarlane, L. (2003). Cyberstalking: A matter for community safety but the numbers do not add up. *Community Safety Journal, 2*(2), 26–34.

Bowker, A., & Gray, M. (2005). The cybersex offender and children. *FBI Law Enforcement Bulletin, 74*(3), 12–17.

Cooper, A. (1997). The Internet and sexuality: Into the new millennium. *Journal of Sexual Education & Therapy, 22*, 5–6.

Deirmenjian, J. M. (1999). Stalking in cyberspace. *Journal of the American Academy of Psychiatry and Law, 27*(3), 407–413.

Dietz, P. E., Mathews, D. B., Martell, D. A., Stuart, T. M., Hrouda, D. R., & Warren, J. (1991). Threatening and otherwise inappropriate letters to members of the United States Congress. *Journal of Forensic Sciences, 36*, 445–468.

D'Ovidio, R., & Doyle, J. (2003). A study on cyberstalking: Understanding investigative hurdles. *FBI Law Enforcement Bulletin; 72*(3), 12–17.

Finkelhor, D., Mitchell, D. J., & Wolak, J. (2000). *Online victimization: A report on the nation's youth.* Alexandria, VA: National Center for Missing & Exploited Children.

Fisher, B. S., Cullen, F. T., Belknap, J., & Turner, M. G. (1999). Being pursued: Stalking victimization in a national study of college women. Washington, DC: U.S. Department of Justice.

Fisher, B. S., Cullen, F. T., & Turner, M. G. (2002). Being pursued: Stalking victimization in a national study of college women. *Criminology and Public Policy, 1*, 257–308.

Fox Headline News. (2004, November 6).

Fremouw, W. J., Westrup, D., & Pennypacker, J. (1997). Stalking on campus: The prevalence and strategies for coping with stalking. *Journal of Forensic Science, 42*(4), 666–669.

Harmon, R. B., Rosner R., & Owens H. (1998). Sex and violence in a forensic population of obsessional harassers. *Psychology, Public Policy and Law, 4*, 236–239.

Hitchcock, J. A. (2003, December). Cyberstalking and law enforcement. *The Police Chief* (Canada), 17–27.

Kamphuis, J. H., & Emmelkamp, P. G. (2001). Traumatic distress among support-seeking female victims of stalking. *American Journal of Psychiatry, 158*, 795–798.

Knott, L. (1999, November 30). Woman files suits against ex-eBay worker. *Detroit News.*

Laycock, G. (2004). New challenges for law enforcement. *European Journal on Criminal Policy And Research, 10*, 39–53.

Leblanc, J. J., Levesque, G. J., Richardson, J. B., & Berka, L. H. (2001). Survey of stalking at WPI. *Journal of Forensic Science, 46*(2), 367–369.

Lee, C., & Lynch, P. (2005). *Cyberstalking—Is it covered by current antistalking laws?* Retrieved March 12, 2006, from http://gsulaw.gsu.edu/lawand/papers/su98/cyberstalking/

Le Toquin, J. L. (2001). The industry response 1: The Internet industry and illegal content. In C. A. Arnaldo (Ed.), *Child abuse on the Internet: Ending the silence* (pp. 141–144). Paris: Berghahn Books/Unesco.

Lucks, B. D. (2004). *Cyberstalking: Identifying and examining electronic crime in cyberspace. Dissertation Abstracts International: B. The Sciences and Engineering, 65*(2-B), 1073.

Mahoney, D. (2001). Child predators on the Web. In C. A. Arnaldo (Ed.), *Child abuse on the Internet: Ending the silence* (pp. 81–88). Paris: Berghahn Books/Unesco.

Meloy, J. R. (2004). Commentary: Stalking, threatening and harassing behavior by patients—the risk management response. *Journal of the American Academy of Psychiatry and Law, 30,* 230–232.

Meloy, J. R., & Gothard, S. (1995). Demographic and clinical comparison of obsessional followers and offenders with mental disorders. *American Journal of Psychiatry, 152,* 258–263.

Merschman, J. C. (2001). The dark side of the Web: Cyberstalking and the need for contemporary legislation [Electronic version]. *Harvard Women's Law Journal, 24,* 255–292.

Miller, G., & Maharaj, D. (1999, January 23). Chilling cyber-stalking case illustrates new breed of crime. *Los Angeles Times.*

Mitchell, K. H., Finkelhor, D, & Wolak, J. (2005). The Internet and family acquaintance sexual abuse. *Child Maltreatment, 1,* 49–60.

Mullen, P. E., Pathé, M., Purcell, R., & Stuart, G. W. (1999). Study of stalkers. *American Journal of Psychiatry, 156,* 1244–1249.

Pathé, M., & Mullen, P. E. (1997). Impact of stalkers on their victim. *British Journal of Psychiatry, 170,* 12–17.

Reno, J. (1999). *Report on cyberstalking: A new challenge for law enforcement and industry—A report from the U.S. attorney general to the vice-president.* Washington, DC: U.S. Department of Justice.

Ryan, P., Wallace, R. P., Lusthaus, A. M., & Kim, J. (2005). Computer crimes. *The American Criminal Law Review, 42*(2), 223–276.

Schwartz-Watts, D., Morgan, D. W., & Barns, C. J. (1997) Stalkers: The South Carolina experience. *Journal of the American Academy of Psychiatry and Law, 25,* 514–545.

Senan, G. (1999, October 16). Three months jail for Internet stalker: Computer programmer sentenced over banned visit to ex-lover. *The Guardian.*

Working to Halt Online Abuse (WHOA). (2003). *Online harassment/cyberstalking statistics.* Retrieved February 2, 2007, from http://www.haltabuse.org

10   Celebrity and Presidential Targets

Robert T. M. Phillips

Celebrities have become targets of potentially violent stalkers who instill fear by their relentless pursuit and, in some reported cases, threatened risk of violence. Celebrity stalking may evolve to planned, often violent attacks on intentionally selected targets. The causes of these incidents are complex, and frequently involve delusional obsessions concerning a contrived relationship between the target and stalker. Similar dynamics can be at play for presidential stalkers. Becoming the focus of someone's delusional obsession is a risk for anyone living in the public eye. Planned attacks by stalkers, however, are not confined to internationally prominent public officials and celebrities. Some of the same themes emerge on a more local level when public figures become the object of pursuit.

Celebrity and presidential stalkers often do not neatly fit any of the typologies that have evolved to codify our understanding of the motivation and special characteristics of stalking. Clinicians are often unaware of a "zone of risk" that extends beyond the delusional love object and can lead to the injury of others in addition to the attempted or accomplished homicide of a celebrity or presidential target. Most people can resist the temptation to intrude on a celebrity's privacy—celebrity stalkers do not. This chapter explores celebrity status, as seen by the public and in the mind of the would-be assailant, as a unique factor in stalking cases that raises issues of clinical relevance and unique typologies. Special attention is given to the behaviors and motivations of individuals who have stalked the presidents of the United States.

CELEBRITY TARGETS: BACKGROUND AND INTRODUCTION

Many celebrities become targets of stalkers who relentlessly pursue and frighten them and who, in some cases, threaten violence. Though each case of celebrity stalking is unique and complex, such incidents frequently involve delusional obsessions concerning the contrived relationship between the stalker and victim. Stalking is not confined solely to well-known figures, of course. However, it is the

*The views and opinions expressed in this chapter are those of the author and do not necessarily reflect the official position or policies of the U.S. Secret Service or the Department of Homeland Security.

very nature of celebrity—the status and the visibility—that attracts the benign (if voyeuristic) attention of an adoring public and the ominous interest of the stalker.

Obsessional following of celebrities is not a new phenomenon in the United States. In 1949, Ruth Ann Steinhagen shot Philadelphia Phillies first baseman Eddie Waitkus in the chest with a .22-caliber rifle. Infatuated with Waitkus, she had watched him from the stands as he played, collected newspaper clippings of him, made a shrine to him in her bedroom, and fantasized about their marriage (Berkow, 2002). Following her arrest, she told the chief psychiatrist of the county behavior clinic, "I've dreamt and dreamt about killing him and there I was holding him in my arms. Don't you see all of my dreams have come true?" (Theodore, 2002).

For the next 30 years, public officials were the most highly visible victims of celebrity stalkings or attacks, as seen in Oscar Collazo and Griselio Torresola's attempt on the life of President Truman (Fein & Vossekuil, 1998). Then, on the evening of December 8, 1980, while standing outside the Dakota Apartments in New York City, Mark David Chapman gunned down singer/songwriter John Lennon in the presence of Lennon's wife, Yoko Ono. Chapman, a former security guard from Hawaii, had previously traveled to New York City with the intent of shooting Lennon, but reportedly was unable to purchase ammunition (Kotb, 2005). In an interview with talk show host Larry King, Chapman described his state of mind on the night of the incident. "On December 8, 1980, Mark David Chapman was a very confused person. He was literally living inside of a paperback novel, J. D. Salinger's *The Catcher in the Rye*. He was vacillating between suicide, between catching the first taxi home, back to Hawaii, between killing, as you said, an icon" (King, 2000, p. 3).

The fact that American news and entertainment media place celebrities and other public figures in constant view may play a role in the development of celebrity stalking. As psychiatrist Park Dietz observed, "The mentally ill will develop delusions about whatever is in their environment, and television became an important part of the environment, bringing new people and new faces into their lives" (Feldman, 1995, p. 12).

Given the ever-present availability of videotapes, DVDs, digital satellite programming, all-news-all-the-time cable shows, and broadcast network television, little is left to the imagination of those committed to the pursuing the famous. As a result, the nature of, and opportunities for, indulging in a celebrity stalker's obsessions are distinct from those stalkers who become obsessed with noncelebrity victims.

The prominence of celebrities makes them uniquely vulnerable objects of pursuit. As Robert Bardo, who stalked Rebecca Schaefer, himself described: "It happens because they're in the limelight . . . [She] was on TV. She appeared on a commercial advertising her show and her personality came out. I'd read those magazine articles. You feel like you know these people. It's not like they're strangers . . . it's like they've been with you all your life" (Orion, 1997, p. 93).

General stalking classification schemes are discussed in detail in chapter 2. The motivations of celebrity stalkers resemble Mullen and colleagues' intimacy seekers and rejected categories with some modifications (Mullen, Pathé, & Purcell 2000; see Table 10.1). The motivations of predatory celebrity stalkers are precisely the same as described by Mullen and colleagues' predatory category. Intimacy-seeking celebrity stalkers want to establish a relationship with their "true love" regardless of the celebrity's wishes. Although these stalkers are prone to jealousy and can become enraged at their would-be partner's indifference to their approaches, they remain steadfast in the belief that the "relationship" will endure. Some intimacy seekers hold the additional erotomanic delusional belief that their love is reciprocated.

Because the celebrity stalker rarely, if ever, has the opportunity to interact with the celebrity, it is difficult to categorize them behaviorally as falling into the Mullen et al. (2000) category of the incompetent type. However, the distinct characteristic of social ineptness, unique to Mullen et al.'s classification of the incompetent suitor, is a personality construct shared by most celebrity stalkers. Celebrity stalkers may have the delusional belief that their relationships are real. When celebrity stalkers feel they have been rejected, they often begin to engage in stalking behaviors due to irritation, arrogance, or the hope that their behavior will change the celebrity's mind. Rejected celebrity stalkers tend to vacillate between seeking reconciliation and revenge. What sustains them is narcissistic entitlement and the belief that this is the only relationship they are going to have. If fixated on reconciliation, they persist without intent to do harm. However, if they believe they have been humiliated or treated unfairly by the celebrity or the celebrity's entourage and if the feelings of scorn are internalized, they pursue stalking to express their distress or anger. In this state, they more resemble Mullen et al.'s resentful stalker.

Table 10.1. Difference in Stalkers' Motivations

	Mullen et al. (2000)	Celebrity Stalker
Rejected	Pursues ex-intimate Aim is reconciliation, revenge, or both	Relationship is delusional Aim is reconciliation or revenge If revenge, resembles Mullen et al.'s resentful stalker
Intimacy seekers	Seeks realization of relationship Persists despite targets' response Convinced quest will culminate in a relationship	Seeks realization of relationship Encouraged by own misperception of targets' response (answered fan letters, autographed photos, etc.) Believes relationship exists and will endure

Predatory celebrity stalkers pursue their victims in preparation for a physical or sexual attack. Either their beliefs hold the celebrity responsible for some perceived wrongdoing or they are attracted to the celebrity in order to act out their sexually perverse fantasies.

The following case examples that have been extensively reported in the literature illustrate features of each type of celebrity stalker.

Celebrity Intimacy Seekers

CASE EXAMPLE 10.1: MARGARET RAY/DAVID LETTERMAN

Margaret Ray broke into David Letterman's Connecticut home seven times. Each time, she provided detailed explanations of her relationship with Letterman and the legitimacy of her presence in his home. Her last intrusion occurred 3 days after she had been released from serving a 9-month sentence for trespassing on his property (Simon, 1996). She slept on his tennis courts and even drove his Porsche. Once when she was apprehended in a tollbooth without money, she claimed to be his wife and the mother of their nonexistent son David Jr. (Frey, 2001). After repeated hospitalizations, including treatment at a state psychiatric hospital and the mental health unit of a correctional institution following convictions for trespassing, Ms. Ray committed suicide in 1998.

CASE EXAMPLE 10.2: ATHENA ROLANDO/BRAD PITT

Athena Rolando, a 19-year-old woman, climbed through an unlocked window at the Hollywood Hills home of Brad Pitt in January 1999 ("Woman found," 1999). She slept in Pitt's clothes and remained in the residence for 10 hours before a housekeeper discovered her and called the police. Rolando's infatuation with Pitt dated back to 1996 when she began leaving letters for him at the gates of his residence.

Rejected Celebrity Stalkers

Not all delusional stalkers desist from pursuing targets or turn their frustrations inward. Of greatest clinical concern is a delusional relationship that, in the celebrity stalker's mind, has gone sour.

CASE EXAMPLE 10.3: ROBERT BARDO/REBECCA SCHAEFFER

Robert Bardo stalked actress Rebecca Schaeffer for 2 years. Schaeffer became the subject of Bardo's delusional obsession in 1986 after she answered one of his many fan letters ("Longing, obsession," 1990).

He wrote letters to her and even traveled to California to try to gain access to the studio where Schaeffer's television show, *My Sister Sam*, was in production. His infatuation with Schaeffer dominated his life. He videotaped every episode of *My Sister Sam*, collected photographs of her, and even wrote songs about the two of them ("Man accused," 1990). Unable to clear security, Bardo hired a detective agency to obtain Schaeffer's home address from the California Department of Motor Vehicles (Saunders, 1998).

Bardo became disillusioned after seeing a movie portraying Schaeffer in bed with another actor. He wrote to his sister: "I have an obsession with the unattainable and I have to eliminate [something] that I cannot attain" (Saunders, 1998). Bardo subsequently went to her home in Los Angeles. On the morning of Ms. Schaeffer's death, he visited her twice. The first time, she talked patiently with him, but when he returned, the actress, who was preparing for a meeting with director Francis Ford Coppola, told Bardo she was busy. Infuriated, Bardo shot and killed her. After his arrest, Bardo described how Schaeffer stood in her doorway with "a cold look on her face" (Saunders, 1998).

What a celebrity stalker believes often affects his behavior. Perceived rejection can evoke intense rage and retaliation, even when the rejection did not come directly from the love object. Many celebrities are surrounded by entourages, which, in addition to personal security guards, often include assistants, production staff, agents, publicists, and other fans. As is the case with the President of the United States or other heavily guarded individuals, the advances of many celebrity stalkers are frequently rebuffed or ignored without the target's knowing that the approach took place. Despite this, stalkers often experience the rejection as if it came directly from the love object.

CASE EXAMPLE 10.4: ROBERT DEWEY HOSKINS/MADONNA

Robert Dewey Hoskins repeatedly appeared at the Hollywood Hills residence of pop diva Madonna, according to Rhonda Saunders, a deputy district attorney who prosecuted both Bardo and Hoskins and headed the Stalking and Threat Management Team affiliated with the LAPD (Saunders, 1998). In an effort to deliver written love messages containing proposals of marriage, Hoskins twice appeared at the home in April 1995. The first time, Hoskins managed to scale the wall of the home and place a note on the front door before being scared away by Madonna's personal bodyguard, Basil Stephens (Saunders, 1998). When Hoskins returned the next day, Madonna's personal assistant, Caresse Henry, intercepted him (Saunders, 1998). When instructed to leave, Hoskins became angry, threatened to kill Henry, and said he would slice Madonna's throat if she did not agree to marry him. Hoskins also left a pamphlet pinned to

Madonna's gate with the phrases "Defiled," "I love you," and "Will you be my wife for keeps?" (Saunders, 1998).

On May 29, 1995, Hoskins again climbed over the wall of the house and was confronted by Basil Stephens. Hoskins unsuccessfully tried to take Stephens' holstered gun and was shot in the arm and lower abdomen after a struggle (Saunders, 1998). In January 1996, Hoskins was tried and found guilty of stalking Madonna, assaulting Stephens, and making terrorist threats against Madonna, her bodyguard, and her personal assistant ("Man is found," 1996). Hoskins received a 10-year sentence.

Predatory Celebrity Stalkers

CASE EXAMPLE 10.5: JONATHAN NORMAN/STEPHEN SPIELBERG

In the summer of 1997, Jonathan Norman, a 31-year-old bodybuilder/actor, made several attempts to enter the estate of filmmaker Stephen Spielberg. Norman had learned the filmmaker's address by buying a tourist map of stars' homes and had spent a month watching the mansion (Mullen et al., 2000). On June 28, 1997, he drove up to the gate and pressed the intercom saying that he worked for one of Mr. Spielberg's associates and needed to speak to him. Security officers chased Norman away (Court TV, 1997).

At around 1:00 A.M. on July 11, 1997, Norman was observed in a vehicle across the street from the residence. When he became aware that he had been detected, he moved his vehicle, but not before he butted the gate with his car as if he were testing its strength. Six hours later, Norman was apprehended in Spielberg's backyard. Norman said he was running through the property because Spielberg's jackal was chasing him. He also claimed that he was Spielberg's newly adopted son (Court TV, 1997).

A search of Norman following his arrest revealed a day planner containing a list of the names of Spielberg's seven children and a "rape kit" containing a knife blade, razor blades, tape, and handcuffs (Mullen et al., 2000). In Norman's car were two more pairs of handcuffs. Police also discovered a book with a shopping list of tools they say Norman planned to use on Spielberg, including three eye masks, three sets of handcuffs, four pairs of nipple clips, and three dog collars (Mullen et al., 2000).

A Los Angeles police officer testified before a grand jury that during questioning Norman claimed that he had written a screenplay about "a man raping another man," which he had wished to show to Spielberg. Prosecutors argued that Norman's ultimate goal was to tie up Spielberg's actress wife, Kate Capshaw, and make her watch him rape the filmmaker

(Erico, 1998). It took a jury less than 4 hours to find Norman guilty of felony stalking in March 1998.

PRESIDENTIAL TARGETS

There is no celebrity that is more visible in American society than the President of the United States. Understanding the unique nature of presidential celebrity and the psychopathology of the stalkers and assassins who target the occupant of that office are essential when performing a forensic psychiatric evaluation of these individuals.

Considerable research exists on stalking that has helped to codify our understanding of the motivation and special characteristics of these behaviors. Stalking typologies have evolved from this work along two themes: empirical (derived from systematic evaluation of stalkers and or their victims) and theoretical (derived out of experience in reviewing the literature and/or direct experience with a population of stalkers; see chapter 2). These typologies fall short, however, when one attempts to use them to understand the unique circumstances of stalkers who pursue the President of the United States.

Developing classification typologies for various celebrities and public figures presents challenges. Often information available about the stalker's behavior is limited or not a matter of public record. Clarke (1982), in his archival study of 17 American assassins and would-be assassins, described four "types" based upon a consideration of the cultural, political, and social context of their behavior, as well as the immediate situation or circumstance in which the behavior occurs.

The Secret Service Exceptional Case Study Project (ECSP) provided a behavior-based case review and analysis of "the thinking and behavior of all 83 persons known to have attacked or approached to attack a prominent pubic official or figure in the United States from 1949 to 1996," thereby dispelling many myths about assassination (Fein & Vossekuil, 1998, p. 4). This project operationalized how the idea of assassination develops into lethal or near lethal action by focusing on motive, target selection, plan of attack, communications, and whether mental illness or life circumstances contributed to the assassination interest or behavior. However, no typology was offered as they concluded that there is no profile of an assassin.

In an effort to integrate what has been learned from the existing pool of research and taxonomies in this area and influenced by the typology of stalkers published by Mullen and colleagues (2000), and the efforts of our Group for the Advancement of Psychiatry (GAP) Committee on Psychiatry and the Law in producing this book, I have searched for a framework that would codify these actions based on motive, the presence or absence of delusions, active psychosis, and the intent to do harm. By drawing upon the Exceptional

Case Study Project (ECSP; Fein & Vossekuil, 1998) and integrating the Clarke (1982) classification with modifications, I have conceptualized five descriptive categories that attempt to capture the various motivations of presidential stalkers and assassins and the clinical context in which presidential stalking occurs: resentful, pathologically obsessed, infamy seeking, intimacy seeking, and nuisance or attention seeking (Phillips, 2006). These are described further in Table 10.2. These categories have evolved and currently represent what appears to fit most, based on actual experience consulting on cases of presidential stalkers. As new data and case material emerge, these categories and our understanding of patterns they reveal may evolve.

The Resentful Presidential Stalker or Assassin

While resentful stalkers comprise a minority of general cases that arise in workplace settings (Mullen et al., 2000), they appear to account for a significant number of presidential stalkings and most of the attempted or completed assassinations. The stalking arises from a quest for retribution. Resentful presidential stalkers or assassins feel justified in their actions and are driven by anger without delusions. Their targeting behavior arises from political disagreement, displaced rage, or perceived narcissistic injury. They are committed to eliminating the target to achieve retribution and not as a means of attaining a platform to make

Table 10.2. Five Descriptive Categories of Presidential Stalkers or Assassins

Stalker or Assassin Type	Motive	Delusional Thinking or Active Psychosis	Harm Intent	Animus Toward POTUS*
Resentful	Retribution	None	Yes	Yes
Pathologically obsessed	Retribution or Personal gain	Persecutory or Grandiose	Yes	Yes No (personal gain)
Infamy seeker	Political statement	None	Yes	Not necessarily
Intimacy seeker	Realization of fanaticized relationship	Erotomanic	No	No
Nuisance	To provide help to or seek help from the President	Grandiose, narcissistic, or dependent; may be actively psychotic	No	No
or				
Attention seeker	To see or be seen with the President	None	No	No

*President of the United States

a grand statement or to attain fame. They feel justified in their actions to the point of righteous indignation. While they may have some paranoid personality traits, they do not suffer from delusional thinking.

The Pathologically Obsessed Presidential Stalker or Assassin

Pathologically obsessed presidential stalkers and assassins are characterized by a severe psychosis of a persecutory or grandiose nature that places the President in peril due to a persistent resolve to do harm. Their delusions can often be characterized as divinely inspired or of idiosyncratic importance. Most often, they incorporate the unshakeable belief that the President is responsible for their life problem and therefore they seek redress for some imagined wrongful act. In those instances, their purpose in assassination may be seen as retributive.

In others, the psychosis is without any animosity toward the President or desire for retribution. Instead, assassination services their intense narcissistic fantasies. Though they may resemble infamy seekers in their desire to attract attention, the psychosis distinguishes them. Their focus is actually not the President but on others for whom their actions are intended as a statement of love or disdain.

The Presidential Infamy Seeker

Presidential infamy seekers are a special class of individuals whose presidential targeting is generally for a grand political statement or for personal reasons outside of politics. Though not delusional, the intensity of their characterologic disturbance is often palpable. Their primary characterologic construct is antisocial. Political zealotry is the common thread that binds these individuals together. It is their zealotry and willingness to sacrifice themselves at any cost for the cause that makes them so dangerous. Their intent to do harm is clear, but it is often only a means to an end and not necessarily the primary motivation for their actions. While the act of attempted or successful assassination constitutes by definition a negative direction of interest, infamy seekers may not bear any animosity toward the target. They seek only the opportunity to act out their particular drama on a world stage.

The Presidential Intimacy Seeker

Presidential intimacy seekers manifest the same characteristics as other intimacy seekers, as described by Mullen et al. (2000). They desire to realize a relationship with a person they delusionally believe is already interested in or in love with them. Erotomanic delusions are pathognomonic of this classification. Primarily seeking fulfillment of a fantasized sexual intimacy, an imagined platonic friendship, or role as a special confidant can also be the primary motivation. They persist with their approach and attempts at personal contact oblivious to any attempts to deter their advances. Their pursuit of the President can, at times, be reckless and unbridled, creating a "zone of risk" extending beyond the delusional love object that places many others in jeopardy.

The Presidential Nuisance or Attention Seeker

Presidential nuisances include those who approach the President or appear at the White House gate driven by delusional thinking without having any intent to do harm. The individuals who comprise these "White House Cases" are often quite different from those reflected in the Exceptional Case Study Project. They usually experience a thought disturbance but have no nefarious intent. The nature of their delusional experience appears far less paranoid and threatening. The reasons stated by the subject for the visit appear more grandiose, narcissistic, or dependent (seeking help for a problem), rather than in response to fear or driven by anger with an intent to do harm or seek revenge (Coggins, Pynchion, & Phillips, 1998). It is the nature and character of their delusional thinking that attracts them to the President or the White House and therefore to the attention of the U.S. Secret Service.

The absence of nefarious intent separates them from resentful presidential stalkers just as the absence of a fanaticized delusional relationship distinguishes them from presidential intimacy seekers. One might actually characterize these individuals as creating more of a nuisance than posing a threat of imminent danger.

Presidential attention seekers, by contrast, approach the President driven by the notice that it garners, whether in sole service to their narcissism and sense of entitlement or because the media attention provides personal financial benefit. They are not delusional. Generally these individuals have no history of violence. They do not make threats to persons or property, nor do they attempt to gain access or close proximity to the President for nefarious purposes. At best they can be characterized as a "wannabes"—people whose primary desire is to "see and be seen" with the leader of the free world in a manner that attracts attention to them.

Whether the stalkers are seen as nuisances or as attention seekers, agents on the scene must determine if such individuals pose a threat to the President, other Secret Service protectees, and/or whether their behavior suggests the need for emergency psychiatric evaluation.

Consider the following case illustrations from history and from cases on which I have consulted as demonstration of how my proposed classification system fits.

The Resentful Presidential Stalker

CASE EXAMPLE 10.6: SAMUEL BYCK/RICHARD NIXON

Samuel Byck was the oldest of three boys born and raised in Philadelphia by Jewish immigrant parents. Despondent over a deteriorating marriage, jealous of the success of his brothers, and frustrated by his failure in numerous business ventures, the retired tire salesman became convinced that the American political system was corrupt. The Small Business Administration had rejected a loan application intended to support the start of his own business, and he held the President responsible for his failures (Clarke, 1982).

Byck became a person of interest with the U.S. Secret Service in 1972 for sending threatening letters to President Nixon (White House Security Review, 1995b). It is reported that on Christmas Eve in 1973 he picketed the White House dressed in a Santa suit carrying a sign that read: "Santa Sez: All I want for Christmas is my constitutional right to peaceably petition my government for redress of grievances" (Clarke, 1982).

Byck developed a plan that he called "Operation Pandora's Box," a plot to hijack a commercial airliner and crash it into the White House with the intention of killing President Nixon (White House Security Review, 1995b). Troubled that his actions might be misconstrued as those of a "maniac or madman," Byck recorded an audiotape describing his planned assault and rationale and sent copies to scientist Jonas Salk, columnist Jack Anderson, Senator Abraham Ribicoff, and composer Leonard Bernstein (Clarke, 1982).

Byck traveled to Baltimore-Washington International Airport on February 22, 1974, with a handgun and a gasoline bomb secreted in a briefcase. He shot and killed an officer who was screening passengers for a Delta Airlines flight headed for Atlanta and boarded the jet. Byck then stormed the cockpit and ordered the two pilots to take off. They told him that they could not depart without removing the wheel blocks (Clarke, 1982). An angry Byck shot the pilot twice and the copilot three times (White House Security Review, 1995b).

He reportedly then grabbed a terrified passenger, demanding that she help him fly the plane (Clarke, 1982). Byck was shot and wounded through the cabin window by a police officer on the ground outside of the plane. Aware that his plan was in shambles, Byck killed himself with his own gun (White House Security Review, 1995b).

Byck meets the criteria for a resentful presidential stalker because the motive for his stalking was retributive. He felt justified in his actions and was driven by anger without delusions. His targeting behavior was born of political dissatisfaction and displaced rage.

The Pathologically Obsessed Presidential Stalker

CASE EXAMPLE 10.7: CHARLES GUITEAU/
JAMES GARFIELD

Charles Guiteau was a self-proclaimed lawyer, theologian, and politician who wrote and delivered speeches on New York City street corners during the 1880 presidential election campaign. He developed the delusion that his speeches were responsible for Garfield's success in the presidential election and as a consequence he believed that he was owed a political patronage position.

In Guiteau's mind it was not a question of whether he would be appointed but where—Paris or Vienna—and most importantly, when! He began writing to President Garfield and Secretary of State Blaine incessantly (Clarke, 1982). Guiteau often appeared unannounced at the White House seeking an audience with the President and Secretary. Despite his persistence, he was unsuccessful in convincing them of his responsibility for the President's success or of his value to the administration.

Rebuffed by the Secretary during an exchange in which he reportedly told Guiteau "never to bother me again with the Paris consulship for as long as you live!" (Rosenberg, 1968, p. 39). Guiteau's admiration turned to animosity. A despondent and narcissistically wounded Guiteau began to plan his assassination attempt.

He purchased a revolver and began stalking the President (Clark, 1982). On the morning of July 2, 1881, Guiteau placed a package containing his writings at a nearby newsstand for intended delivery to the press and entered the Baltimore and Potomac Railroad Station (Rosenberg, 1968). Guiteau shot and mortally wounded President Garfield at the train station, firing twice at the President's back as he headed for the train (Clarke, 1982). Guiteau was subsequently tried for murder of the President of the United States.

Despite a 72-day "trial of the century" involving a "Who's Who" of American psychiatry of the time presenting testimony about his sanity, Guiteau was found guilty and sentenced to death. On June 30, 1882, he was executed by hanging after reciting a hymn he had written for the occasion (Clarke, 1982; Rosenberg, 1968).

In retrospect, the evidence presented of Guiteau's insanity included more than his grandiose behaviors and expansive delusions. His correspondence both before and after the fateful day provides a trail of his deteriorating mental state. Prior to the instant offense, his writings characterized his intent, "This is not murder. It is a political necessity" (Clarke, 1982, p. 207). Later he added, "The President's nomination was an act of God. The President's election was an act of God. The President's removal is an act of God" (p. 207).

Guiteau was psychotic, held idiosyncratic delusions, blamed the President for his current life circumstances, and sought retribution. He meets the criteria for a pathologically obsessed presidential stalker.

CASE EXAMPLE 10.8: JOHN W. HINCKLEY JR./
RONALD REAGAN

John W. Hinckley Jr. shot and wounded President Ronald Reagan on March 30, 1981, at the Washington Hilton Hotel as the President headed toward his limousine. Three other individuals were inadvertently struck by gunfire, among them Press Secretary James Brady, who sustained a debilitating head injury. Hinckley's belief that his actions would lead to fulfillment of his romantic delusions was an uncanny example of life imitating art.

Hinckley had become fascinated with the 1976 movie *Taxi Driver*, in which actor Robert De Niro played Travis Bickle, an alienated schizoid taxi driver who began stalking a young woman who works for a senator-turned-presidential-candidate. Failing to win the woman's affection, Bickle turned his anger toward the senator and began methodically plotting his assassination, only to have his scheme foiled by the heavy presence of Secret Service agents. Bickle subsequently fixated on "Iris," a young prostitute played by a young and then-little-known actress, Jodie Foster. In the film, Bickle became a hero when he rescued Iris from her pimp in violent gun battle.

Hinckley became obsessed with Travis Bickle and began to emulate him in dress and manner. Most importantly, he became obsessed with Jodie Foster. Hinckley traveled to New Haven in August 1980 to make contact with Foster, who was then a freshman drama student at Yale University. He left poems and letters in her mailbox and spoke to her twice by telephone, recording the conversations (Bonnie, Jefferies, & Low, 2000).

Unsuccessful in his efforts to win Foster's affection, Hinckley began stalking President Jimmy Carter on the campaign trail in the belief that assassinating the President would bring Foster closer to him. Hinckley continued leaving correspondence for Foster. Concerned that he was despondent and suicidal, his parents arranged an appointment with a psychiatrist (Bonnie et al., 2000). Although Hinckley saw the psychiatrist episodically over the next 4 months, he never disclosed appearing at presidential campaign sites, his plans of assassination, or his love of Foster.

In November 1980, Hinckley's interest shifted from President Carter to President-elect Reagan, as evidenced by Hinckley's traveling to Reagan's transitional residence in Washington, DC. He also made several additional trips to New Haven and left more notes for Foster. Finally, on March 30, 1981, one day after he checked into the Park Central Hotel in Washington, DC, Hinckley wrote a letter to Jodie Foster outlining his assassination plan (Bonnie et al., 2000). He then went to the Washington Hilton and attempted to execute it.

Mr. Hinckley's stalking behaviors began with President Carter and then shifted to President Reagan. This change in target selection is not uncommon among presidential stalkers. Many attackers and near lethal approachers consider multiple potential targets and change their primary target several times before settling on their final choice (Fein & Vossekuil, 2000).

John W. Hinckley Jr.'s psychosis was without any animosity toward the President or desire for retribution. Instead, his planned assassination serviced his intense narcissistic fantasies. Though he may resemble an infamy seeker in his desire to attract attention, it is the psychosis that is distinguishing. His focus was actually not on the President but on another for whom his actions were intended as a statement of love. As such, he too meets the criteria for pathologically obsessed presidential stalker and assassin.

Following what was arguably the most influential insanity defense case of the twentieth century, a jury acquitted John W. Hinckley Jr. of 13 assault, murder, and weapons counts, finding him not guilty by reason of insanity. He was committed to St. Elizabeth's Hospital for the criminally insane in Washington, DC.

PRESIDENTIAL INFAMY SEEKERS

CASE EXAMPLE 10.9: FRANCISCO MARTIN DURAN/ WILLIAM JEFFERSON CLINTON

Francisco Martin Duran was an avid supporter of antigovernment ideologies who saw gun control as a Big Brother conspiracy. He was angry with the government and the President for signing the assault weapons ban of 1994 and for failing to reconsider his courts martial and dishonorable discharge from the United States Army. He left work on September 30, 1994, without contacting his family or employer, and began his cross-country journey to Washington, DC with an arsenal of weapons (Locy, 1994; *United States v. Francisco Martin Duran*, 1995). Before leaving Colorado he told several people of his intention to kill the President and gave one person a card bearing his signature that he said would be "valuable" someday.

En route, he passed the clock tower at the University of Texas in Austin, the site where Charles Whitman killed 13 and wounded many others, and the book depository in Dallas, Texas, the site where

Lee Harvey Oswald is believed to have fired upon President Kennedy. Between October 10 and 29, he stayed at various hotels in the Washington area, including the Washington Hilton Hotel, the site of the attempted assassination of President Ronald Reagan (Locy, 1995b; *United States v. Francisco Martin Duran*, 1996).

On October 28, 1994, Mr. Duran wrote a letter to his wife that included a will. On that same date, he was in a hotel room watching television and saw a news report that the president was arriving in Washington the next day.

On the morning of October 29, wearing a trench coat and carrying his shotgun and an SKS assault weapon, Duran headed for Pennsylvania Avenue. He walked up and down Pennsylvania Avenue in front of the White House for several hours, passing the various entrances for tourists (White House Security Review, 1995a).

While Duran was standing in front of the north side of the White House fence in the early afternoon, two eighth-grade students on a field trip ran to nearby spot along the fence. Pointing toward a small group of men dressed in dark business suits in the vicinity of the north portico of the White House, one of the excited students remarked, "That man looks a lot like Bill Clinton," to which his friend replied, "Yeah, it does" (Locy 1995a; *United States of America v. Francisco Martin Duran*, 1996). The man they saw, Dennis Basso, was on a tour of the White House and did bear some resemblance to the President.

Hearing this, Duran fired at least 29 shots at the White House. Eleven rounds found their mark on the north façade. Additionally, a window in the Press Briefing Room in the West Wing was breached by a round (White House Security Review, 1995a). Remarkably, no one was injured by the storm of gunfire.

Duran began running east along the fence while continuing to fire in the direction of the White House (*United States of America v. Francisco Martin Duran*, 1996). When he stopped, apparently trying to reload a second 30-round clip, a passerby tackled him (Locy, 1995a). Soon thereafter Secret Service agents arrived to help subdue Duran and confiscate his rifle.

A search of Duran's truck after his arrest revealed a rifle, ammunition, and a nerve gas antidote (Locy, 1994; White House Security Review, 1995a). Several documents were found, including a letter in which he had written, "Can you imagine a higher moral calling than to destroy someone's dreams with one bullet?"; a road atlas on which he had written, "Kill the Pres."; a cover torn from a telephone book bearing a picture of President Clinton, which Mr. Duran had defaced by drawing a circle around Clinton's head and an "X" on his face; a handwritten document with the heading, "Last will and words"; an order form for the book *Hit*

Man; and several books about out-of-body experiences (Locy, 1994; White House Security Review, 1995a). When they searched his house and office, law enforcement agents found a business card on the back of which Duran had written, "Kill all government offices [*sic*] and department heads," and assorted other pieces of antigovernment literature (*United States v. Francisco Martin Duran,* 1996; White House Security Review, 1995a, pp. 32).

Admittedly, Duran did not exhibit typical stalking behavior in his approach to the White House. He was not on record with the Protective Intelligence Division of the U.S. Secret Service before the attack (White House Security Review, 1995a). It could be argued that his path through the sites of previous assassinations such as the Dallas Book Depository and the Washington Hilton were vicarious stalking behaviors. He was stalking the idea if not the experience of assassinating a President. However, Duran does meet the criteria for presidential infamy seekers because his actions targeted the President in order to make a grand political statement. Notably, when examined pretrial by a government's expert, Mr. Duran's first question upon introduction was "Doc, are we going to be on *Hard Copy?*" (Phillips, 1996). Duran's actions emerged out of a desire to become famous. He exhibited extreme character pathology but not psychosis. His political zealotry was palpable.

Presidential Intimacy Seekers

CASE EXAMPLE 10.10: JANE DOE/WILLIAM JEFFERSON CLINTON

Ms. Doe first came to the attention of the U.S. Secret Service in the spring of 1995 when she appeared at a Presidential site with flowers that she intended to give to President Clinton. When interviewed, she spoke of a great affection for the President and indicated that she had sent many small gifts and letters to him in the past. At that time, after a full factual investigation was conducted by the Secret Service, she was deemed not to present a threat or danger to any protectee of the Service or to herself.

Subsequently, she again returned to the presidential site and was again interviewed by U.S. Secret Service agents. This time she said that she loved the President and that she returned with the hope of jogging with him. Ms. Doe said that had she known she would not be allowed to jog with the President, she would not have returned. Again, following additional investigation, the Secret Service agents thought that she did not show any threatening attitudes and no further action was taken.

Upon returning to her hometown, Ms. Doe repeatedly sent the President numerous letters expressing her love and affection, in addition to sending many small gifts, some that she purchased, others that she made, as tokens of her affection for him. It is believed that Ms. Doe made repeated visits to Washington, DC, in a hopes of seeing and meeting the President.

Months later, Presidential Protection Detail agents observed a woman behaving strangely along a rope line as the President was shaking hands at a political fund-raiser at a Washington, DC, hotel. When the woman greeted the President, she was tongue-tied and acted somewhat bizarrely. It was noted that she broke the receiving line and returned to a position that would allow her to shake the President's hand again.

Agents interviewed the woman and determined that she was Ms. Doe, who apparently had a legitimate ticket to attend the event. Her behaviors were not deemed to be threatening to the President, and she returned to her hometown. Over the course of the next several years, Ms. Doe began to radically change her appearance. She continued to legitimately gain entry to presidential functions.

Finally, during a presidential visit to her hometown, Ms. Doe carried a cell phone while breaching the secure perimeter surrounding the presidential limo. Entering a secure site with an object in hand that could have easily been mistaken for a weapon demonstrated the greater danger she posed to herself and others when her delusional thoughts became so intense she could not control them. Ms. Doe was subsequently civilly committed.

Presidential intimacy seekers manifest the same characteristics noted to be found among other intimacy stalkers. They desire to realize a relationship with a person they believe is already interested or in love with them. They persist with their approach and attempts at personal contact oblivious to any attempts to deter their advances.

Ms. Doe meets the criteria for an intimacy seeking presidential stalker because she possessed a delusional love interest in the President. She sought fulfillment of a fantasized relationship and made repeated attempts at approach or contact. In so doing, she recklessly created a "zone of risk," placing in jeopardy herself, the target, and his protectors, as well as innocent bystanders.

Presidential Nuisance or Attention Seekers

CASE EXAMPLE 10.11: RICHARD WEAVER/ GEORGE W. BUSH

In 1991, Richard Weaver attended a prayer breakfast at the Washington Hilton Hotel. According to his website, Weaver is the founder and president of the Spiritual Revolution Thru Christ, Inc., in Sacramento,

California (http://www.richardweaver.org.). He mingled in the grand ballroom with senators and dignitaries, as is customary. What distinguishes Rev. Weaver is that he managed to follow a VIP into the holding room of then-President George H. W. Bush and have his picture taken shaking hands with the President.

Richard Weaver had succeeded in meeting celebrities, sports figures, presidents, and other politicians with great ease for nearly 3 decades. He enjoyed the media attention and often used the photographs taken with celebrities to promote his ministry. Three weeks before the 2001 inauguration of George W. Bush, Mr. Weaver reported that he felt a strong inner sense that God wanted him to deliver a message to the President: "Your miracle election is to remind you to stand for Christ daily without political compromise. Keep Christ first and God will give you another miracle election in four years" (Montgomery & Santana, 2001, p. B1). Armed with the typed message on a laminated blue card and carrying a medallion bearing the image of former president George H. W. Bush, Mr. Weaver headed to Washington.

In an interview, Mr. Weaver stated that on the morning of Inauguration Day he was given a blue standing-room ticket by a woman who had an extra one (Montgomery & Santana, 2001). As he approached the entry, he came upon a group of VIPs and overheard one of them talking about a special entrance (Montgomery & Santana, 2001). Mr. Weaver's distinguished appearance and impeccable dress allowed him to blend in with the group as they entered the Capitol grounds.

Once inside, he asked a guard for directions to the nearest restroom. He was directed through a metal detector at the entry of a VIP seating area. Rev. Weaver claims to have taken a seat only 20 rows away from the podium to hear the Inaugural Address. Following the ceremony, he walked into the Capitol and began to wander around upstairs.

When challenged by a U.S. Capitol Police officer, Rev. Weaver said he was lost and searching for an exit. The officer escorted him to an exit, which happened to be in close proximity to the President's awaiting motorcade. Mr. Weaver then presented Mr. Bush with the medallion and card (Grove, 2003).

On February 6, 2003, Mr. Weaver again gained entrance without invitation to another prayer breakfast at the Washington Hilton. After clearing magnetometers, he entered the ballroom and went from table to table socializing. When he happened upon the table of a distinguished senator at prayer, he joined in and asked if he could be seated there. The senator agreed. The table was located in front of the stage where the President spoke. As the President came down a set of stairs leaving the stage, Mr. Weaver came from behind a rope line and stanchion, shook the President's hand, and handed him an eight-page, typed "Message from

God" about Iraq. When questioned by authorities, Rev. Weaver stated, "I don't try to sneak in. I just go where I think God wants me to go" (Grove, 2003, p. C1).

Rev. Weaver was not so successful during George W. Bush's second inauguration on January 23, 2005. Although he had previously told journalists that God made him "invisible and undetectable by security," he was apprehended at a checkpoint on First Street and Pennsylvania Avenue and never made it to the Capitol (Haskell, 2005, p. 1).

Rev. Weaver was the quintessential example of a presidential attention seeker. Narcissistic and entitled, he was driven by the need to be noticed. With no history of violence and having displayed no evidence of intent to do harm, he is best characterized as a "wannabe." He wanted to be seen, to be noticed, and to be in the presence of the President.

MANAGEMENT OF CELEBRITY AND PRESIDENTIAL STALKERS

The issue of risk assessment and management of stalkers in general is described in detail in chapters 3 and 4, and the approaches identified in those chapters should be considered as well when a clinician is managing someone who is stalking a public figure. For stalkers who pursue celebrities and presidential targets, several unique issues are raised related to their management. Essentially, clinicians will be required to think about psycholegal issues, such as confidentiality, involvement in criminal justice systems, and violence risk assessment, as they would with any person engaging in stalking or obsessional harassment types of behaviors. In doing so, it is important that treatment providers not be intimidated by the fame of stalker's identified target. When consultation is needed, seeking such guidance from a person with forensic expertise may be helpful.

Involvement of special agencies, such as the Secret Service, may occur when the President has been threatened or when members of the particular agency have concerns about the well-being of their protectees. In these cases, treating clinicians may find themselves working to help the patient, but also coordinating efforts at assessment with Secret Service agents. Legal and forensic consultation along the way may be critical, as clinicians at times may inadvertently provide information to law enforcement when it may not be indicated to do so (Zonana, 2005).

However, the need to report credible threats to the life of a president or some other protectee should never be ignored. In deciding whether to report a presidential threat, the *Tarasoff* principle applies, just as it does when a patient poses a danger to another person. Clinicians must balance their obligation to protect the President with their duty to uphold a patient's rights to confidentiality and to freedom from self-incrimination (Griffith, Zonana, Pinsince, & Adams, 1998).

Interesting research has been done to examine nuances of management and assessment of celebrity and presidential stalkers. Given the frequency of repetitive or disturbing contact with public figures, studies have attempted to examine differences between those who write letters, follow, or otherwise present themselves to public figures without harming them, and those who attack. Data available have indicated that direct threats toward public figures are not altogether common, and when they do occur, they are negatively correlated with an approach or attack (Meloy, James, Farnham, Pathé, Darnley, et al., 2004; Meloy, 2001). Generally, attacks that do occur are thought to be premeditated and undertaken to achieve some goal, rather than the reflection of a sudden emotional outburst as is seen with stalkers who may have had a real relationship with their victim at one time. Most frequently, when a weapon is used against a public figure such as a president, it involves a firearm (Meloy, 2001). Assailants also have often shown some history of mental illness and a recent decompensation.

Dietz and colleagues (1991) reviewed letters to members of the U.S. Congress that contained threats or were otherwise inappropriate. Of the 86 subjects, 20 had threatened assassination. In that study, persons with mental disorders writing to public figures were at times found to mention and even threaten other public figures in their letters. The authors concluded that this raised important questions related to notification of third parties who may be endangered and the issue of sharing information with certain protective agencies. On a more local level, Noffsinger and Saleh (2000) described a case of a patient who had developed ideas of reference toward a local newscaster. They found that clinicians often did not take actions to protect potential victims in a manner that was delineated by the law in their jurisdiction. Their experience led them to conclude that letters written by clinicians to identified victims at risk of harm by others can be a nuanced approach. Specifically, because letters with content related to being identified as at risk of being harmed engender anxiety, the authors suggested that a specific personal communication from a member of the treatment staff may be more helpful. Interestingly, they also found that notification of potential victims at risk did not adversely affect the treatment relationship with the patient.

Hoffman and Sheridan (2005) also recognized that public figures are at a higher risk than the general population to receive unusual contacts. In their work, they have identified the need to develop a flexible approach to managing individuals who may be fixated on public figures. They emphasize the need to understand the motivations and underlying psychiatric issues that a particular stalker may be presenting. In this way, the typology described above can be helpful in looking at motivational and psychiatric factors.

Extrapolating from available research findings, clinicians, either in a forensic evaluative or treating role, would do well to conduct a thorough assessment of a patient's motivations, access to weapons, and psychiatric status, among other aspects of their history. Furthermore, an understanding of any communications and the content of those communications can also help in risk management approaches. Finally, exploration of legal duties, such as the duty to protect identified potential victims, should be undertaken.

CONCLUSIONS

Although high-profile celebrity stalking cases generate considerable media attention, they do not comprise the majority of cases. Most stalking occurs between people who truly know each other. While the need for love and recognition often propels the successful actor or aspiring politician, they quickly discover that excessive or unwelcome intrusion by the public is a tax on their fame. With increased media attention comes the loss of privacy in daily life. Most people can resist the temptation to intrude on the celebrity's privacy; celebrity stalkers cannot.

The existing typologies of stalking have helped clinicians codify their understanding of the motivation and special characteristics of stalking. Yet, the behavior of celebrity stalkers often does not neatly fit into any existing typological category. However, it does appear that Mullen et al.'s (2000) classification with some modification provides the closest fit and best clinical description. The motivation and special characteristics of those who focus on presidential targets are even more difficult to fit into existing classifications. These concepts have been discussed at length within our GAP Committee on Psychiatry and the Law, and although the complexity of stalking behavior is difficult to precisely define in stalking classification schemes, these approaches can be useful in generating treatment and risk management decision tree analyses.

This chapter has presented a framework that integrates what I have learned from evaluating presidential stalkers and assassins with the existing pool of research and stalking taxonomies (Phillips, 2006). This framework attempts to categorize the actions of would-be and actual assassins based on motive, the presence or absence of delusions and/or active psychosis, and the intent to do harm. The framework is one that should be familiar to physicians. It attempts to utilize the signs and symptoms manifested by the subject and consider this information in the context of a diagnostic nomenclature. It has permitted me to provide a uniquely clinical perspective to the risk assessment process when consulting on U.S. Secret Service Protective Intelligence cases.

I have found this to be of great assistance to the clinical assessment of risk when consulting to the Secret Service, as well as considering treatment options, case management issues, and prevention strategies when providing opinions to the United States Attorney, the Federal Public Defender, or to private counsel. It may also be useful when developing a therapeutic plan for the treatment of such persons by forensic clinicians who are responsible for their care.

Becoming the focus of someone's delusional obsession is a risk for anyone living in the public eye, more so for celebrities and politicians than for anyone else. Being the object of stalking, obsessive love, or hate from a stranger can generate enormous anxiety and realistically based fear. The fact that these stalkers have moved from private obsession to actions that have brought them to our attention warrants the need for a better clinical understanding of their behavior. Through an understanding of these unique stalking behaviors, we are better able to provide useful strategies to protect potential celebrity and political targets and hopefully deter their stalkers.

REFERENCES

Berkow, I. (2002). *Baseball natural: The story of Eddie Waitkus* (Foreword). Carbondale and Edwardsville, IL: Southern Illinois University Press.

Bonnie, R., Jefferies, J., & Low, P. (2000). *A case study in the insanity defense: The trial of John W. Hinckley, Jr.* New York: Foundation Press.

Clarke, J. W. (1982). *American assassins: The darker side of politics.* Princeton: Princeton University Press.

Coggins, M., Pynchion, M., & Phillips, R. T. M. (1998, May). *White House cases: Risk assessment and management.* Issue workshop presentation conducted at the 154th Annual Meeting and Scientific Assembly of the American Psychiatric Association, Toronto, Ontario, Canada.

Court TV. (1997, October 8–9). *The Stephen Spielberg stalker grand jury hearing summary.* Retrieved July 10, 2006, from http://www.courttv.com/legaldocs. newsmakers/spielberg

Dietz, P. E., Matthews, D. B., Martell, D. A., Stewart, T. M., Hrouda, D. R., & Warren, J. (1991). Threatening and otherwise inappropriate letters to members of the United States Congress. *Journal of Forensic Science, 36,* 1445–1468.

Erico, M. (1998). *Spielberg stalker sent away.* Retrieved April 1, 2006, from http://www.eonline.com /newsitems/Pf/0,1527,33170.00.html

Fein, R., & Vossekuil, B. (1998). Preventing attacks on public officials and public figures: A Secret Service perspective. In J. R. Meloy (Ed.), *The psychology of stalking: Clinical and forensic perspectives* (pp. 175–191). San Diego: Academic Press.

Fein, R. A., & Vossekuil, B. (2000). *Protective intelligence and threat assessment investigations: A guide for state and local law enforcement officials.* Washington, DC: U.S. Department of Justice.

Feldman, H. (1995, Summer). Stalking: Everything you hoped you'd never have to know. *Aftra Magazine, 28*(2), 12.

Frey, D. (2001). *Answers from Margaret Ray's mother.* Retrieved July 20, 2006, from http://www.newyorkcityvoices.org/jan01u.html

Griffith, E. E., Zonana, H., Pinsince, A. J., & Adams, A. K. (1988). Institutional response to inpatients' threats against the President. *Hospital and Community Psychiatry, 39,* 1166–1171.

Grove, L. (2003, February 7). Gate crasher hands Bush "message from God." *The Washington Post*, p. C1.

Haskell, B. (2005, January 25). Virginia Guard soldier helps nab "handshake man." *News Archive Virginia National Guard*. Retrieved April 1, 2006, from http://www.VirginiaGuard.com

Hoffman, J. M., & Sheridan, L. P. (2005). The stalking of public figures: Management and intervention. *Journal of Forensic Science, 50,* 1459–1465.

King, L. (Executive Producer). (2000, September 30). A look back at Mark David Chapman in his own words [Television Broadcast]. In *Larry King live weekend*. Retrieved July 20, 2006, from http://transcripts.cnn.com/TRANSCRIPTS/0009/30/lklw.00.html

Kotb, H. (Correspondent). (2005, November 18). *The man who shot John Lennon* [Television Broadcast]. New York: NBC Dateline.

Locy, T. (1994, November 18). Duran charged with trying to assassinate the president. *The Washington Post*, p. A1.

Locy, T. (1995a, March 23). Tourist tells how shooter was tackled. *The Washington Post*, p. B4.

Locy, T. (1995b, April 5). Duran convicted of trying to kill President Clinton. *The Washington Post*, p. D1. Longing, obsession and an actress' death. (1990, July 18). *The Oregonian*. Retrieved July 10, 2006, from http://www.OregonLive.com/webarchive

Man accused in killing feels "guilty." (1990, July 18). *Los Angeles Times*, p. 8.

Man is found guilty of stalking Madonna. (1996, January 9). *New York Times*. Retrieved July 17, 2006, from http://www.newyorktimes.com/archives

Meloy, J. R. (2001). Communicated threats and violence toward public and private targets: Discerning differences among those who stalk and attack. *Journal of Forensic Science, 46,* 1211–1213.

Meloy, J. R., James, D. V., Farnham, F. R., Pathé, M., & Darnley, B., et al. (2004). A research review of public figure threats, approaches, attacks, and assassinations in the United States. *Journal of Forensic Science, 49,* 1086–1093.

Montgomery, D., & Santana, A. (2001, January 26). Inaugural intruder credits God: Minister offered president medallion, spiritual boost. *The Washington Post*, p. B1.

Mullen, P. E., Pathé, M., & Purcell, R. (2000). *Stalkers and their victims.* Cambridge, UK: Cambridge University Press.

Noffsinger, S. G., & Saleh, F. M. (2000). Ideas of reference about newscasters. *Psychiatric Services, 51,* 679.

Orion, D. (1997). *I know you really love me: A psychiatrist's journal of erotomaina, stalking and obsessive love.* New York: Macmillan.

Phillips, R. T. M. (1995). Trial testimony in *United States v. Francisco Martin Duran* (1995). No. 95–3096, 94cr00447–01 No. 95–3096 (U.S. Ct. App. D.C. 1996).

Phillips, R. T. M. (2006). Assessing presidential stalkers and assassins. *Journal of the American Academy Psychiatry and the Law, 34,* 154–164.

Rosenberg, C. (1968). *The trial of the assassin Guiteau.* Chicago: University of Chicago Press.

Saunders, R. (1998). The legal perspective on stalking. In J. Meloy (Ed.), *The psychology of stalking: Clinical and forensic perspectives* (p. 25). San Diego: Academic Press.

Simon, R. (1996). *Bad men do what good men dream*. Washington, DC: American Psychiatric Press.

Richard Weaver. (n.d.). Spiritual revolution thru Christ. Retrieved April 1, 2006, from http://www.richardweaver.org

Theodore, J. (2002). *Baseball natural: The story of Eddie Waitkus.* Carbondale, IL: Southern Illinois University Press.

United States of America v. Francisco Martin Duran, No. 95–3096, 94cr00447–01 No. 95–3096 (U.S. Ct. App. D.C. 1996).

White House Security Review. (1995a). *The October 29, 1994 shooting*, p. 32–38.

White House Security Review. (1995b). *Air incursions and attempted air incursions*, p. 100.

Woman found in Brad Pitt's home wearing clothes. (1999, January 8). *Los Angeles Times*, p. B5.

Zonana, H. (2005). Physicians should not be agents of the police. *Psychiatric Services, 56*, 1021.

INDEX

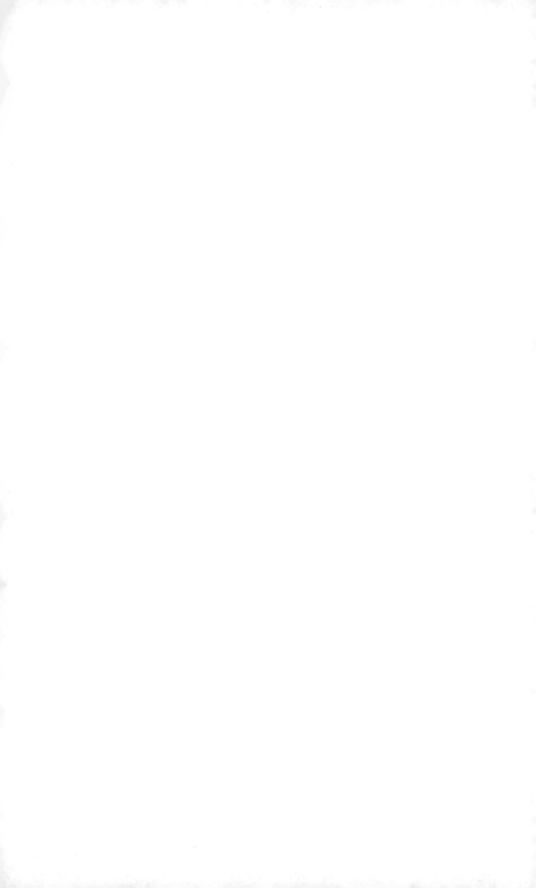